Dermatology
Fundamentals of Practice

Robin Graham-Brown, BSc, MB, FRCP, FRCPCH
Consultant Dermatologist, Leicester Royal Infirmary;
Honorary Senior Lecturer in Dermatology,
University of Leicester School of Medicine;
Director of Services for Older People,
University Hospitals of Leicester,
Leicester, UK

Johnny Bourke, MD, FRCPI
Consultant Dermatologist,
South Infirmary, Victoria Hospital, Cork, Ireland;
Clinical Lecturer in Medicine,
University College, Cork, Ireland

Tim Cunliffe, MD, MBBS, MRCGP
GPwSI in Dermatology,
Middlesbrough Primary Care Skin Service,
One Life Centre, Middlesbrough, UK

D1342574

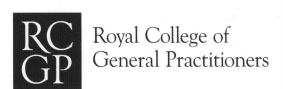

Royal College of
General Practitioners

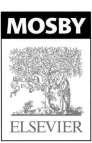

MOSBY

ELSEVIER

EDINBURGH   LONDON   NEW YORK   OXFORD   PHILADELPHIA   ST LOUIS   SYDNEY   TORONTO   2008

MOSBY
ELSEVIER

© 2008, Elsevier Limited. All rights reserved.

First published 2008

ISBN: 978-0-7234-3447-4

British Library Cataloguing in Publication Data
A catalogue record for this book is available from the British Library.

Library of Congress Cataloging in Publication Data
A catalog record for this book is available from the Library of Congress.

Note
Knowledge and best practice in this field are constantly changing. As new research and experience broaden our knowledge, changes in practice, treatment and drug therapy may become necessary or appropriate. Readers are advised to check the most current information provided (i) on procedures featured or (ii) by the manufacturer of each product to be administered, to verify the recommended dose or formula, the method and duration of administration, and contraindications. It is the responsibility of the practitioner, relying on their own experience and knowledge of the patient, to make diagnoses, to determine dosages and the best treatment for each individual patient, and to take all appropriate safety precautions. To the fullest extent of the law, neither the Publisher nor the Authors assumes any liability for any injury and/or damage to persons or property arising out of or related to any use of the material contained in this book.

The Publisher

The Publisher's policy is to use **paper manufactured from sustainable forests**

Typeset by IMH(Cartrif), Loanhead, Scotland
Printed in China

Contents

Preface

Surveys over many years have indicated that skin disease accounts for 10–15% of GP consultations in the United Kingdom. Many books have been produced, aimed at helping clinicians in primary care deal rapidly and effectively with dermatological problems – both in making the correct initial diagnosis and in deciding on the most appropriate therapeutic option(s).

This book is a new departure. It has been written and illustrated in the light of the publication of the curriculum statement on dermatology that forms part of the wider new curriculum for general practice training published by the Royal College of General Practitioners in 2007,* and therefore attends directly and specifically to improving knowledge and understanding of those disorders that have been marked out by the College as being essential to all GPs.

To assist in this process most effectively, we have divided the book into two parts. In the first (Section 1), we have used illustrated algorithms which outline a simple approach to the common presenting features of skin disease. Some sample photographs are provided for each diagnosis, and there is a reference to the appropriate chapter(s) in the second part (Sections 2 and 3), where the reader will find more detailed descriptions of the disorders and management issues specified in the RCGP curriculum, together with further pictures.

We hope the 'road map' provided by the RCGP, together with our long experience as practising dermatologists (Robin Graham-Brown and Johnny Bourke), GP/GPwSI (Tim Cunliffe) and educators (all three of us) has given us the necessary insight into the needs of the audience we seek to address.

Robin Graham-Brown
Johnny Bourke
Tim Cunliffe

*http://www.rcgp-curriculum.org.uk/PDF/curr_15_10_skin_problems.pdf

Acknowledgements

Our thanks to Dr Fergus Lyons and Dr Michelle Murphy for allowing us to use photographs of some of their patients.

The following figures are courtesy of Dr W. T. Bailie: 1.10c, 1.34d, 1.36b, 1.37b, 1.37c, 1.48b, 1.52b, 2.9d, 2.9e, 2.14b, 2.18b, 2.19c, 2.19d, 2.20, 2.28a, 2.28b, 2.29a, 2.29b, 2.29c, 2.29d, 3.4t, 3.4u, 3.8, 3.16i, 3.16j, 3.16k, 3.16l, 4.5b, 4.5c, 4.6b, 4.9b, 4.10b, 4.12, 4.14b, 4.24c, 6.11a, 6.12b, 7.5, 7.6, 7.15b, 7.16b, 7.16c, 8.13f, 8.19i, 8.27b, 8.28a, 8.28b, 8.29a, 8.29b, 9.3c, 9.8a, 9.9a, 9.9b, 9.22b, 9.25e, 9.30f, 9.30i, 9.30j, 9.30k, 9.31c, 9.31d, 10.2, 10.3, 10.4, 10.5, 10.6, 10.7, 10.8, 10.9, 10.11, 10.12, 10.13, 10.14, 10.15, 10.16, 10.17, 10.18, 10.19, 10.20, 10.21, 10.22, 10.23, 10.25, 10.26, 10.28, 11.1, 11.2, 11.3, 11.4, 11.5, 11.6, 11.7, 11.8, 11.9, 11.10, 11.11, 11.12, 11.13, 12.4, 13.1, 14.5, 14.6, 14.7, 14.8, 14.10, 14.12, 14.14, 14.16, 15.2, 15.3, 15.4, 15.5, 15.6, 15.7, 15.9, 15.10, 15.11, 15.12, 15.13, 15.14, 15.15, 15.16, 15.17, 15.18, 15.19, 15.20, 15.21a, 15.21b, 15.21c, 15.22, 15.23, 15.24, 15.25, 15.27, 15.28, 15.29, 15.30, 15.33, 15.35, 15.36, 15.38, 15.39, 15.41, 15.43, 15.45, 15.46, 15.47, 15.48, 16.2, 16.3, 16.4c, 17.3, 17.27, 17.28, 17.29, 17.35, 17.45, 18.7, 19.1, 19.2, 20.2, 20.3, 20.4, 20.6, 20.8, 20.12, 20.16a, 20.19a, 20.19b, 20.20, 21.2, 21.4, 21.5, 21.9a, 21.9b, 22.2, 23.1, 23.8, 23.9, 23.11, 25.3, 25.4.

Figures are reproduced with permission from Graham-Brown and Bourke, *Mosby's Color Atlas and Text of Dermatology* 2nd edition.

We are grateful to Dr D. A. Burns who supplied many of the photographs used throughout the book.

Symptoms and Signs

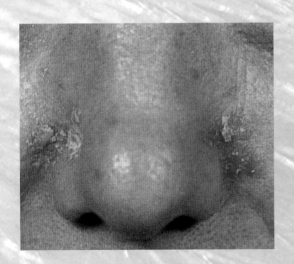
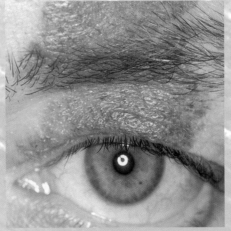
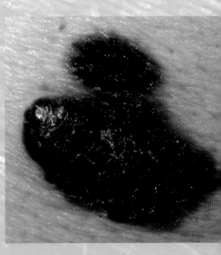

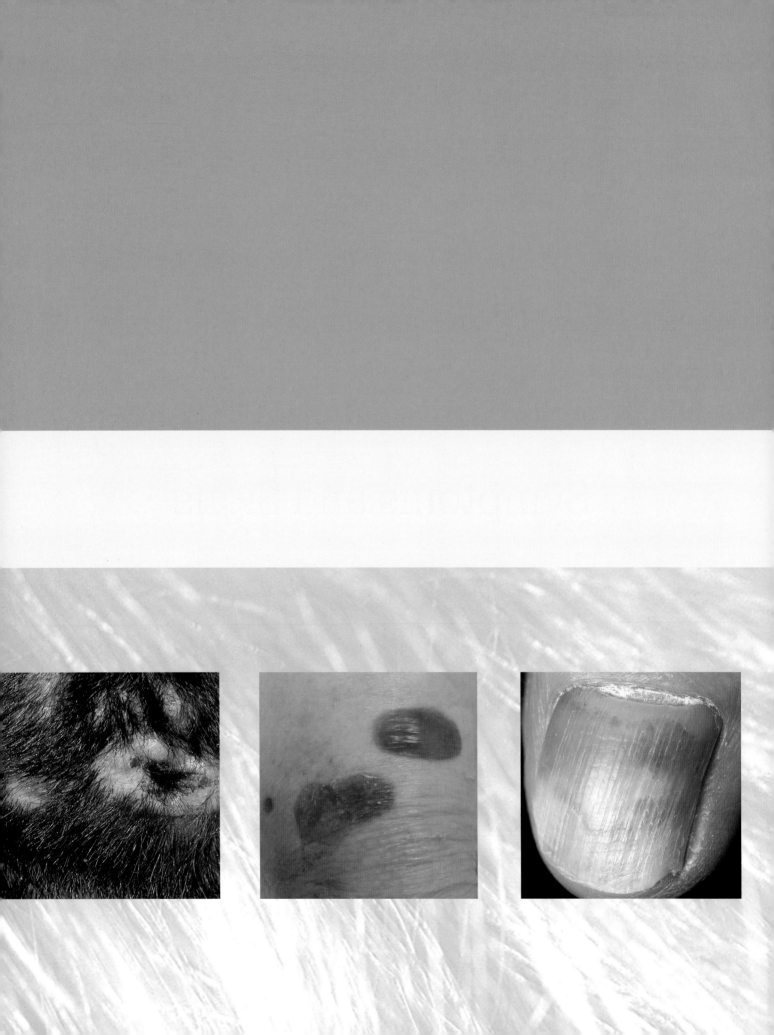

Chapter 1

Rashes

Summary

- Itchy v. non-itchy rashes
- Scaly v. non-scaly rashes
- Painful rashes

Generalized rashes can roughly be divided in a number of ways: itchy v. non-itchy v. painful; scaly v. non-scaly. Facial rashes are worth considering separately mainly because of the acne group of disorders and photosensitivity. Common itchy conditions include dermatitis, many infections and urticaria. Psoriasis, seborrhoeic dermatitis, pityriasis rosea, drug rashes and viral rashes tend to be relatively less itchy, although this is not absolute. Itch can be a significant problem in as many as 20% of cases of psoriasis, for example. Painful rashes include cellulitis and herpetic infections in particular. Scale is another useful way of classifying rashes as outlined below. The reader is directed to Chapters 10, 11, 15, 19 and 21 in Section 2 for more detailed descriptions of these conditions.

Algorithm 1.1 Itchy v. non-itchy

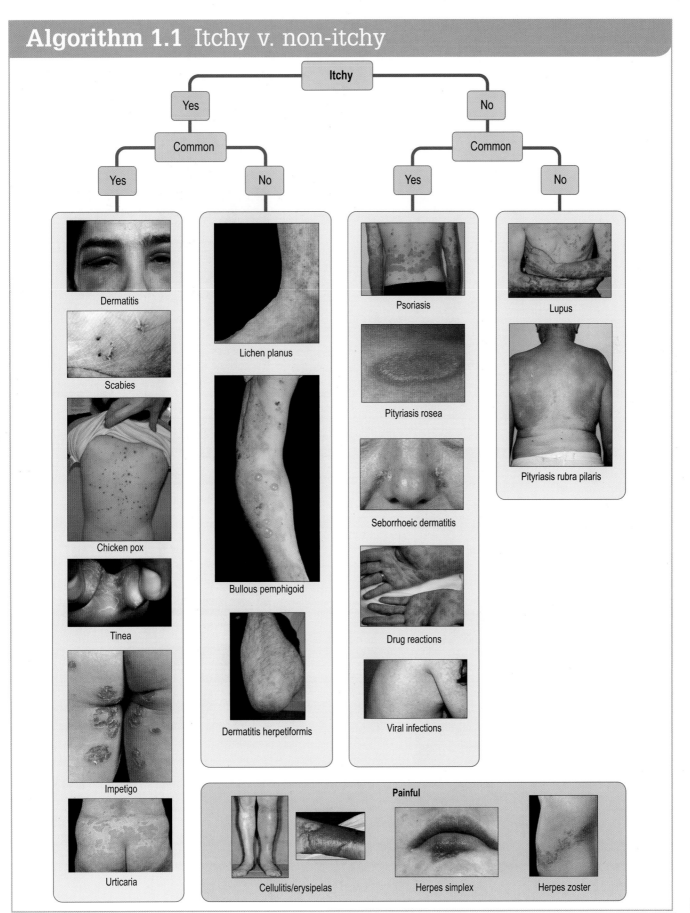

Itchy
- Yes
  - Common
    - Yes
      - Dermatitis
      - Scabies
      - Chicken pox
      - Tinea
      - Impetigo
      - Urticaria
    - No
      - Lichen planus
      - Bullous pemphigoid
      - Dermatitis herpetiformis
- No
  - Common
    - Yes
      - Psoriasis
      - Pityriasis rosea
      - Seborrhoeic dermatitis
      - Drug reactions
      - Viral infections
    - No
      - Lupus
      - Pityriasis rubra pilaris

Painful
- Cellulitis/erysipelas
- Herpes simplex
- Herpes zoster

Algorithm 1.2 Scaly v. non-scaly

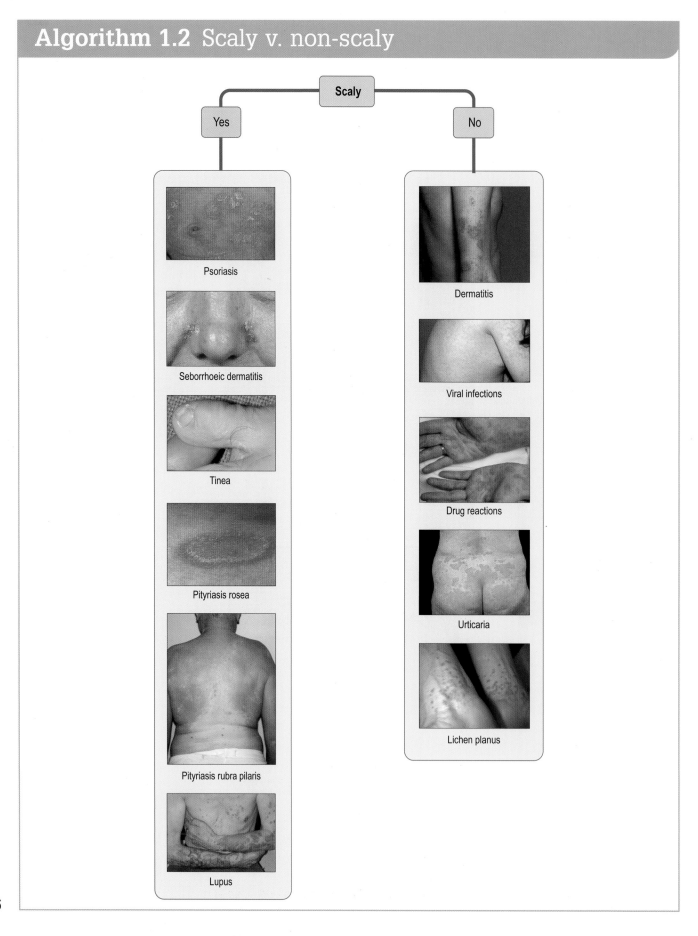

Scaly

Yes

No

Psoriasis

Seborrhoeic dermatitis

Tinea

Pityriasis rosea

Pityriasis rubra pilaris

Lupus

Dermatitis

Viral infections

Drug reactions

Urticaria

Lichen planus

ITCHY RASHES Dermatitis *Endogenous*

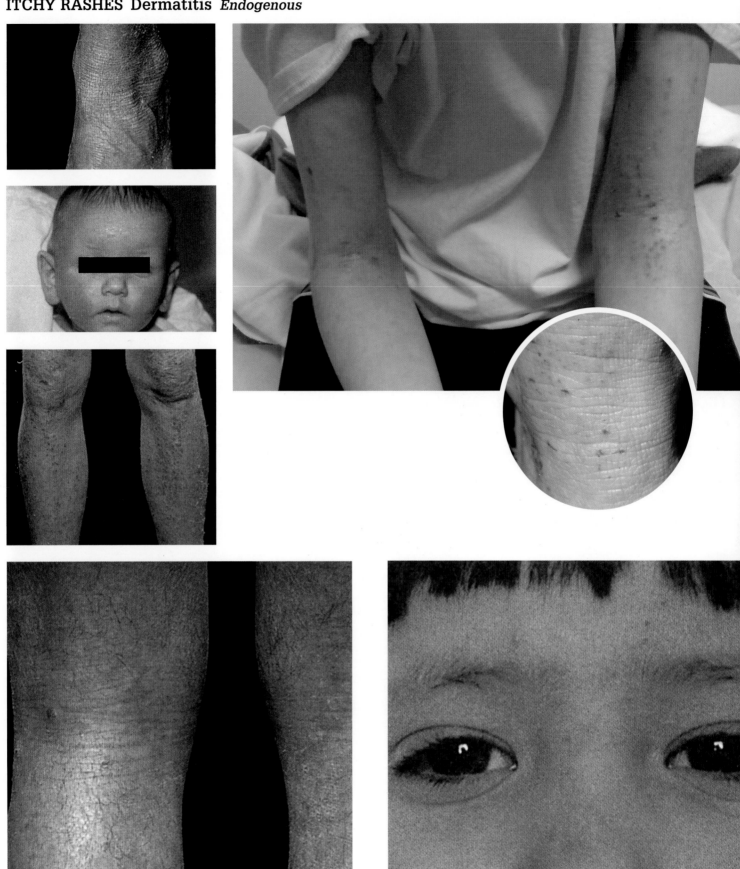

FIGURE 1.3 Atopic dermatitis affecting the face, trunk, ankles, antecubital and popliteal fossae

ITCHY RASHES Dermatitis *Endogenous*

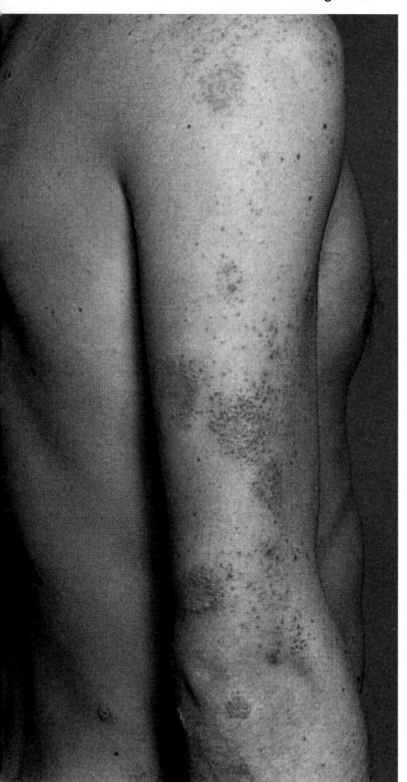

FIGURE 1.4 Discoid eczema

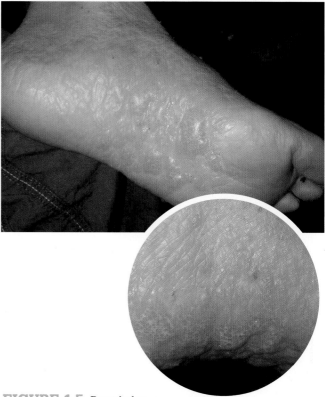

FIGURE 1.5 Pompholyx

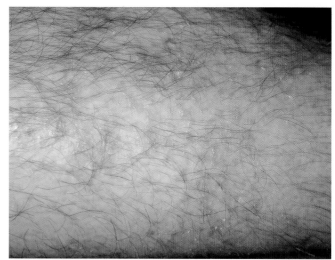

FIGURE 1.6 Asteatotic eczema

ITCHY RASHES Dermatitis *Endogenous*

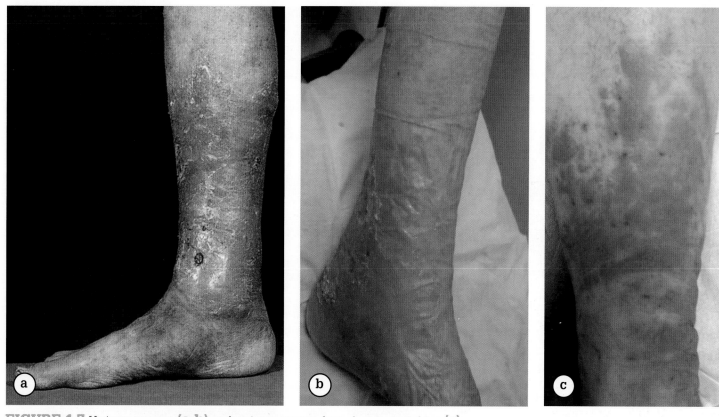

FIGURE 1.7 Varicose eczema (a,b) and varicose exzema from chronic scratching (c)

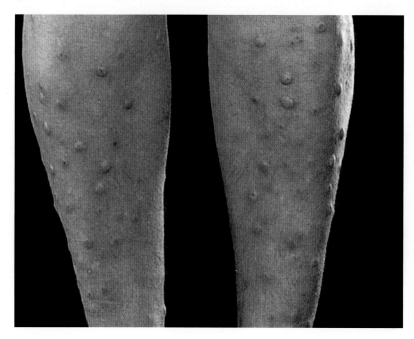

FIGURE 1.8 Nodular prurigo

ITCHY RASHES *Allergic Contact Dermatitis*

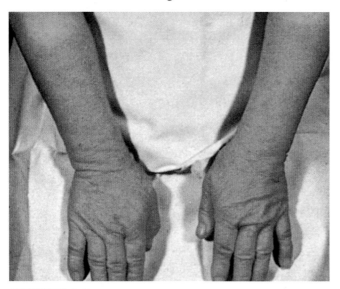

FIGURE 1.9 Allergic contact dermatitis due to thiuram in rubber gloves

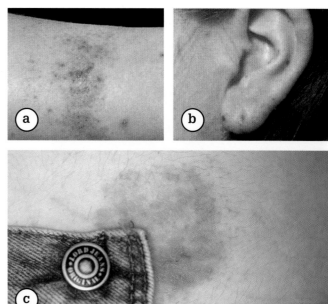

FIGURE 1.10 Allergic contact dermatitis due to nickel in **(a)** watch strap, **(b)** earrings, **(c)** jeans

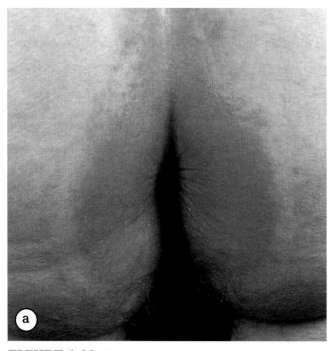

FIGURE 1.11 Allergic contact dermatitis due to neomycin in **(a)** haemarrhoids cream, **(b)** ear drops

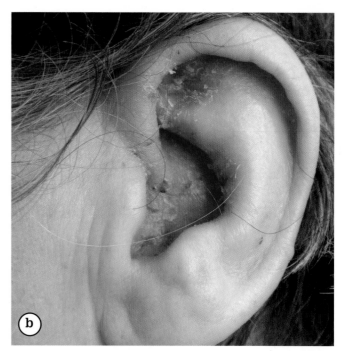

ITCHY RASHES *Allergic Contact Dermatitis*

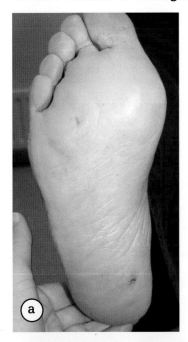

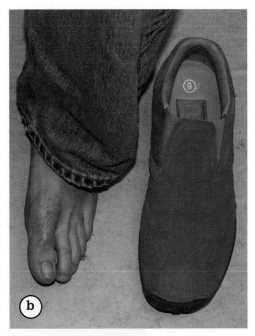

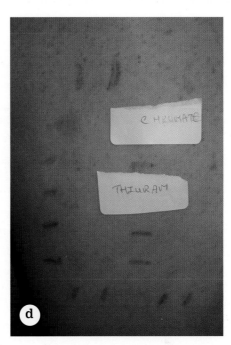

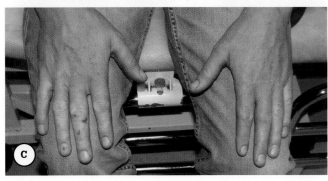

FIGURE 1.12 (a) (b) (c) (d) Allergic contact dermatitis due to chromate (leather) and thiuram (rubber) in shoes and gloves with positive patch test

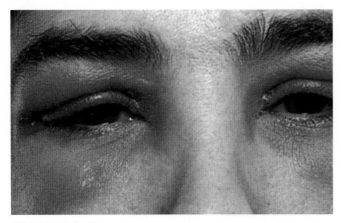

FIGURE 1.13 Allergic contact dermatitis due to cosmetics

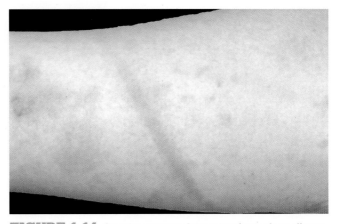

FIGURE 1.14 Streaky contact dermatitis from plant allergy

ITCHY RASHES *Irritant Contact Dermatitis*

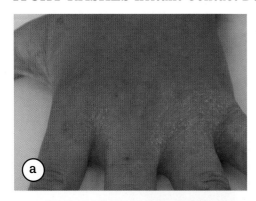
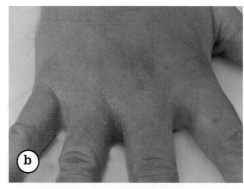

FIGURE 1.15 Irritant contact dermatitis commonly starts in the web spacs between the fingers

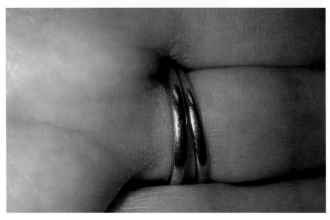
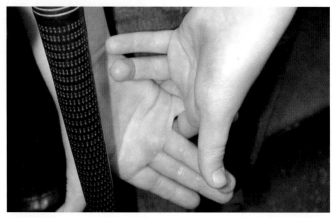

FIGURE 1.16 Irritant contact dermatitis due to soap and detergent lodged underneath rings

FIGURE 1.17 Traumatic irritant contact dermatitis from a golf club grip

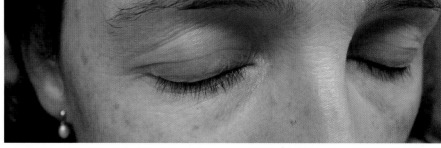

FIGURE 1.18 Cosmetics may also cause irritant dermatitis particularly on the eyelids

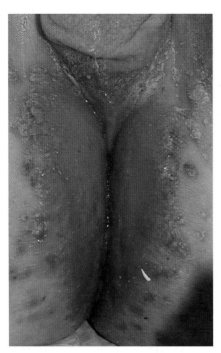
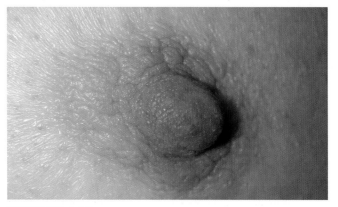

FIGURE 1.19 Irritant nappy dermatitis from alkaline urine and faeces

FIGURE 1.20 Irritant dermatitis of the nipple from clothing ('jogger's nipple')

ITCHY RASHES Infections

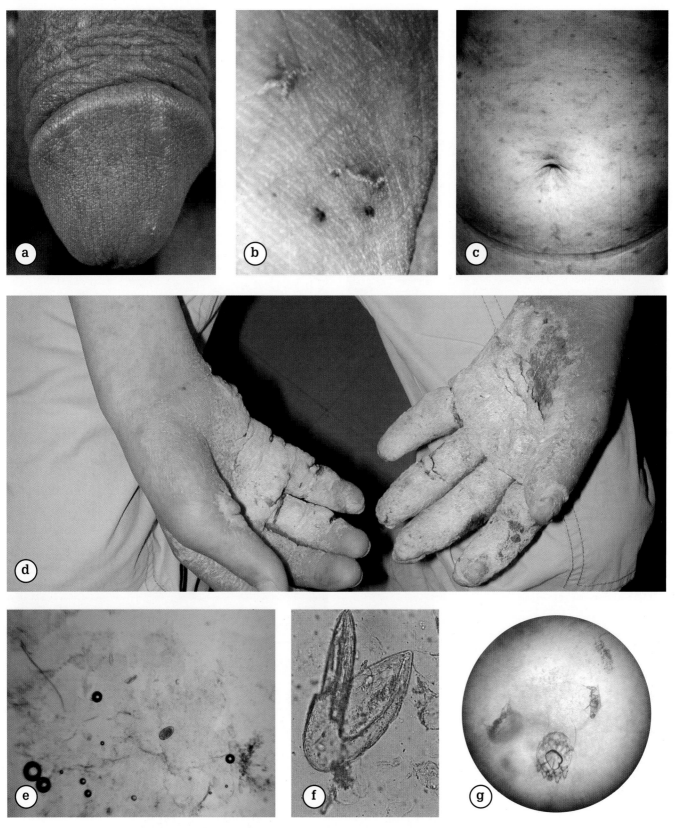

FIGURE 1.21 Scabies: **(a)** burrows on the glans penis, **(b)** burrows on the back of the hand, **(c)** generalized scabies mimicking dermatitis, **(d)** Norwegian crusted scabies due to massive numbers of mites (seen in the elderly and mentally retarded), **(e)** low power microscopic view of broken egg, **(f)** high power microscopic view of broken egg, **(g)** high power microscopic view of scabies mites

ITCHY RASHES Infections

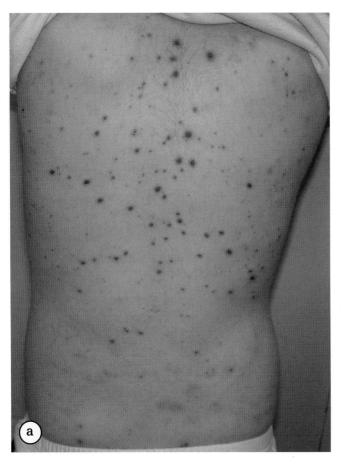

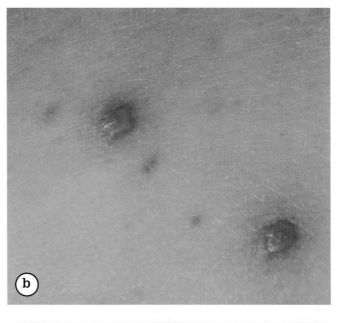

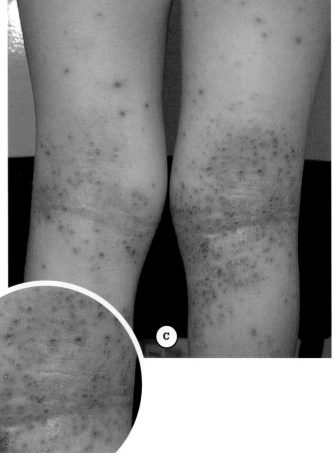

FIGURE 1.22 (a) (b) Chickenpox on the trunk with typical violaceous vesicles on close-up and **(c)** in a child with atopic dermatitis

ITCHY RASHES Infections

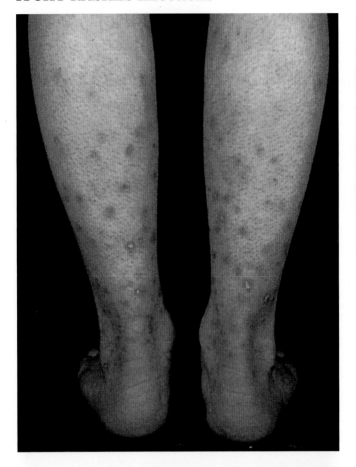

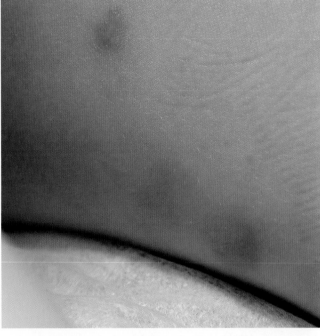

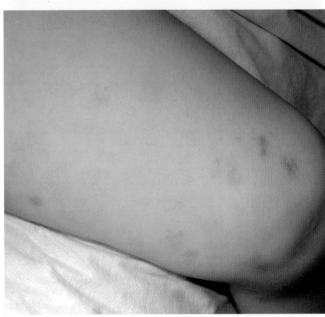

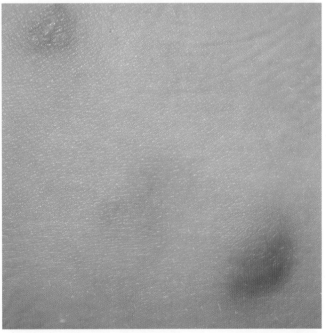

FIGURE 1.23 Insect bites also known as papular urticaria

ITCHY RASHES Infections *Bacterial*

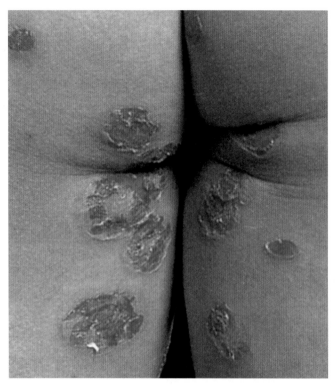

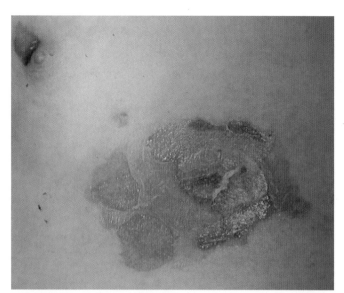

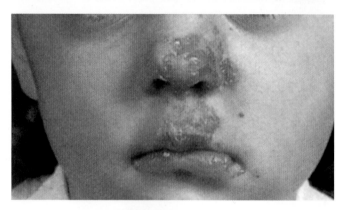

FIGURE 1.24 Typical yellow and golden crusts seen in impetigo. Blistering (above) may also be a feature (bullous impetigo)

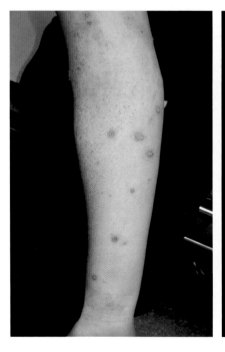

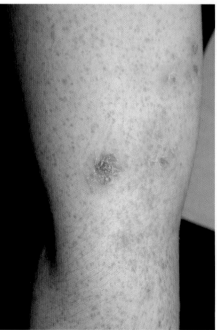

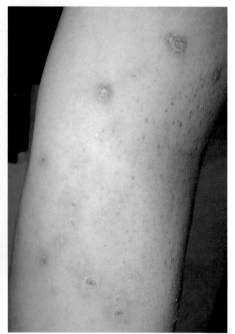

ITCHY RASHES Infections

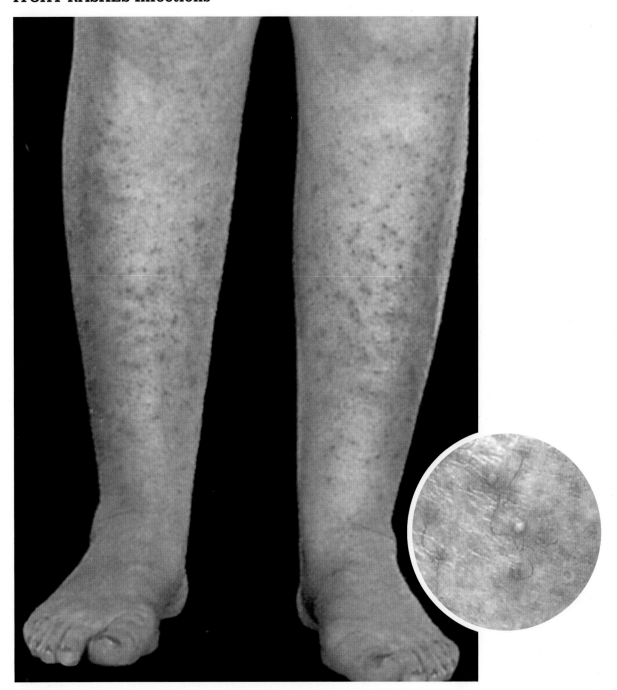

FIGURE 1.25 Folliculitis on the legs with close-up of follicular pustules

ITCHY RASHES Infections *Fungal*

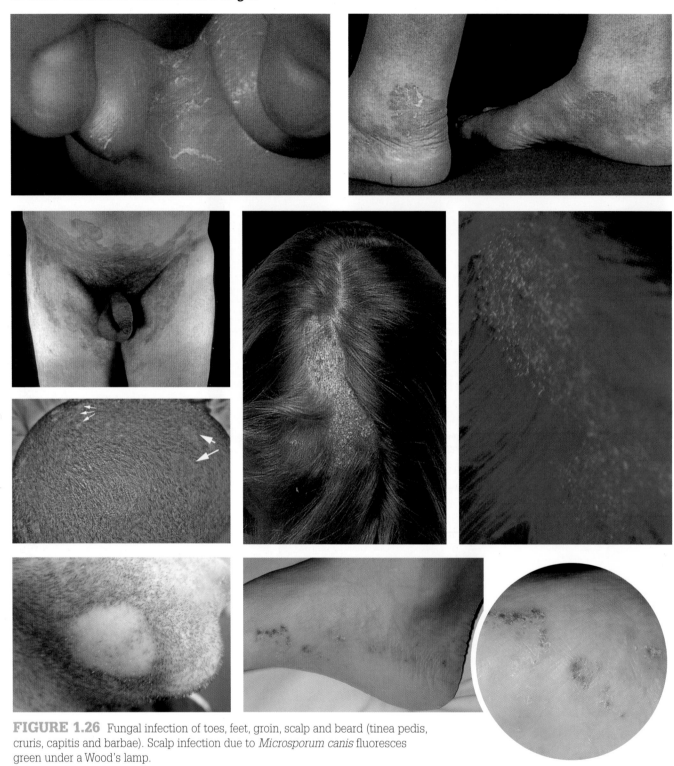

FIGURE 1.26 Fungal infection of toes, feet, groin, scalp and beard (tinea pedis, cruris, capitis and barbae). Scalp infection due to *Microsporum canis* fluoresces green under a Wood's lamp.

ITCHY RASHES Infections

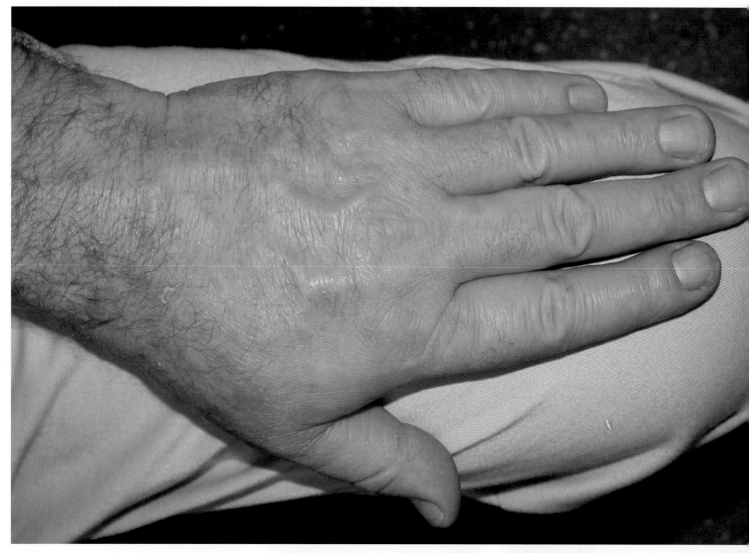

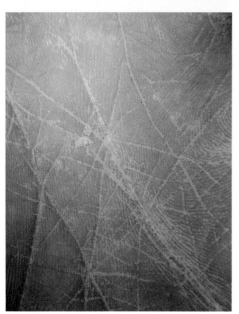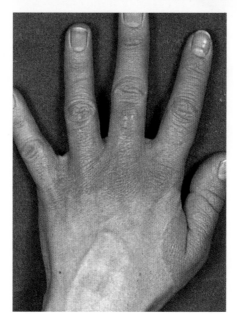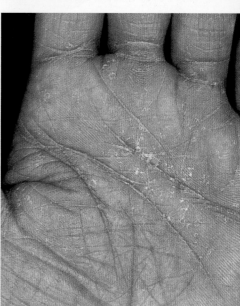

FIGURE 1.27 Fungal infection of hands with typical scaling of the palmar creases and a well-defined edge at the wrist

ITCHY RASHES Infections

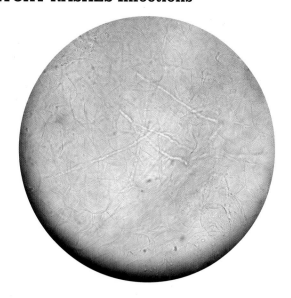

FIGURE 1.28 Microscopy of hyphae in fungal infection

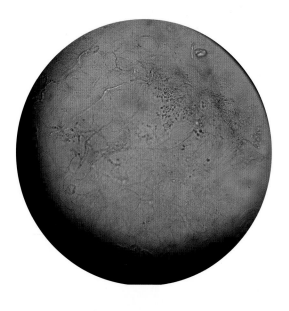

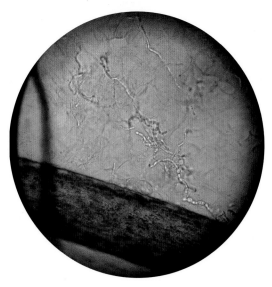

ITCHY RASHES Urticaria

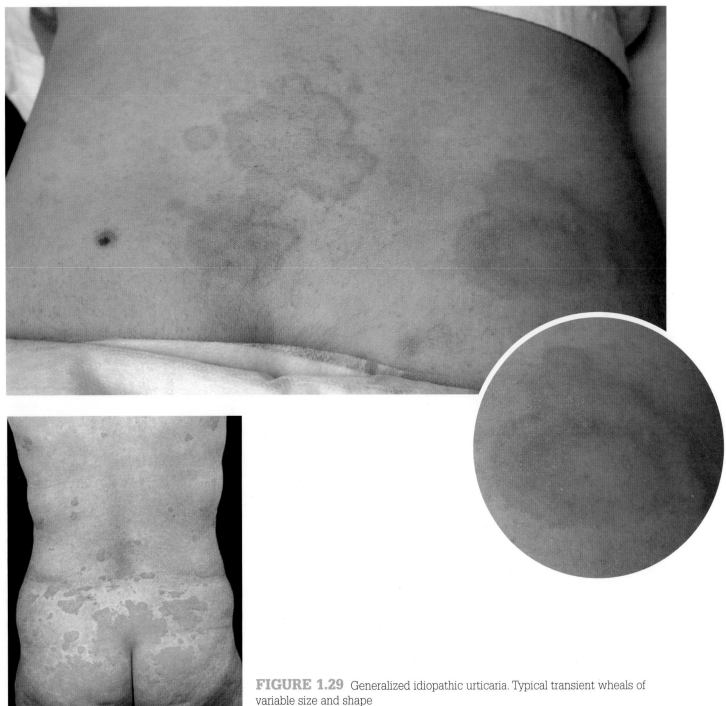

FIGURE 1.29 Generalized idiopathic urticaria. Typical transient wheals of variable size and shape

ITCHY RASHES Urticaria

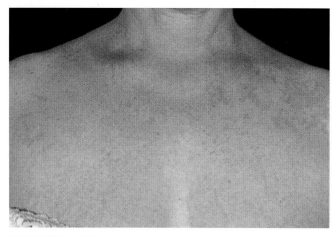

FIGURE 1.30 Delayed pressure urticaria reproduced with weights strapped to the shoulder

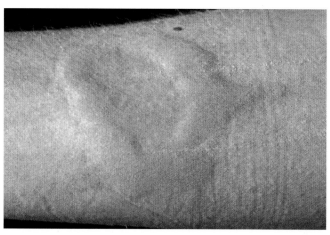

FIGURE 1.31 Cold urticaria reproduced with an ice cube

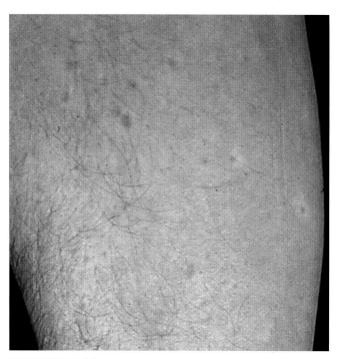

FIGURE 1.32 Tiny urticarial papules induced by sweating in cholinergic urticaria

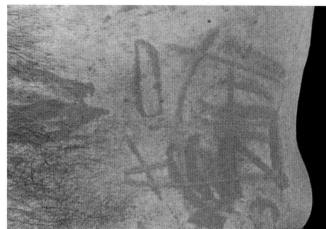

FIGURE 1.33 Dermographism is common, affecting around 15% of the population

UNCOMMON ITCHY RASHES Lichen planus

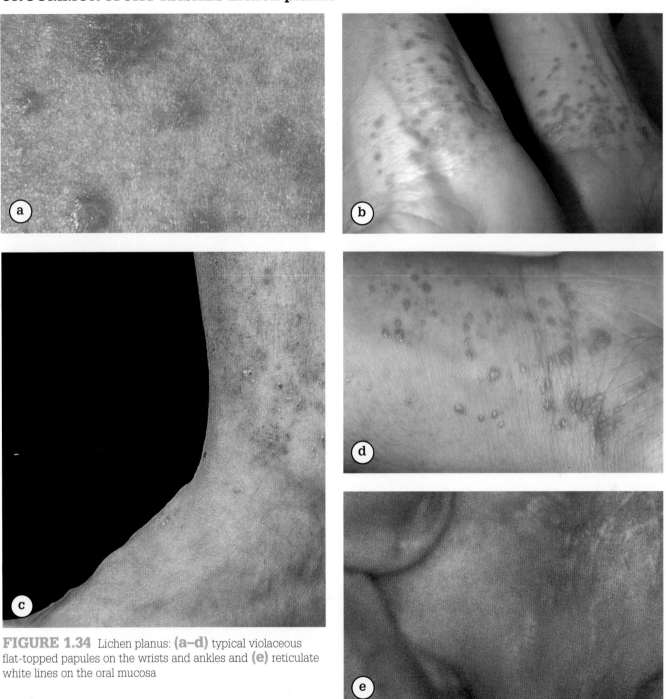

FIGURE 1.34 Lichen planus: **(a–d)** typical violaceous flat-topped papules on the wrists and ankles and **(e)** reticulate white lines on the oral mucosa

UNCOMMON ITCHY RASHES Dermatitis herpetiformis

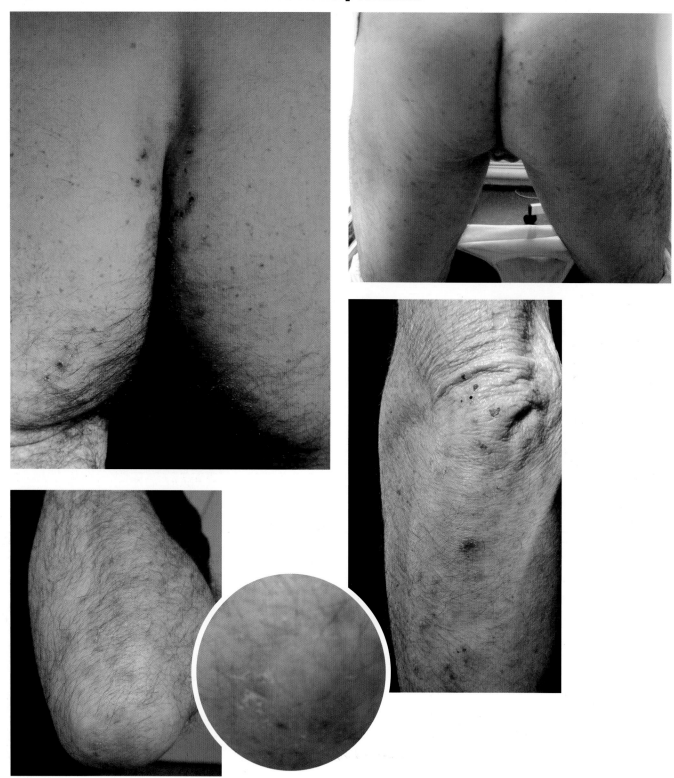

FIGURE 1.35 Excoriated vesicles on the elbows, knees and buttocks in dermatitis herpetiformis

NON-ITCHY RASHES Psoriasis

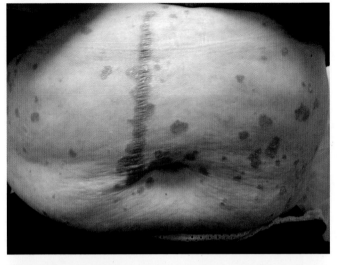

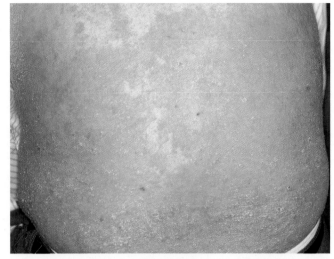

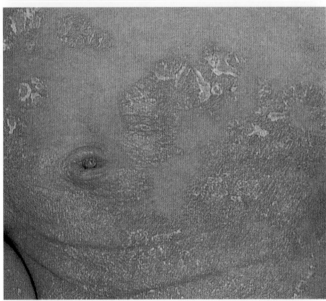

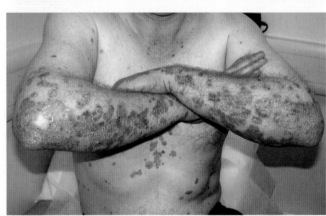

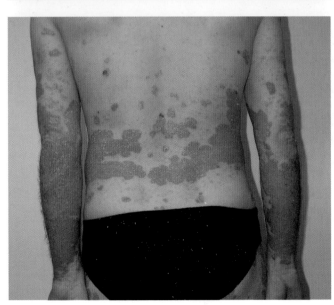

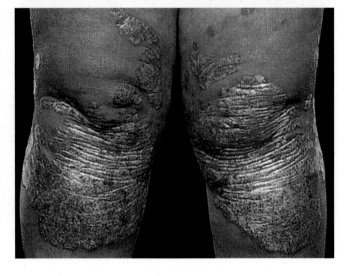

FIGURE 1.36 Psoriasis

NON-ITCHY RASHES Psoriasis

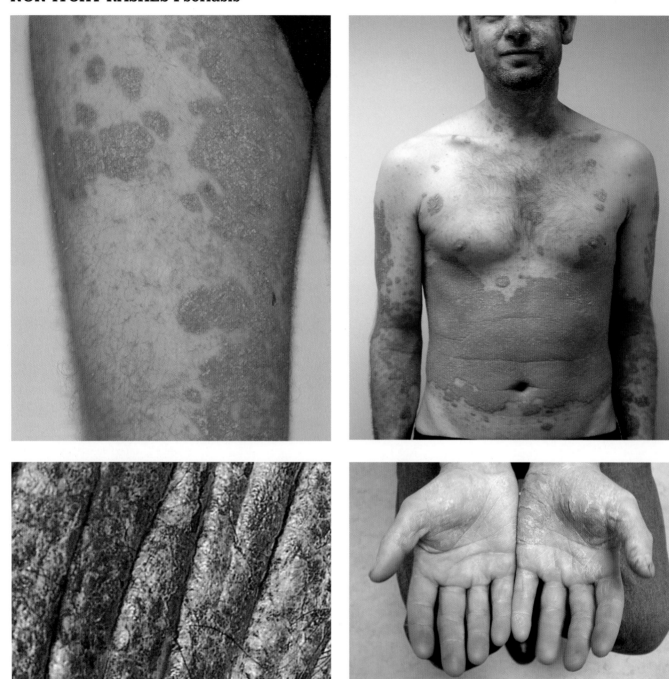

FIGURE 1.36 Psoriasis *(continued)*

NON-ITCHY RASHES Pityriasis rosea

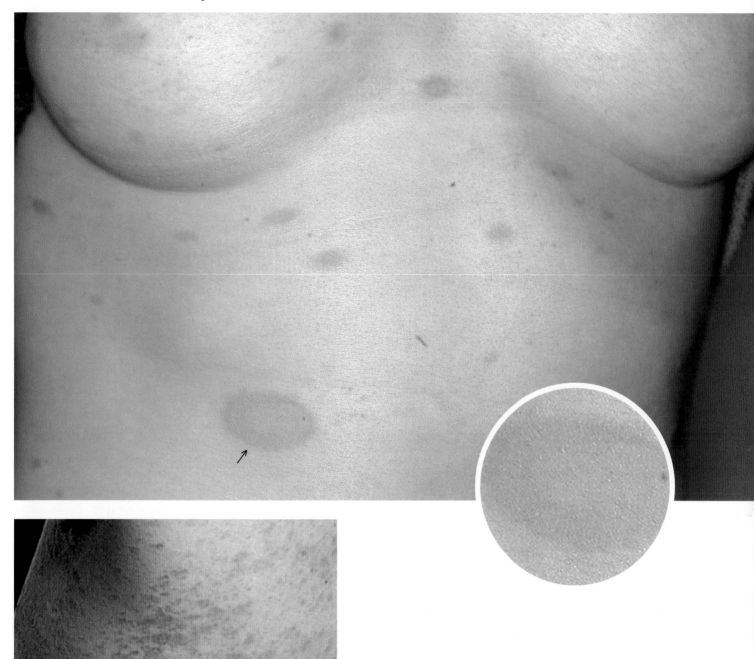

FIGURE 1.37 Pityriasis rosea: thin, annular plaques with peripheral scale following the lines of the ribs. Often preceded by a single, larger lesion, the herald patch (arrow)

NON-ITCHY RASHES Seborrhoeic dermatitis

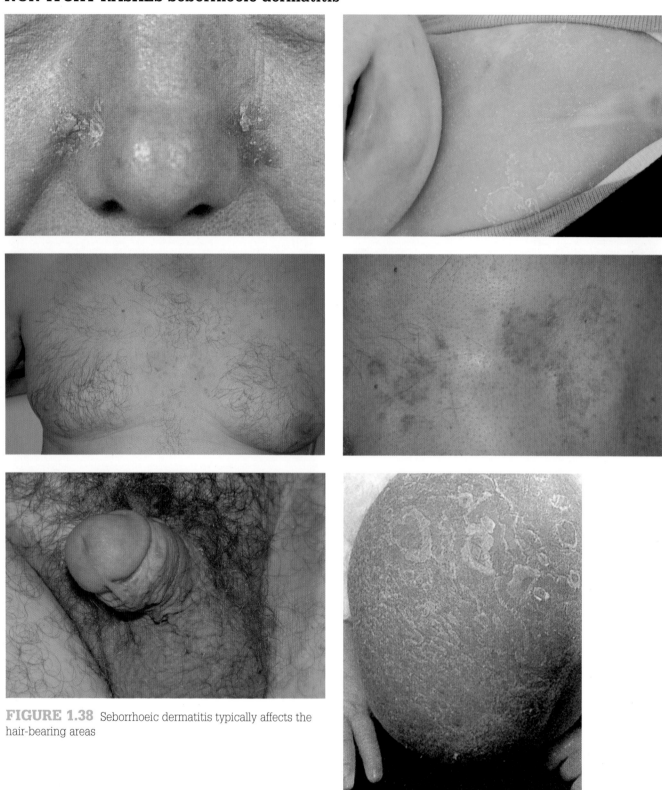

FIGURE 1.38 Seborrhoeic dermatitis typically affects the hair-bearing areas

NON-ITCHY RASHES Drug reactions

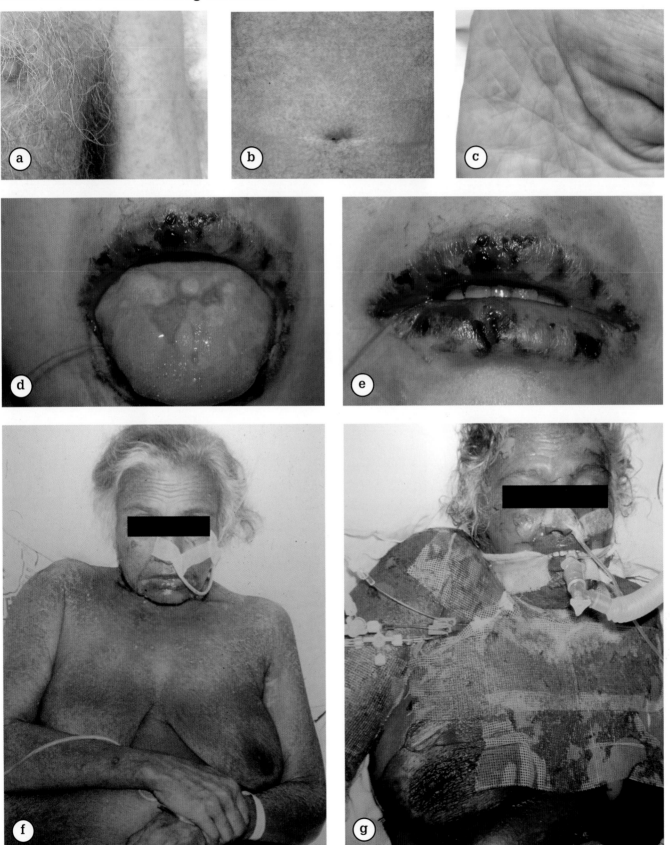

FIGURE 1.39 Drug reactions: **(a–b)** typical morbilliform drug eruption, **(c)** typical target lesions of erythema multiforme, **(d,e)** oral involvement in Stevens–Johnson syndrome, **(f,g)** extensive sloughing of the skin in toxic epidermal necrolysis

NON-ITCHY RASHES Viral infections

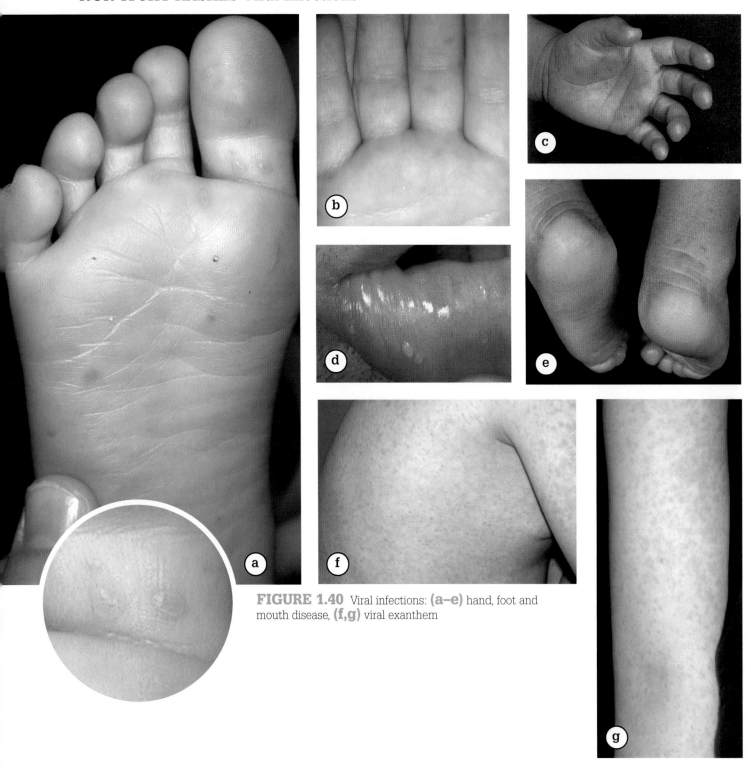

FIGURE 1.40 Viral infections: **(a–e)** hand, foot and mouth disease, **(f,g)** viral exanthem

NON-ITCHY RASHES Acne

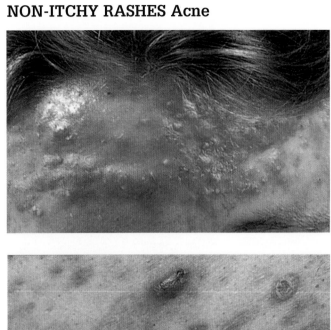

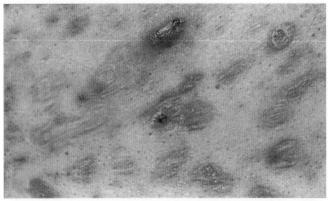

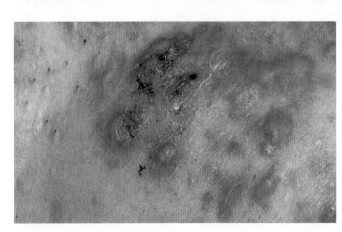

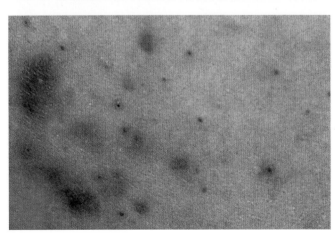

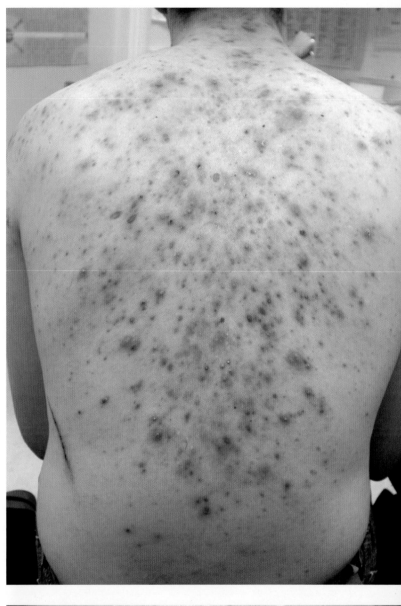

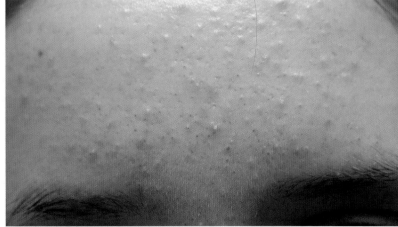

FIGURE 1.41 Acne: papules, pustules, comedones (blackheads and whiteheads) and scars

UNCOMMON NON-ITCHY RASHES Lupus

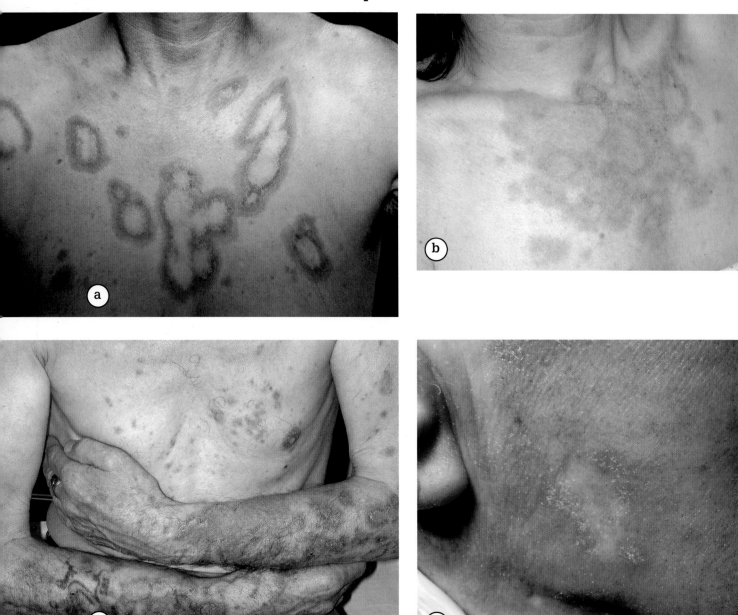

FIGURE 1.42 Lupus: **(a–c)** annular plaques on the chest and arms in subacute lupus, **(d)** typical discoid lupus of the cheek with central scarring

UNCOMMON NON-ITCHY RASHES Lupus

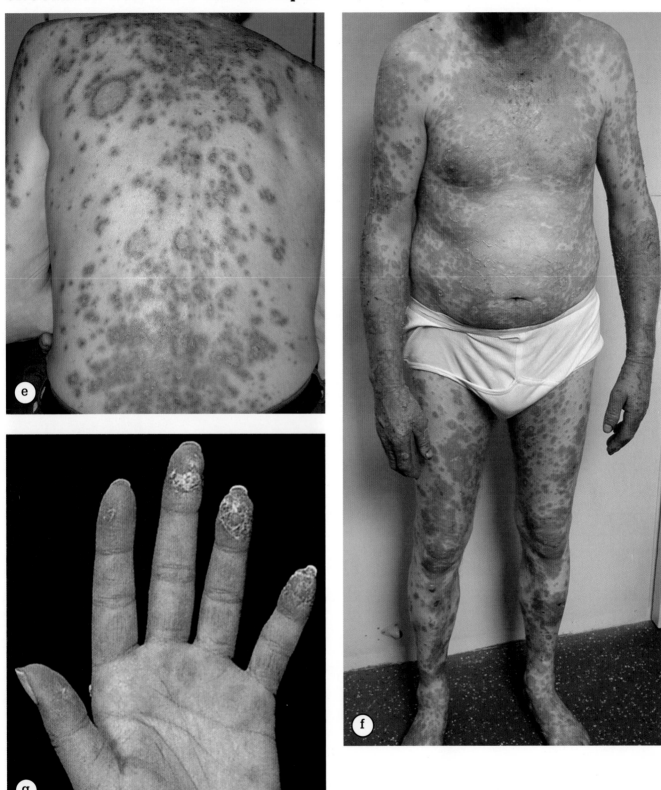

FIGURE 1.42 Lupus (*continued*): **(e,f)** generalized cutaneous lupus, **(g)** chilblain lupus

UNCOMMON NON-ITCHY RASHES Connective tissue disease

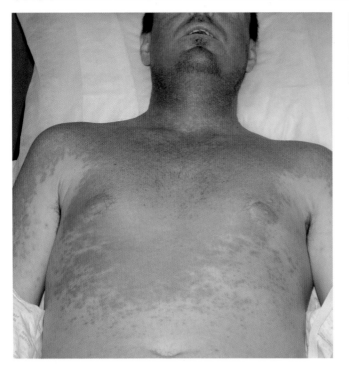

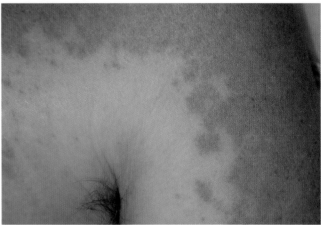

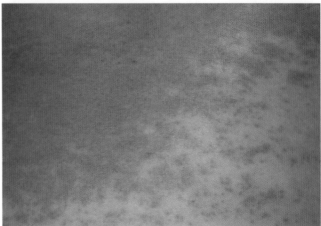

FIGURE 1.43 Photosensitive rash of mixed connective tissue disease

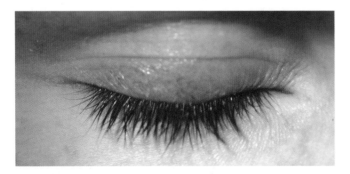

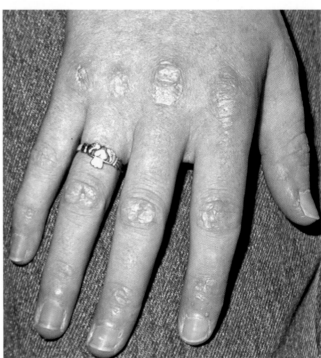

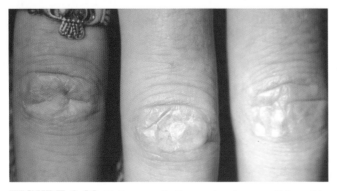

FIGURE 1.44 Violaceous (heliotrope) rash on eyelids and knuckles in dermatomyositis

UNCOMMON NON-ITCHY RASHES

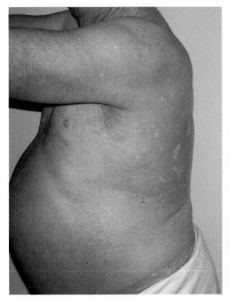
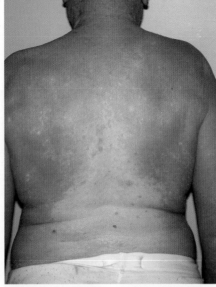
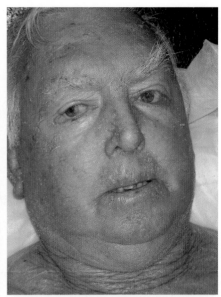

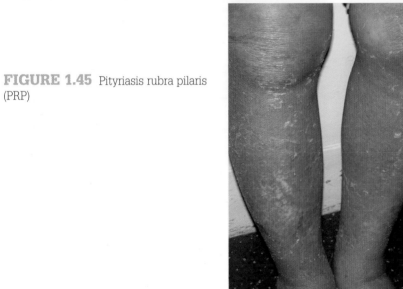
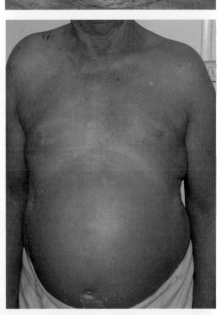

FIGURE 1.45 Pityriasis rubra pilaris (PRP)

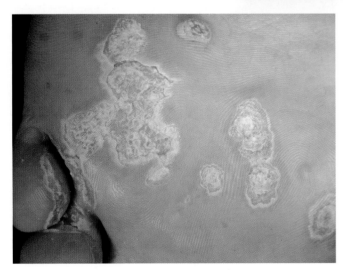
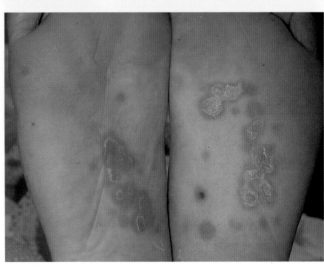

FIGURE 1.46 Reiter's syndrome

FIGURE 1.47 Syphilis

PAINFUL RASHES Infections

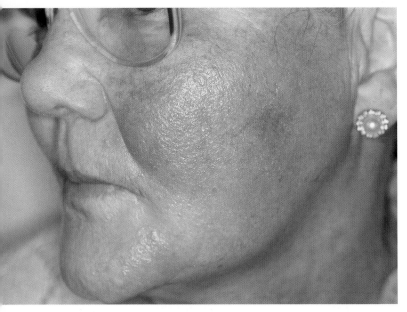

FIGURE 1.48 Cellulitis

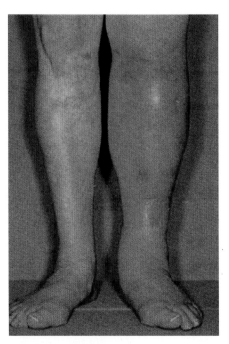

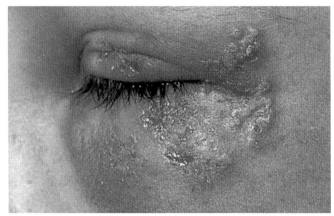

FIGURE 1.49 Erysipelas

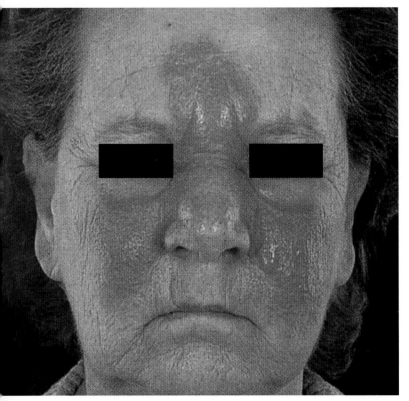

FIGURE 1.50 Herpes simplex with secondary bacterial
infection (impetigo)

PAINFUL RASHES Infections

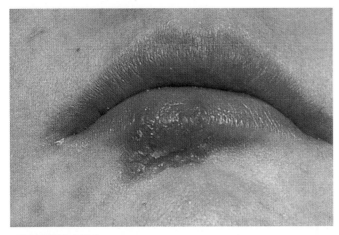

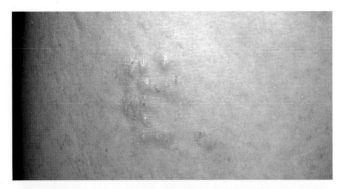

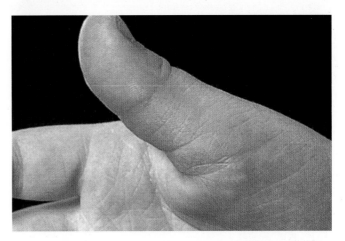

FIGURE 1.51 Herpes simplex infection of the lip, thigh and thumb

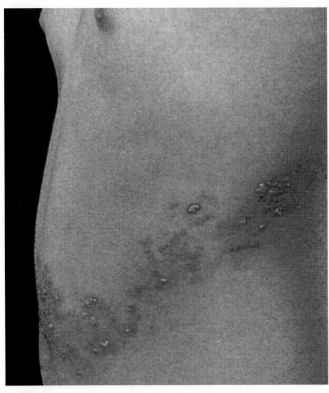

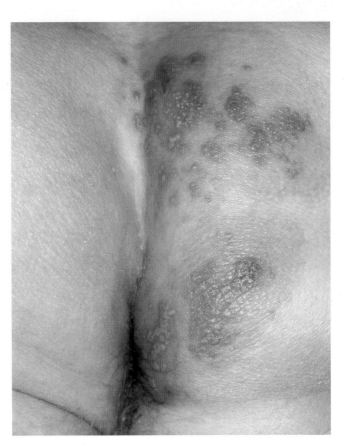

FIGURE 1.52 Herpes zoster

PAINFUL RASHES Infections

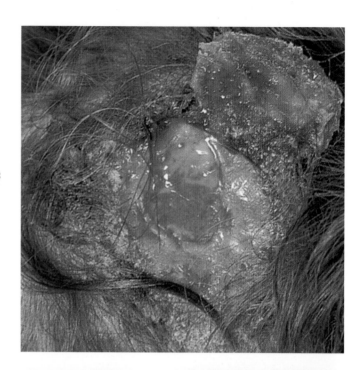

FIGURE 1.53 Painful inflammatory reaction in tinea capitis producing a kerion

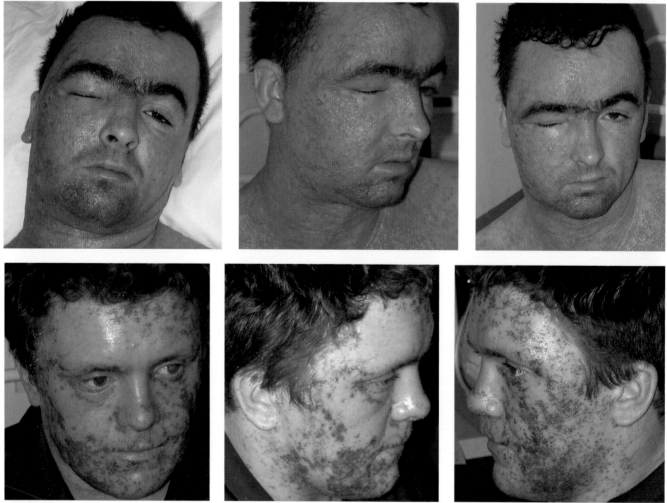

FIGURE 1.54 Atopic dermatitis with widespread herpes simplex infection – eczema herpeticum (Kaposi's varicelliform eruption)

Chapter 2

Facial Rashes

Summary

- Papulopustular rashes
- Scaly rashes
- Itchy rashes
- Painful rashes
- Photosensitive rashes

These can be divided into the papulopustular, scaly, itchy and painful groups. The acne group of disorders are characterized by papules and pustules. The presence of comedones (blackheads and whiteheads) indicates acne vulgaris. Telangiectasia suggests rosacea and occasionally lupus. The most common of the scaly group is seborrhoeic dermatitis, with psoriasis, fungal infection and lupus being much less common. Itchy facial rashes include atopic allergic and perioral dermatitis, while pain usually indicates infection. Photosensitive rashes affect the face, neck and exposed areas of the limbs but are particularly characterized by the areas they spare: the upper eyelids, under the chin, behind the ears, the hairline and the underside (volar) aspect of the arms. The reader is directed to Chapters 10, 11, 15 and 20 in Section 2 for more detailed descriptions of these conditions.

Algorithm 2.1 Facial rashes

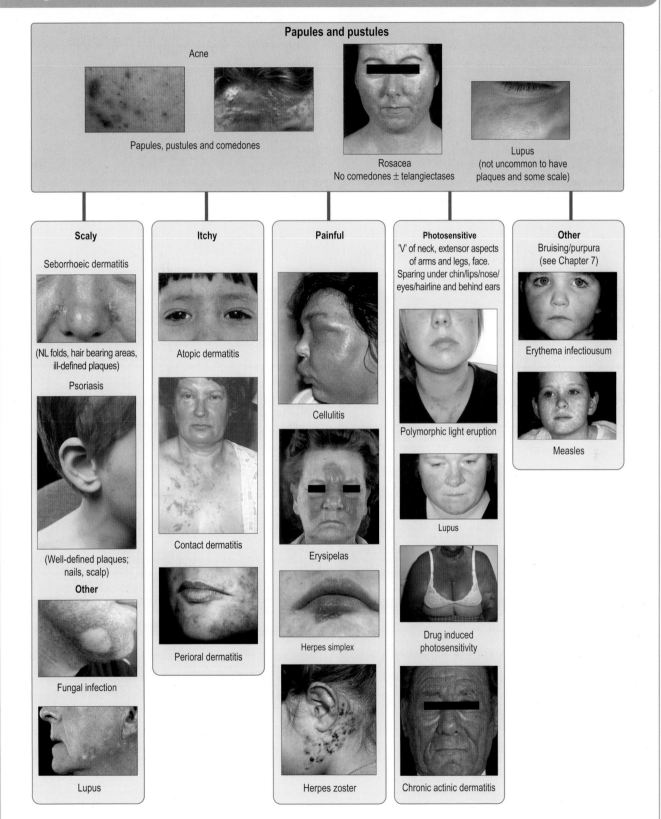

Papules and pustules

Acne

Papules, pustules and comedones

Rosacea
No comedones ± telangiectases

Lupus
(not uncommon to have
plaques and some scale)

Scaly

Seborrhoeic dermatitis

(NL folds, hair bearing areas,
ill-defined plaques)

Psoriasis

(Well-defined plaques;
nails, scalp)

Other

Fungal infection

Lupus

Itchy

Atopic dermatitis

Contact dermatitis

Perioral dermatitis

Painful

Cellulitis

Erysipelas

Herpes simplex

Herpes zoster

Photosensitive
'V' of neck, extensor aspects
of arms and legs, face.
Sparing under chin/lips/nose/
eyes/hairline and behind ears

Polymorphic light eruption

Lupus

Drug induced
photosensitivity

Chronic actinic dermatitis

Other
Bruising/purpura
(see Chapter 7)

Erythema infectiousum

Measles

PAPULES, PUSTULES AND COMEDONES

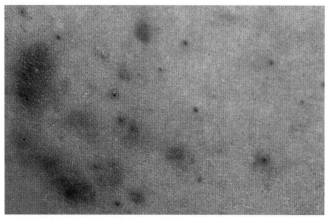 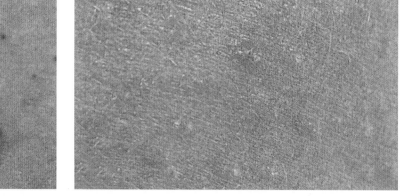

FIGURE 2.2 Comedones (blackheads and whiteheads)

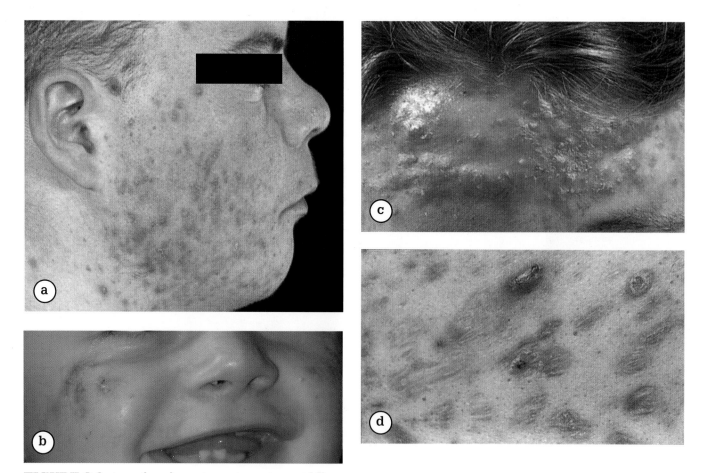

FIGURE 2.3 Acne: (a–c) papules and pustules and (d) atrophic scars

PAPULES, PUSTULES AND TELANGIECTASES

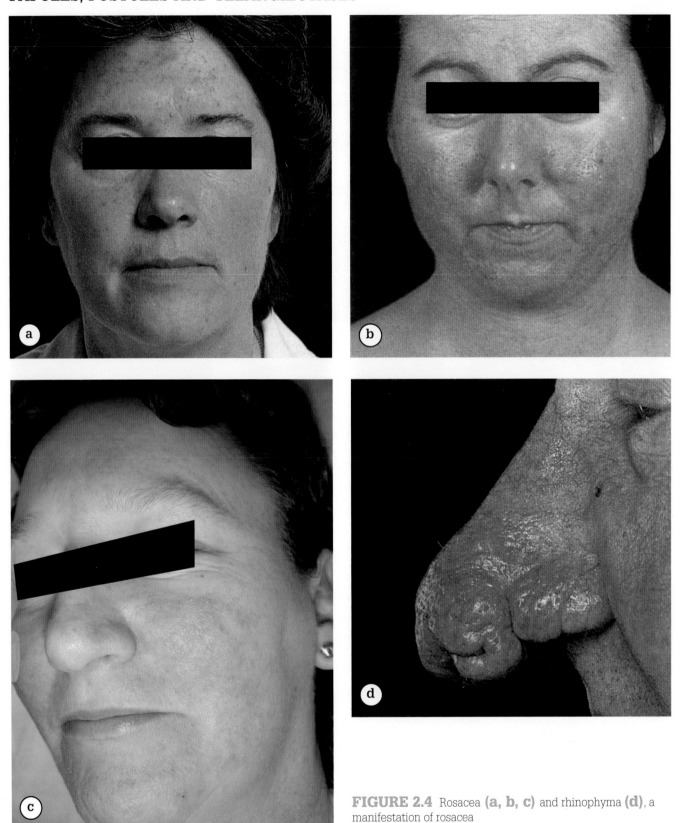

FIGURE 2.4 Rosacea **(a, b, c)** and rhinophyma **(d)**, a manifestation of rosacea

ITCHY PAPULES

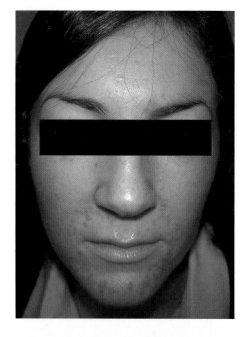

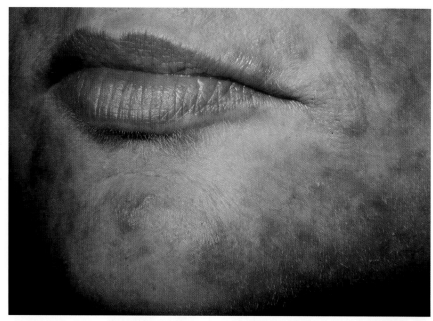

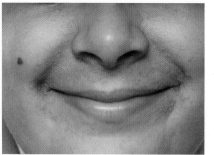

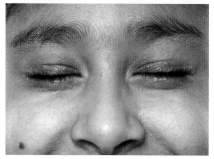

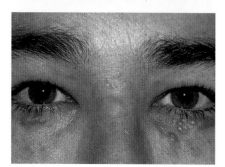

FIGURE 2.5 Perioral dermatitis with and without ocular involvement

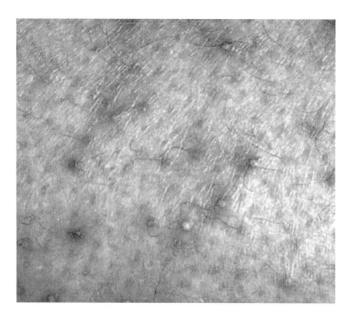

FIGURE 2.6 Folliculitis

SCALY RASH Seborrhoeic dermatitis

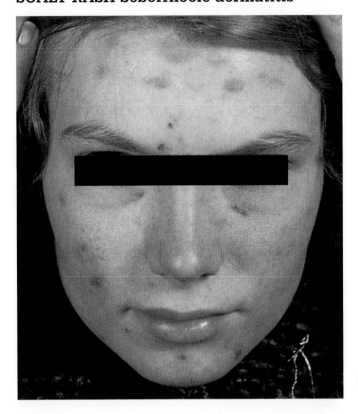

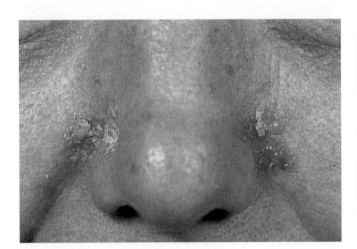

FIGURE 2.8 Seborrhoeic dermatitis

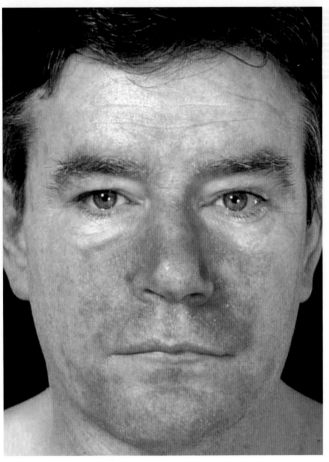

FIGURE 2.7 Acne excoriée

SCALY RASH Psoriasis

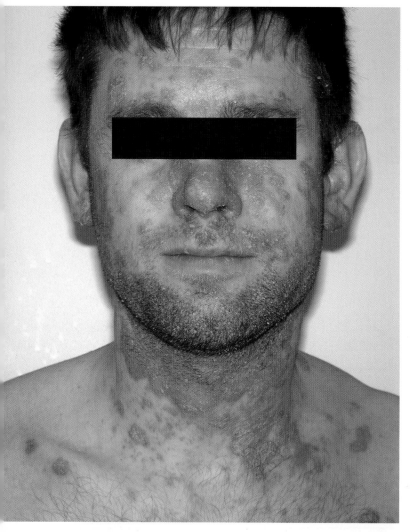
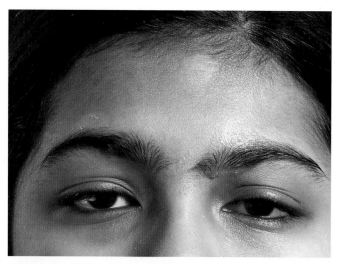
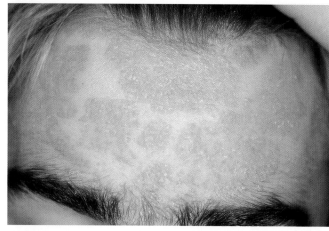
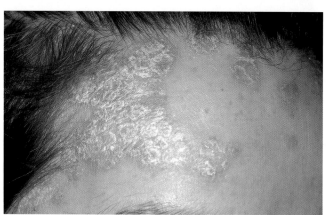
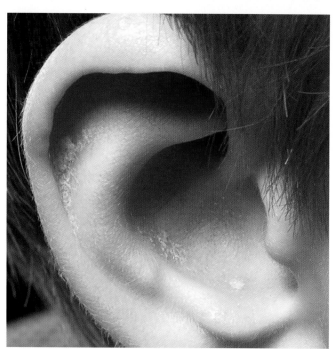

FIGURE 2.9 Psoriasis

SCALY RASH Other

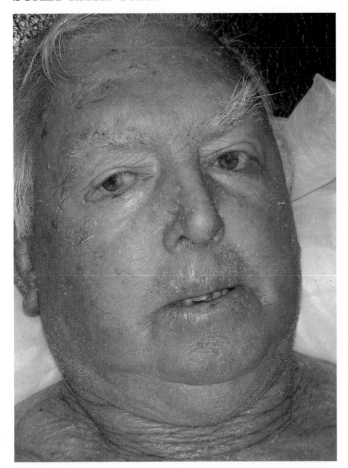

FIGURE 2.10 Pityriasis rubra pilaris

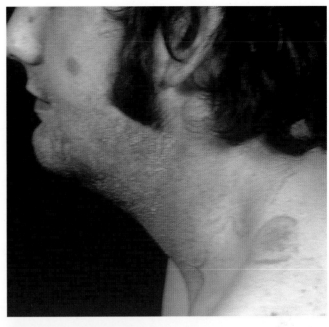

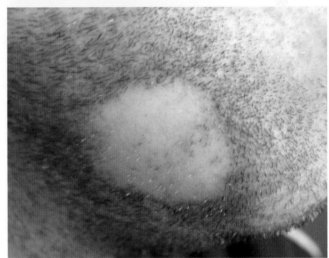

FIGURE 2.11 Tinea facei

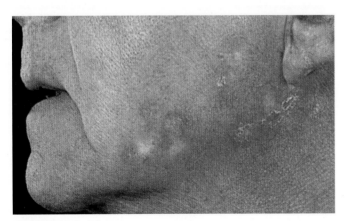

FIGURE 2.12 Lupus

ITCHY RASH Atopic dermatitis

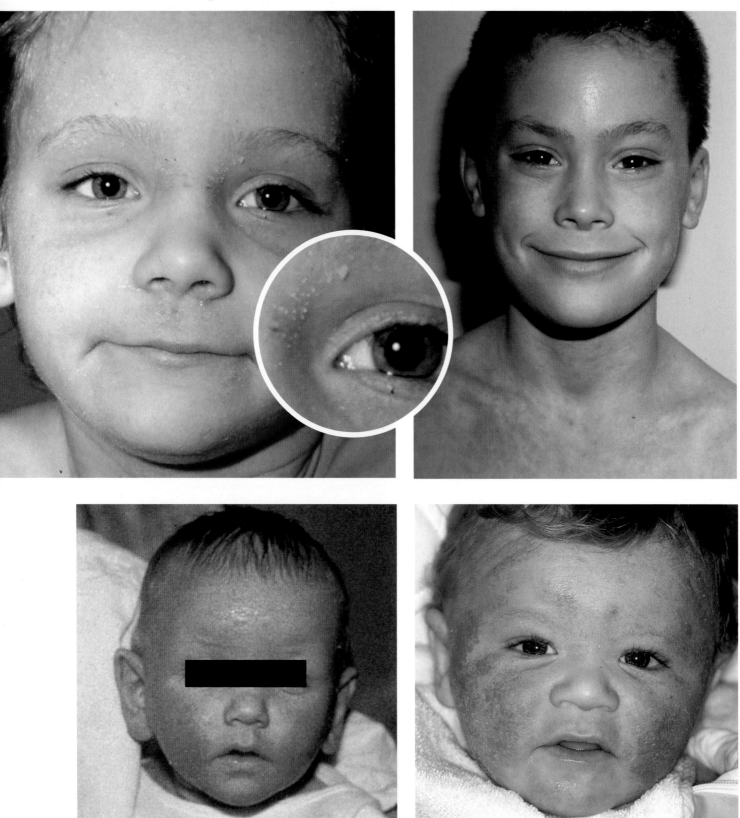

FIGURE 2.13 Atopic dermatitis

ITCHY RASH Allergic contact dermatitis

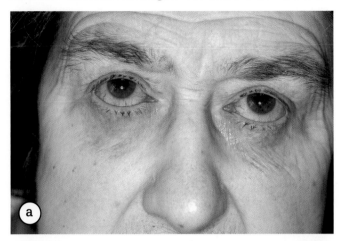

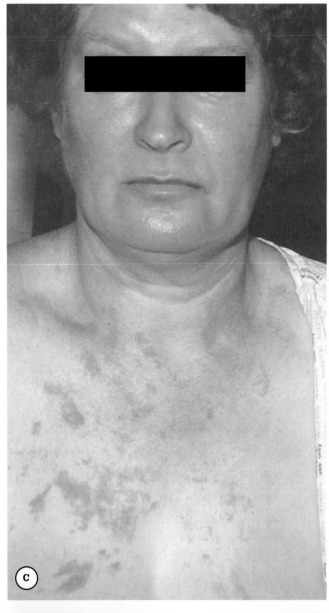

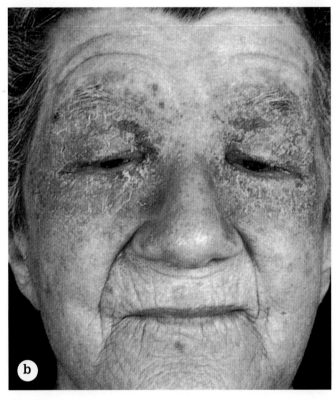

FIGURE 2.14 Allergic contact dermatitis due to eye drops **(a,b)**, plants **(c)** and cosmetics **(d)**

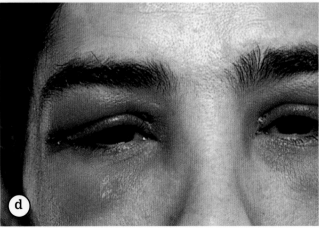

ITCHY RASH Other dermatitis

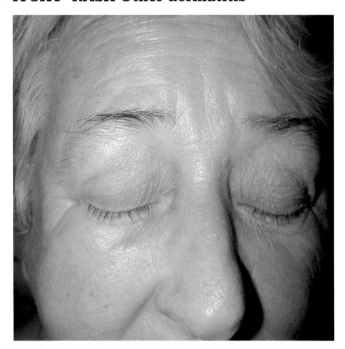

FIGURE 2.15 Alergic contact dermatitis of the eyelids due to allergy to rubber gloves

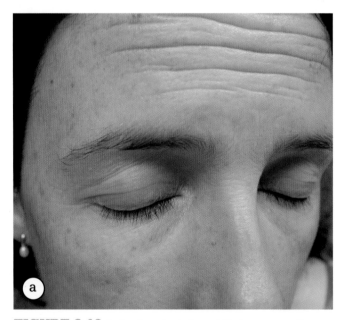

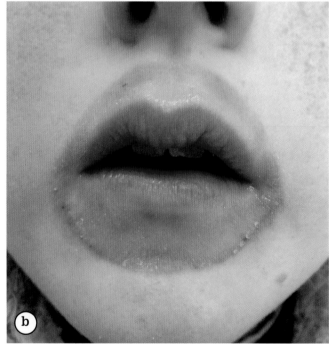

FIGURE 2.16 Irritant contact dermatitis from cosmetics **(a)** and due to repeated lip-licking **(b)**

PAINFUL RASH

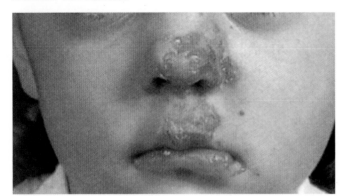

FIGURE 2.17 Impetigo

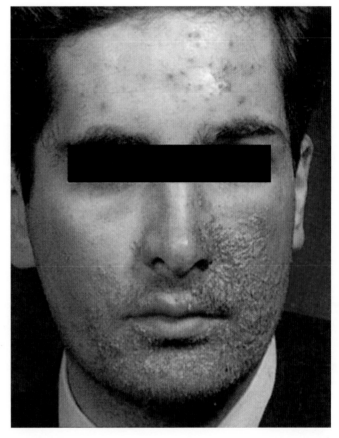

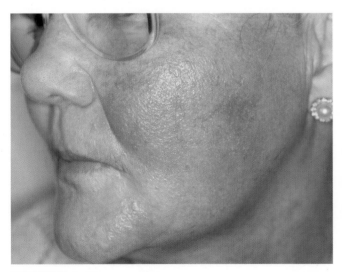

FIGURE 2.18 Erysipelas/cellulitis

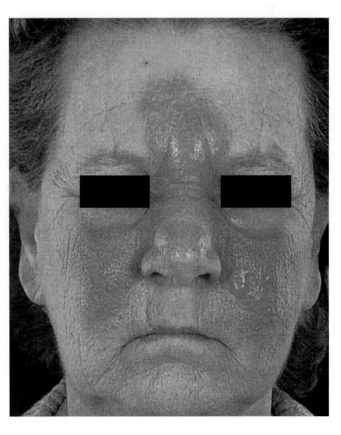

PAINFUL RASH

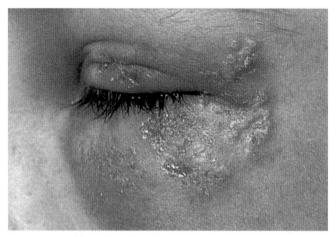

FIGURE 2.19 Herpes simplex virus

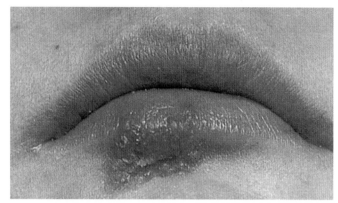

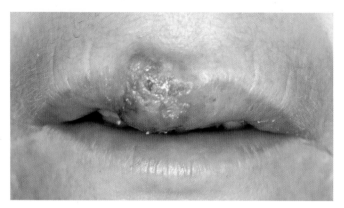

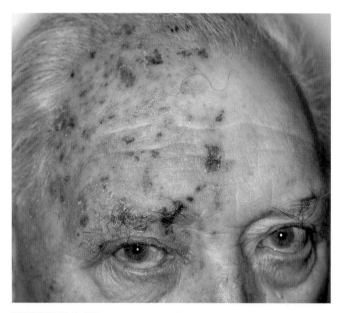

FIGURE 2.20 Herpes zoster virus

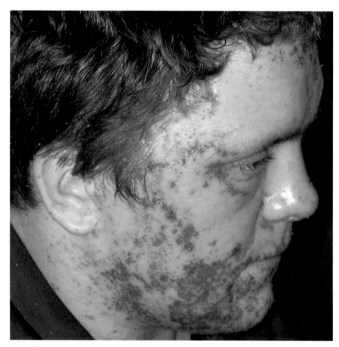

FIGURE 2.21 Eczema herpeticum

PHOTOSENSITIVE RASH

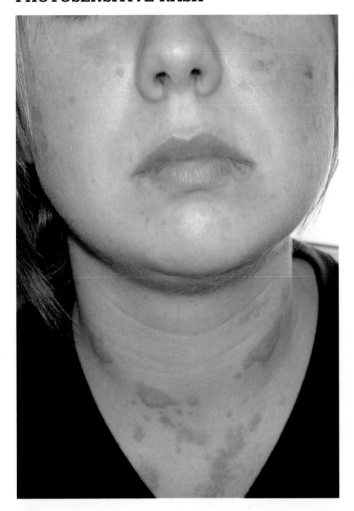

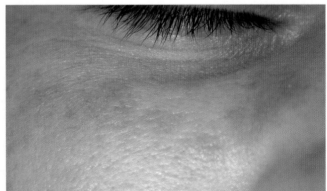

FIGURE 2.22 Polymorphic light eruption (often erroneously called 'prickly heat')

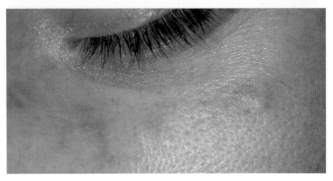

FIGURE 2.23 Butterfly rash of SLE

PHOTOSENSITIVE RASH

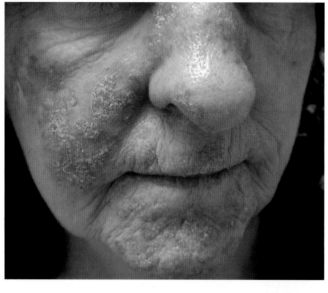

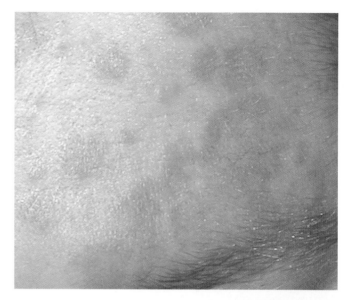

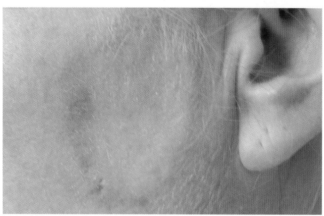

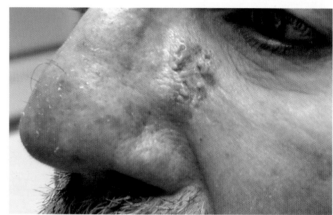

FIGURE 2.24 Discoid lupus in a photosensitive distribution

FIGURE 2.25 Chronic actinic dermatitis

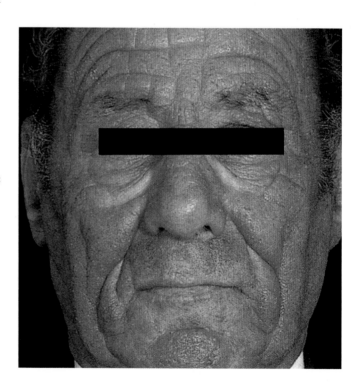

OTHER RASHES

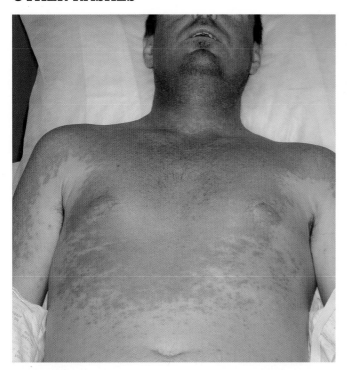

FIGURE 2.26 Mixed connective tissue disease

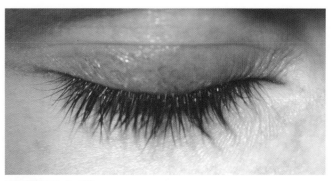

FIGURE 2.27 Dermatomyositis

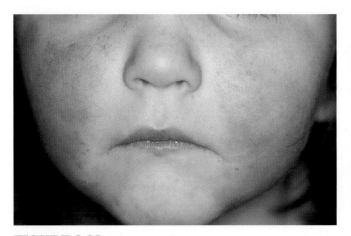

FIGURE 2.28 Erythema infectiosum

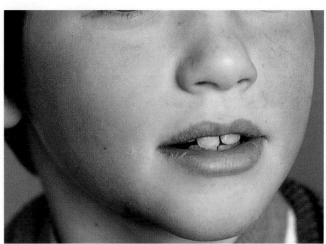

OTHER RASHES

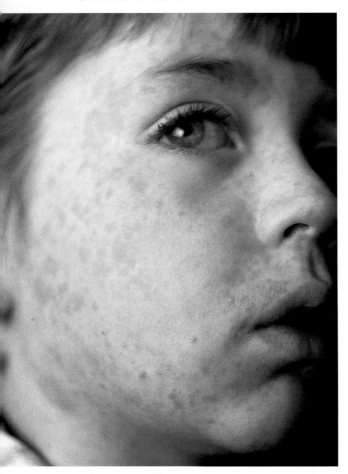

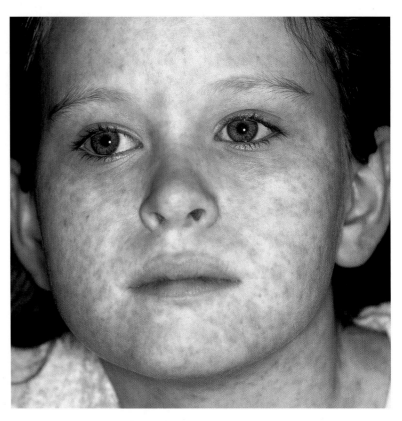

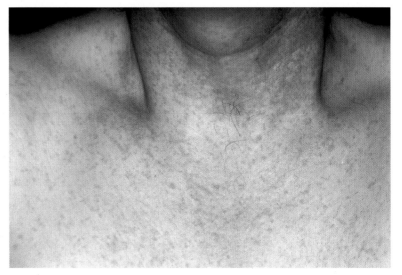

FIGURE 2.29 Measles

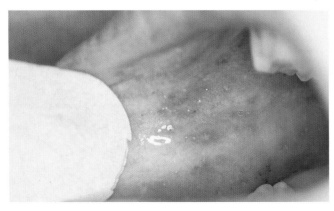

FIGURE 2.30 Koplik spots on the buccal mucosa

Chapter 3

Hair

Summary

- Localized and generalized alopecia
- Scarring versus non-scarring alopecia
- Hirsutism and hypertrichosis

Hair loss

This is a common complaint presenting to general practice. The commonest conditions to consider are male/female pattern (androgenetic) alopecia, tinea capitis and alopecia areata. For diagnostic purposes, hair loss can be divided into localized and generalized and thereafter classified according to whether there is a rash or scarring. The following algorithms outline commoner examples of hair loss with clinical photographs. The reader is directed to Chapter 18 in Section 2 for more detailed descriptions of these conditions.

Excessive hair

This is also a common complaint, particularly with the recent developments in cosmetic procedures. Most people who complain of excessive hair are otherwise normal. They will have facial and/or limb hair without features of androgen excess (deeper voice, increased muscle bulk, virilization, menstrual irregularity, etc.). There is much racial variation, with considerable body hair being the norm for some. These patients do not need further investigation but merely advice on hair removal techniques. If there is concern about androgen excess then ovarian ultrasound and serum/urine hormone profile may be indicated. The reader is directed to Chapter 18 in Section 2 for more detailed descriptions of these conditions.

Algorithm 3.1 Localized hair loss

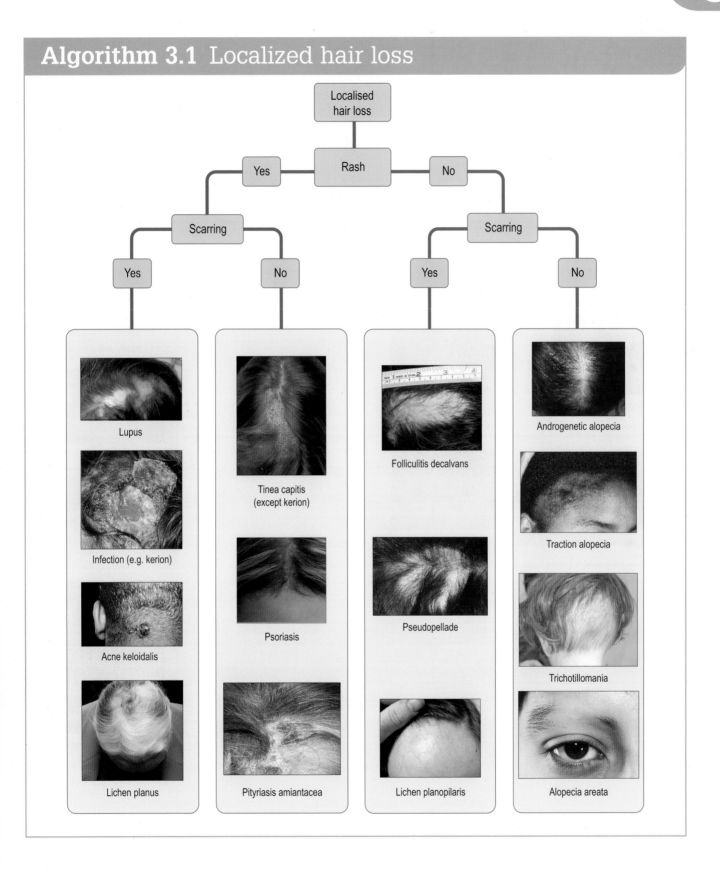

Localised hair loss

Rash — Yes / No

Yes → Scarring → Yes / No

No → Scarring → Yes / No

Rash — Yes — Scarring — Yes:
- Lupus
- Infection (e.g. kerion)
- Acne keloidalis
- Lichen planus

Rash — Yes — Scarring — No:
- Tinea capitis (except kerion)
- Psoriasis
- Pityriasis amiantacea

Rash — No — Scarring — Yes:
- Folliculitis decalvans
- Pseudopellade
- Lichen planopilaris

Rash — No — Scarring — No:
- Androgenetic alopecia
- Traction alopecia
- Trichotillomania
- Alopecia areata

3

Algorithm 3.2 Generalized hair loss

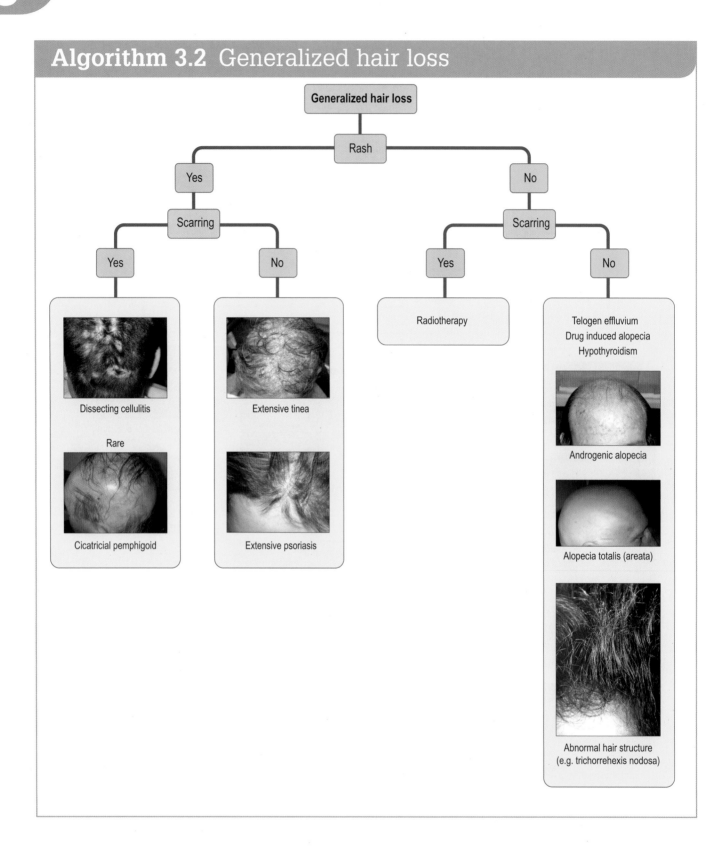

Generalized hair loss

Rash

Yes — No

Scarring (Yes side) — Scarring (No side)

Yes — No | Yes — No

Dissecting cellulitis

Rare

Cicatricial pemphigoid

Extensive tinea

Extensive psoriasis

Radiotherapy

Telogen effluvium
Drug induced alopecia
Hypothyroidism

Androgenic alopecia

Alopecia totalis (areata)

Abnormal hair structure
(e.g. trichorrehexis nodosa)

Algorithm 3.3 Excessive hair

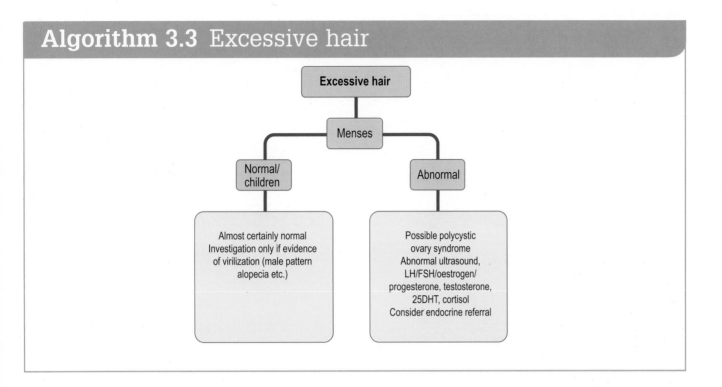

3

LOCALIZED AND GENERALIZED HAIR LOSS WITHOUT SCARRING

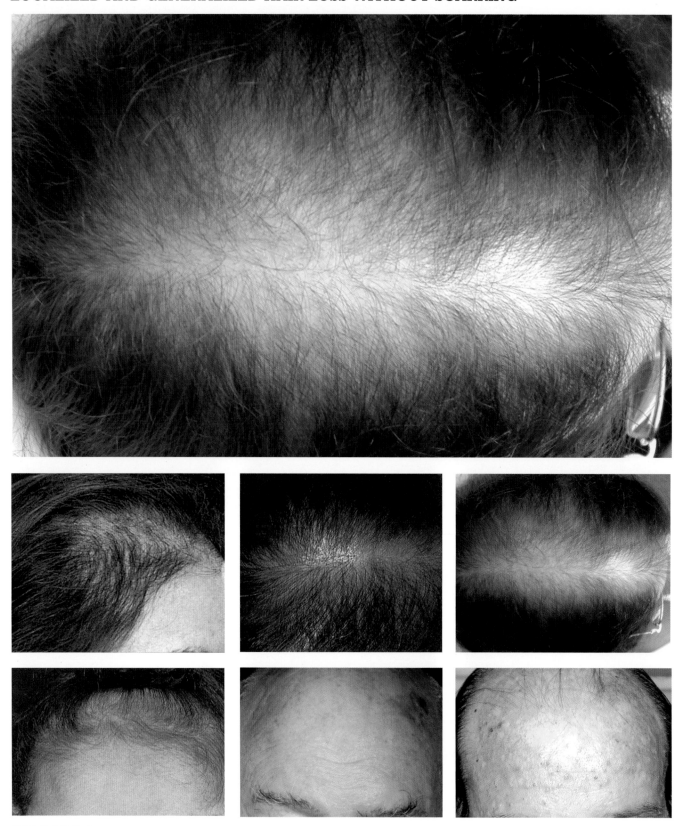

FIGURE 3.4 Androgenetic alopecia. Typical central alopecia on the vertex in female pattern alopecia. Frontal balding in male pattern alopecia

LOCALIZED AND GENERALIZED HAIR LOSS WITHOUT SCARRING

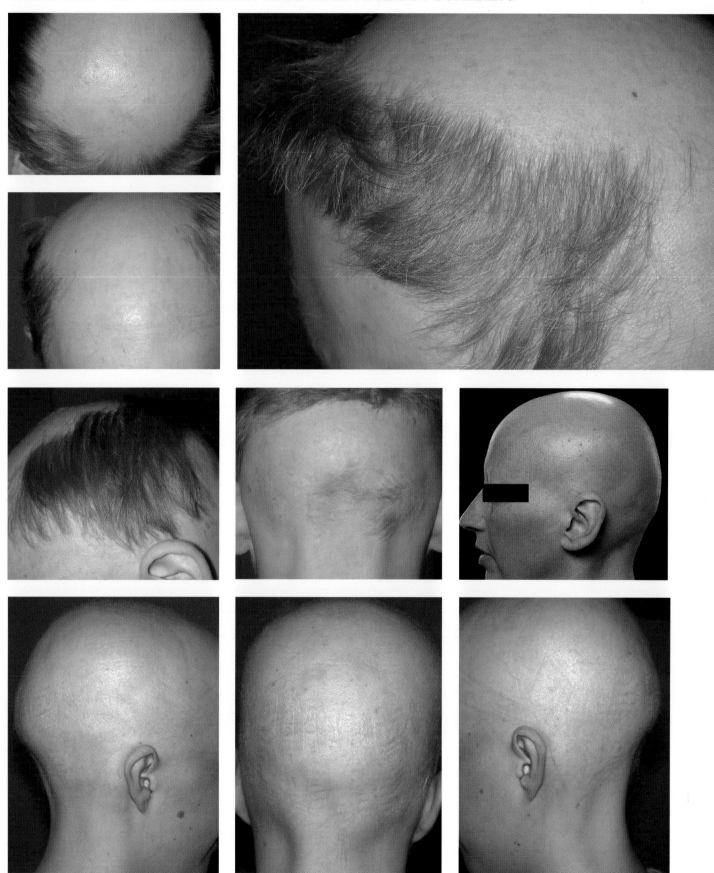

FIGURE 3.5 Alopecia areata partial and total (alopecia totalis)

LOCALIZED AND GENERALIZED HAIR LOSS WITHOUT SCARRING

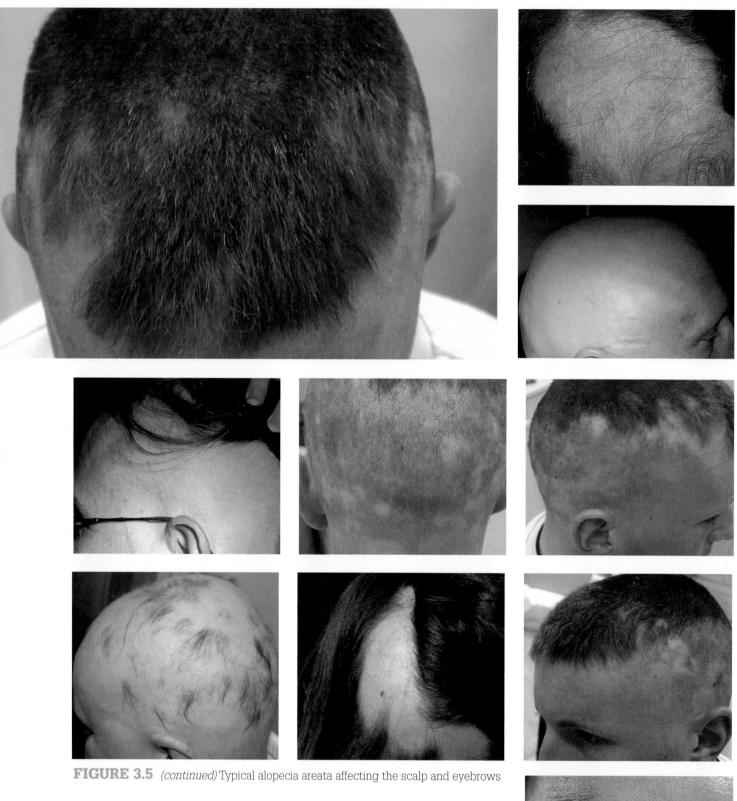

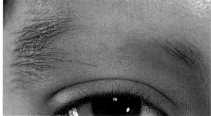

FIGURE 3.5 *(continued)* Typical alopecia areata affecting the scalp and eyebrows

LOCALIZED AND GENERALIZED HAIR LOSS WITHOUT SCARRING

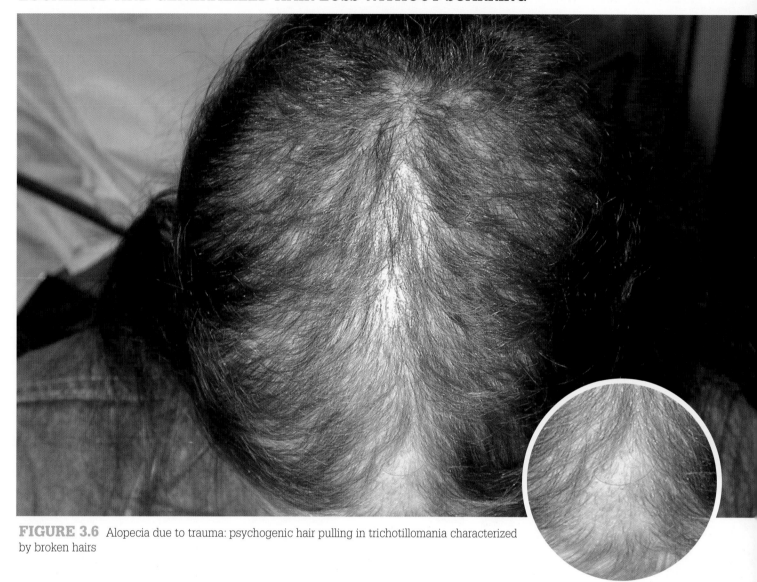

FIGURE 3.6 Alopecia due to trauma: psychogenic hair pulling in trichotillomania characterized by broken hairs

LOCALIZED AND GENERALIZED HAIR LOSS WITHOUT SCARRING

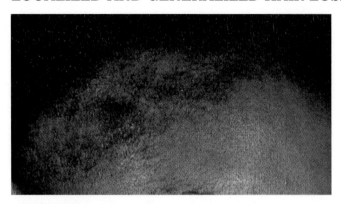

FIGURE 3.7 Traction from tightly bound hair style

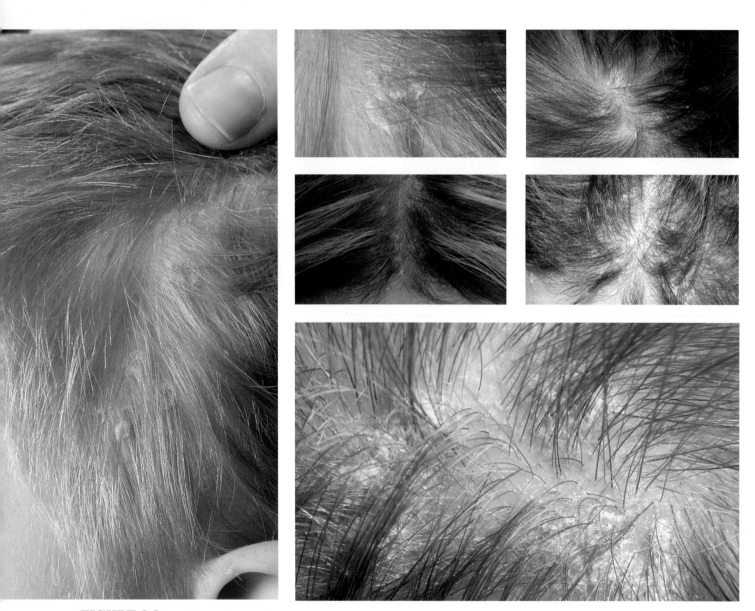

FIGURE 3.8 Mild alopecia associated with extensive psoriasis

LOCALIZED AND GENERALIZED HAIR LOSS WITHOUT SCARRING

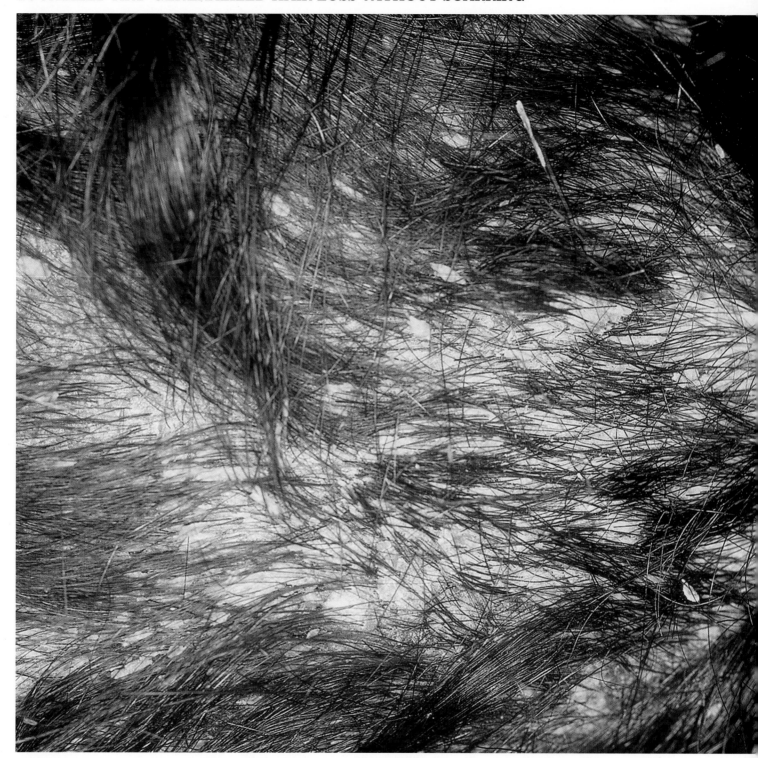

FIGURE 3.9 Alopecia with tinea amiantacea mainly seen in childhood associated with dermatitis and psoriasis

LOCALIZED AND GENERALIZED HAIR LOSS WITHOUT SCARRING

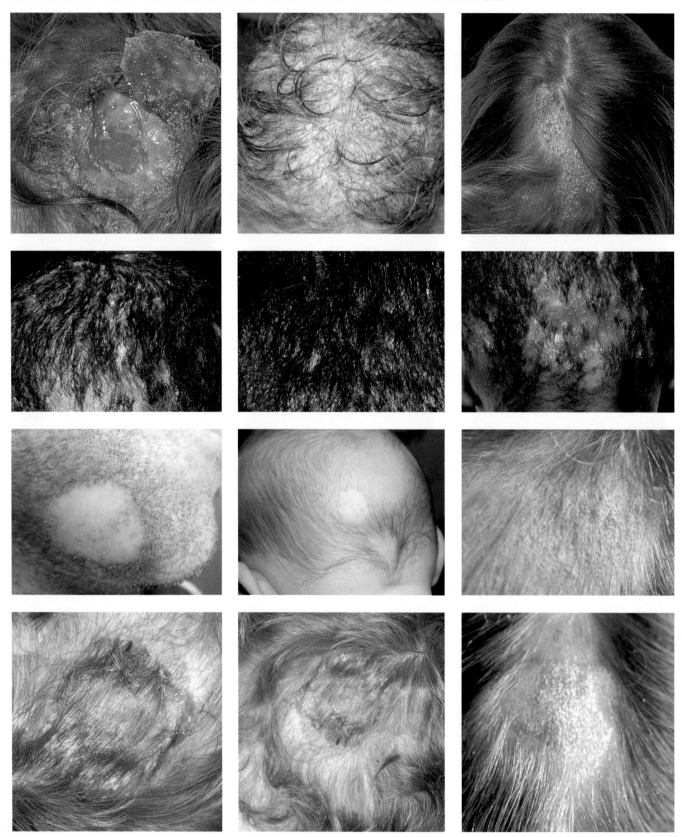

FIGURE 3.10 Localized and extensive alopecia due to tinea

LOCALIZED AND GENERALIZED HAIR LOSS WITHOUT SCARRING

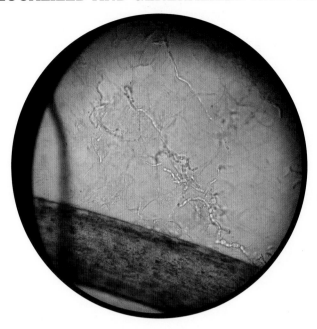

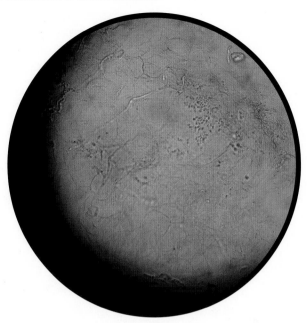

FIGURE 3.11 Microscopy of fungal infection from a scalp scrape

Structural abnormalities of the hair

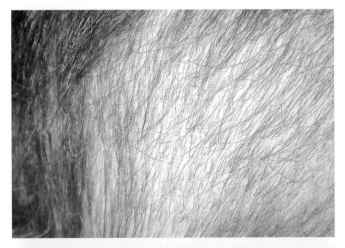

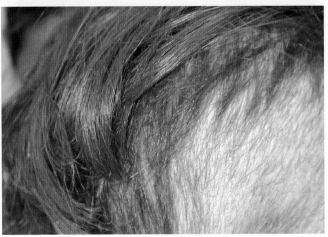

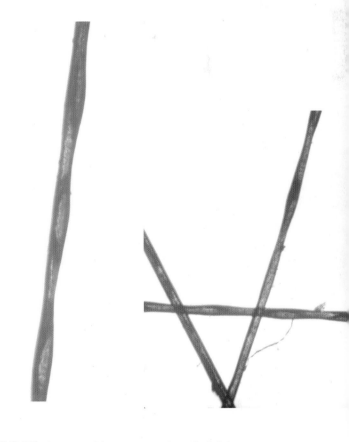

FIGURE 3.12 Congenital hair twisting (monilethrix)

LOCALIZED AND GENERALIZED HAIR LOSS WITHOUT SCARRING

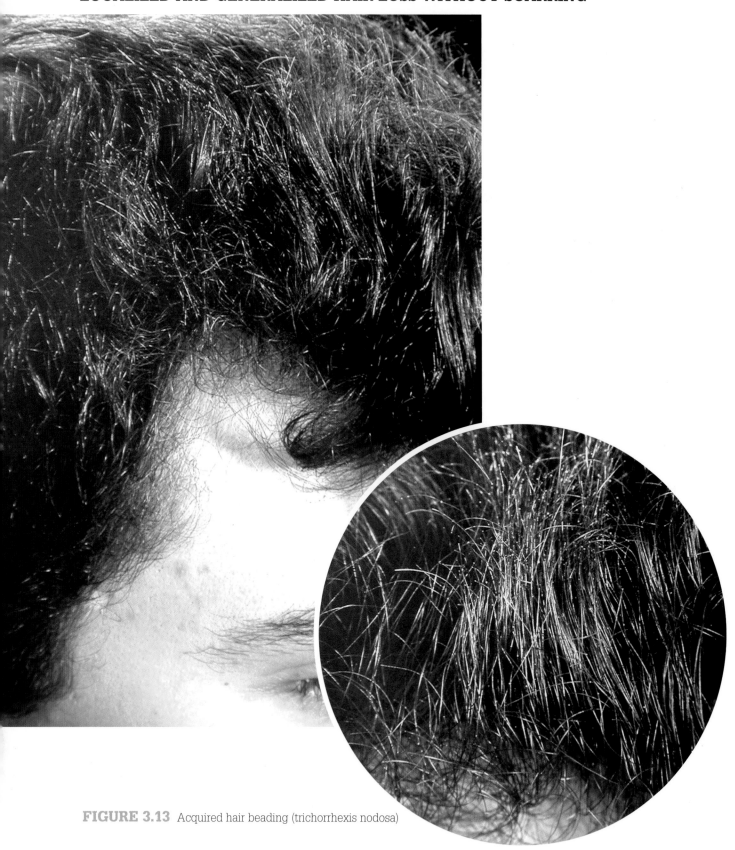

FIGURE 3.13 Acquired hair beading (trichorrhexis nodosa)

LOCALIZED AND GENERALIZED HAIR LOSS WITH SCARRING

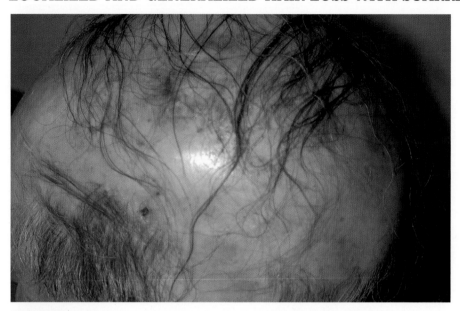

FIGURE 3.14 Blistering and scarring due to cicatricial pemphigoid

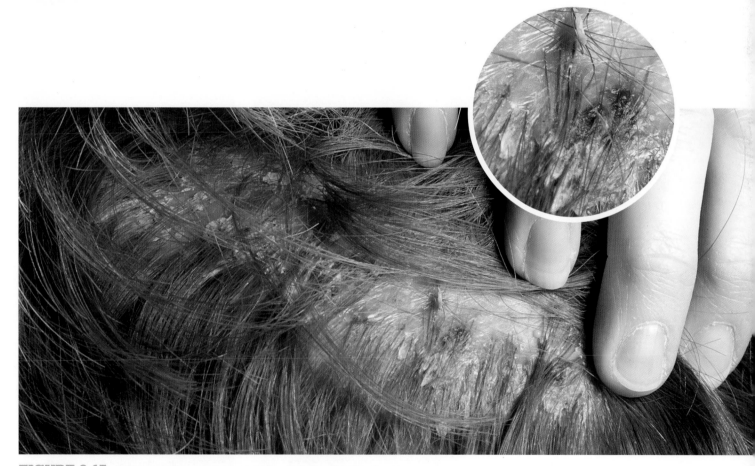

FIGURE 3.15 Follicular tufting and scarring due to folliculitis decalvans

LOCALIZED AND GENERALIZED HAIR LOSS WITH SCARRING

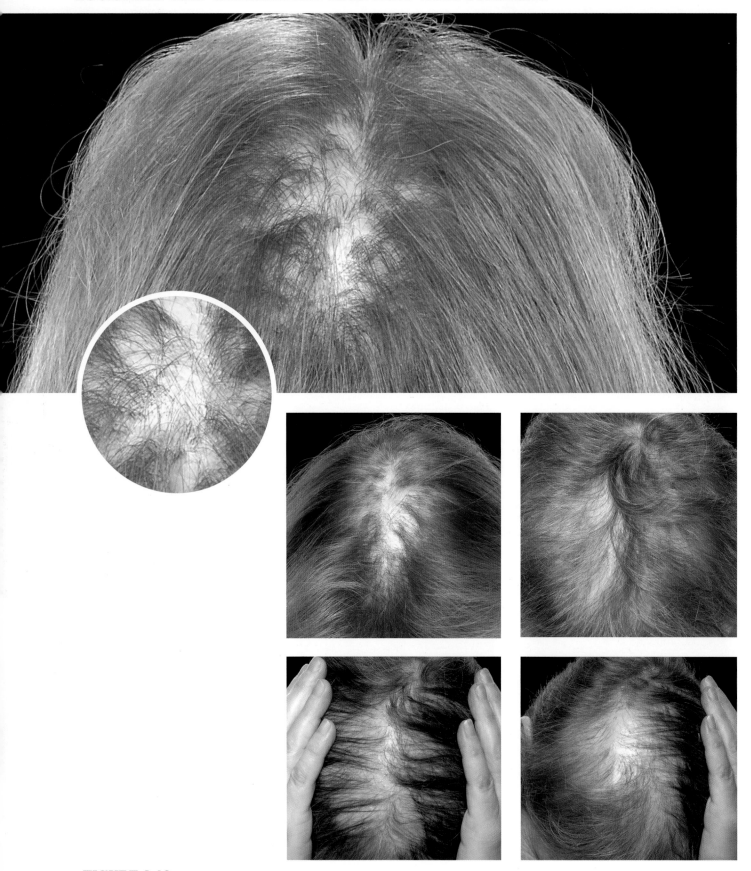

FIGURE 3.16 Scattered patchy scarring without inflammation due to pseudopelade

LOCALIZED AND GENERALIZED HAIR LOSS WITH SCARRING

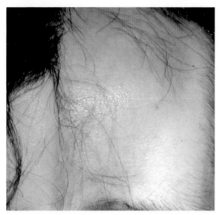

FIGURE 3.17 Scarring alopecia due to linear morphoea

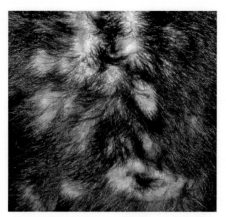

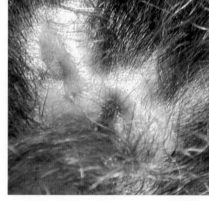

FIGURE 3.18 Localized and generalized scarring alopecia with cystic acne-like lesions in dissecting cellulitis of the scalp

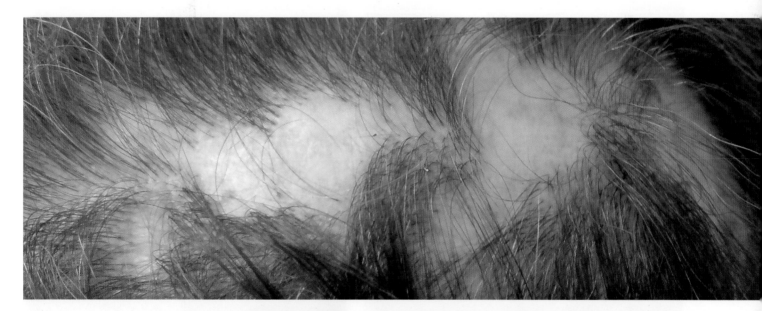

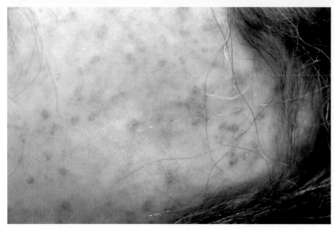

FIGURE 3.19 Alopecia associated with discoid lupus

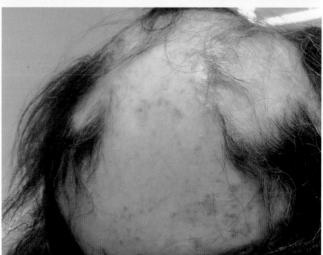

LOCALIZED AND GENERALIZED HAIR LOSS WITH SCARRING

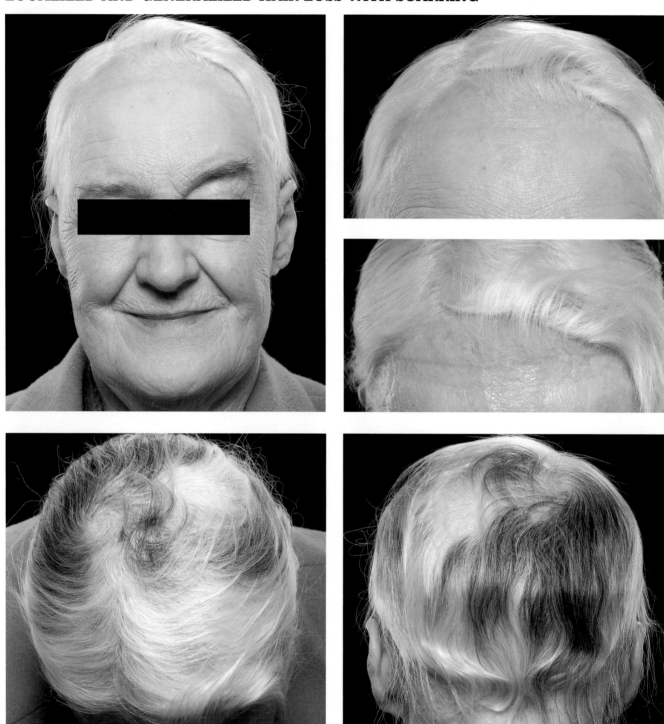

FIGURE 3.20 Alopecia associated with lichen planus

LOCALIZED AND GENERALIZED HAIR LOSS WITH SCARRING

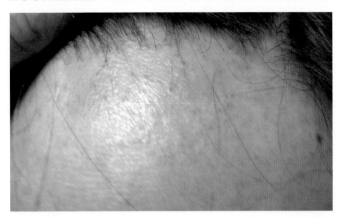

FIGURE 3.21 Frontal fibrosing alopecia (probably a variant of lichen planus (lichen planopilaris)

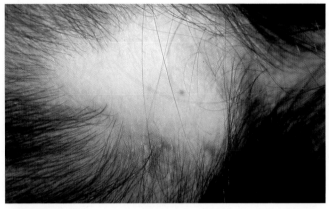

FIGURE 3.22 Alopecia with scarring due to congenital aplasia cutis

Localized naevi and tumours

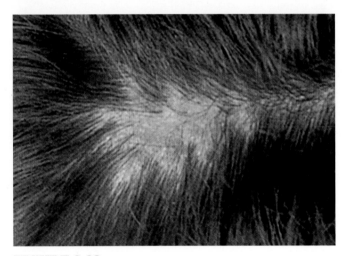

FIGURE 3.23 Naevus sebaceous

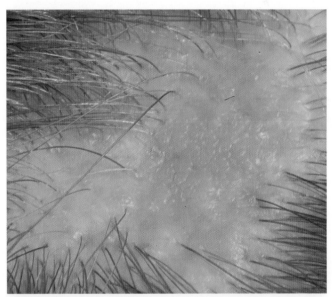

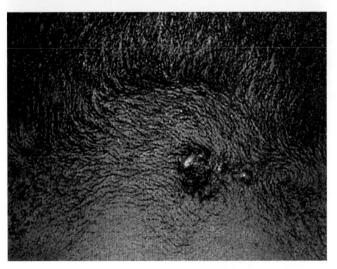

FIGURE 3.24 Acne keloidalis

EXCESSIVE HAIR

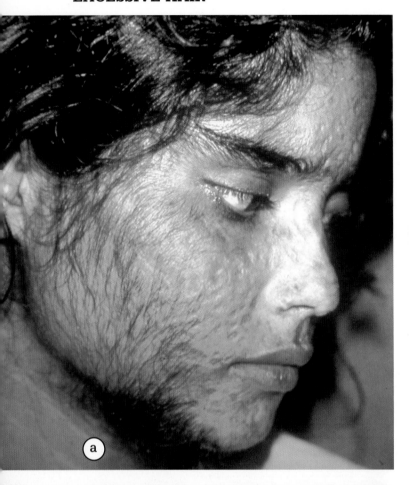

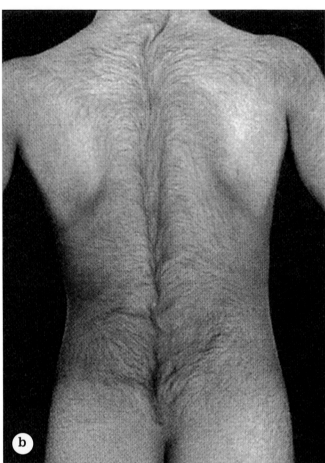

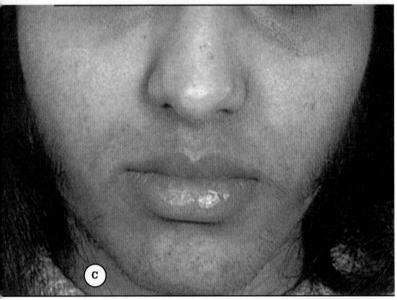

FIGURE 3.25 Excessive hair: **(a)** porphyria cutanea tarda, **(b,c)** normal variants – considerable racial variation

EXCESSIVE HAIR

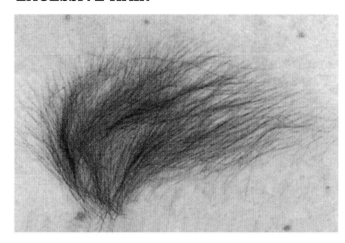

FIGURE 3.26 Hypertrichosis overlying spina bifida occulta (faun tail)

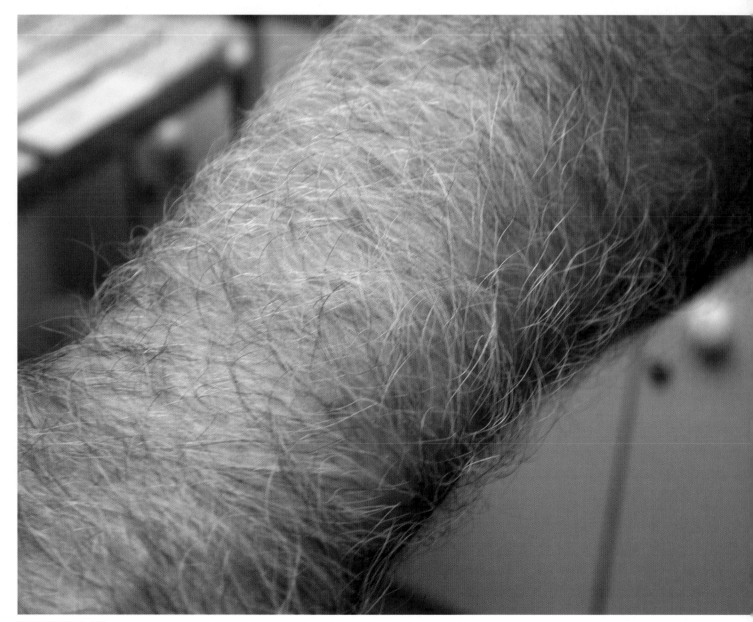

FIGURE 3.27 Hypertrichosis due to ciclosporin

Chapter 4

Nails

Summary

- Nail colour
- Nail dystrophy

It is useful to consider nail abnormalities under a number of headings. The colour of the nails is often diagnostic: for example, green nails in *Pseudomonas* superinfection or red in the case of a subungual haematoma. Brown or black discoloration is usually due to a haematoma but occasionally a melanocytic naevus or even a melanoma. The pattern of nail dystrophy is also helpful, longitudinal depression signalling a myxoid cyst, a central column of transverse furrows indicating repetitive trauma to the cuticle, and a central raised 'Christmas tree' shaped deformity diagnostic of median nail dystrophy. Onycholysis, which involves lifting of the nail from its bed and opacification of that part of the nail, is most commonly seen in psoriasis and fungal infection. Subungual hyperkeratosis is also a feature of psoriasis and fungal infection. Pitting – distinctive tiny depressions in the nail – is seen in psoriasis, alopecia areata and occasionally in other conditions affecting the periungual area, such as chronic dermatitis. The reader is directed to Chapter 18 in Section 2 for more detailed descriptions of these conditions.

Algorithm 4.1 Nail colour

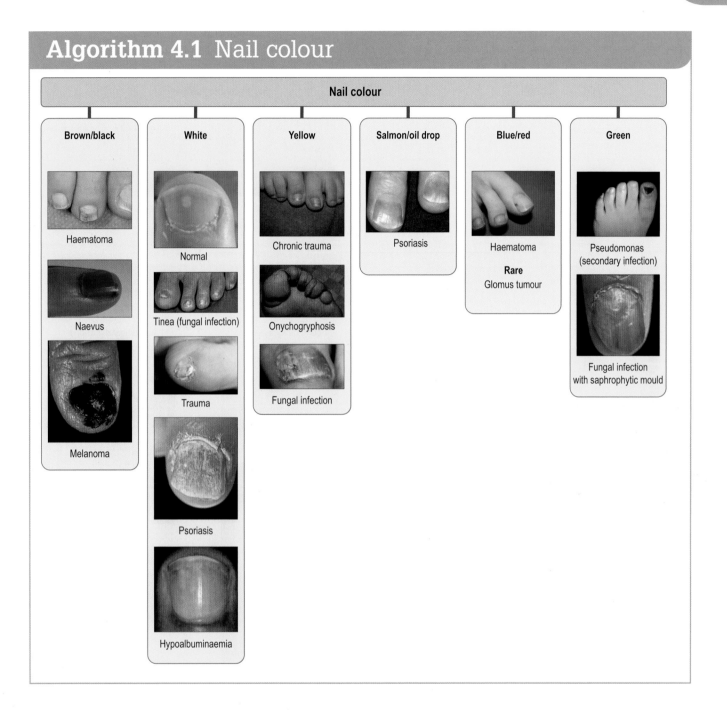

Nail colour

Brown/black
- Haematoma
- Naevus
- Melanoma

White
- Normal
- Tinea (fungal infection)
- Trauma
- Psoriasis
- Hypoalbuminaemia

Yellow
- Chronic trauma
- Onychogryphosis
- Fungal infection

Salmon/oil drop
- Psoriasis

Blue/red
- Haematoma
- **Rare** Glomus tumour

Green
- Pseudomonas (secondary infection)
- Fungal infection with saphrophytic mould

Algorithm 4.2 Nail dystrophy

Transverse nail dystrophy

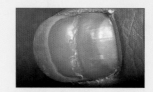

Beau's lines

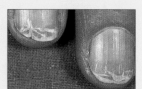

Lamellar dystrophy

Nail dystrophy

Onycholysis

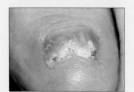

Psoriasis

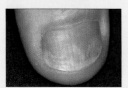

Fungal

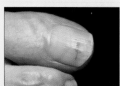

Trauma

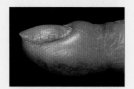

Paronychia

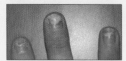

Artificial nails

Other
Drugs e.g. tetracycline

Pitting
Normal (<3 pits)

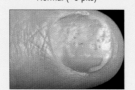

Psoriasis

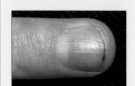

Alopecia areata

Other
Dermatitis
Trauma

Subungual hyperkeratosis

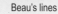
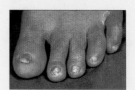

Fungal infection

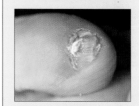

Trauma

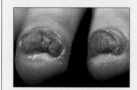

Pachyonychia congenita

Other
Psoriasis

Longitudinal dystrophy

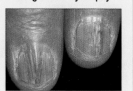

Lichen planus

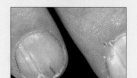

Darier's disease

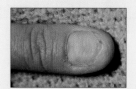

Trauma (habit tic)

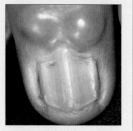

Myxoid cyst

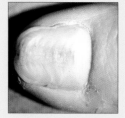

Median nail dystrophy

NAIL COLOUR

Brown/black nails

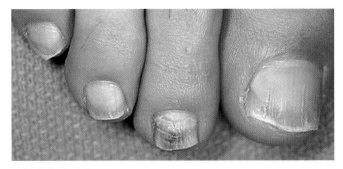

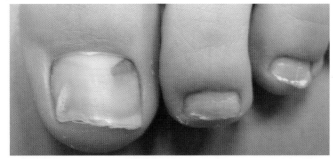

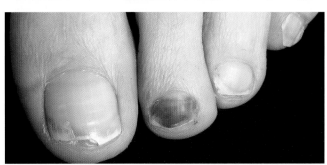

FIGURE 4.3 Brown/black subungual haematoma

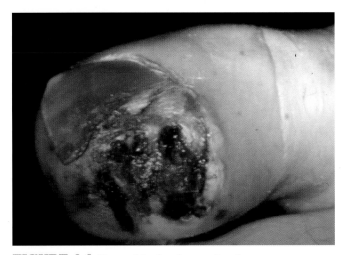

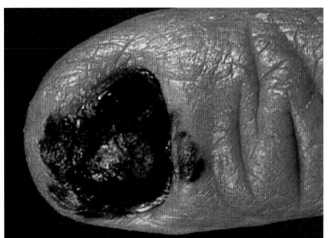

FIGURE 4.4 Brown/black subungual melanoma

NAIL COLOUR

White nails

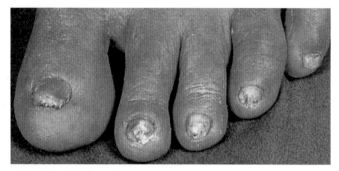 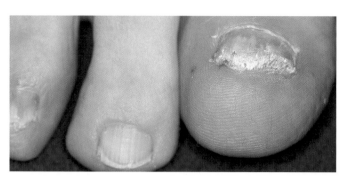

FIGURE 4.5 White nails – fungal

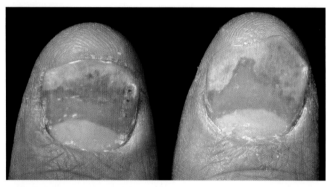 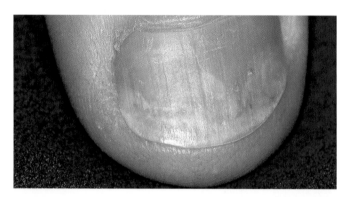

FIGURE 4.6 White nails – psoriasis

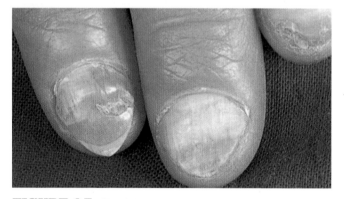

FIGURE 4.7 *Candida* in chronic mucocutaneous candidiasis

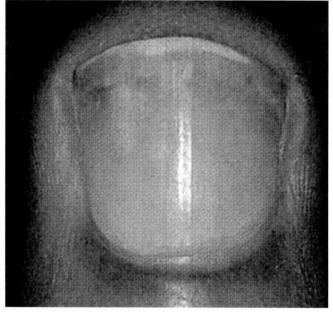

FIGURE 4.8 Pallor due to hypoalbuminaemia

NAIL COLOUR

Yellow nails

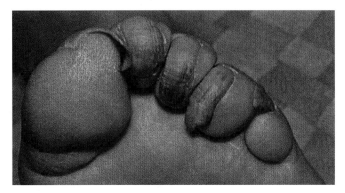

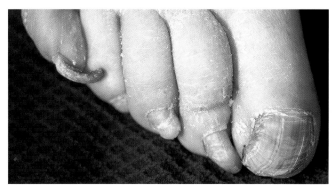

FIGURE 4.9 Onychogryphosis

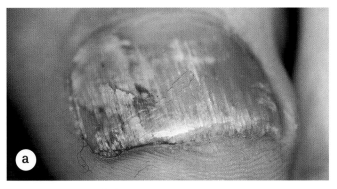

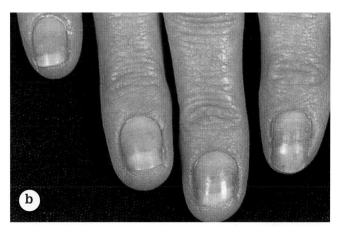

FIGURE 4.10 **(a)** Fungal infection with yellow discoloration, **(b)** yellow nail syndrome

FIGURE 4.11 Congenital dystrophy of great toenail

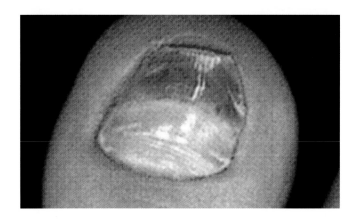

NAIL COLOUR

Salmon/oil drop

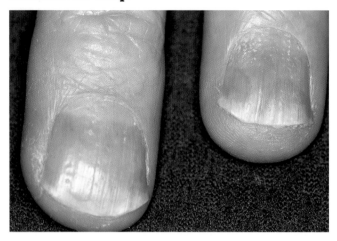

FIGURE 4.12 Salmon/oil drop

Green, red and blue nails

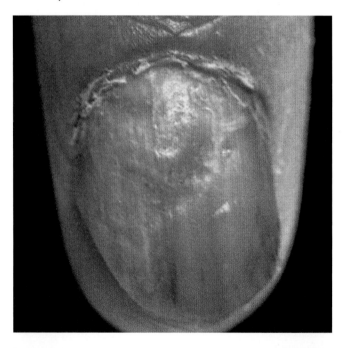

FIGURE 4.13 Green-black discoloration due to infection with saprophytic mould – scopulariopsis

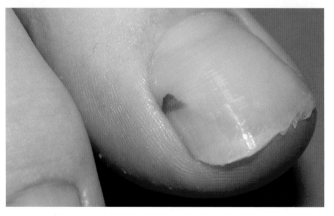

FIGURE 4.14 Red subungual haematoma

NAIL DYSTROPHY

Pitting

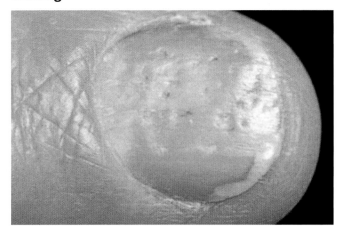

FIGURE 4.15 Pitting – psoriasis

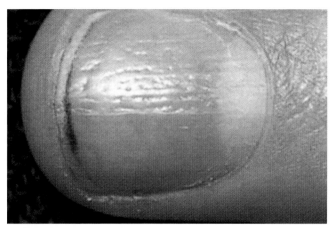

FIGURE 4.16 Alopecia areata

Onycholysis

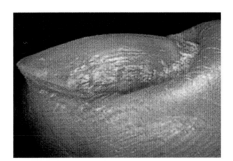

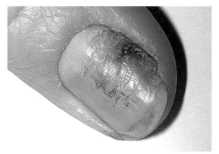

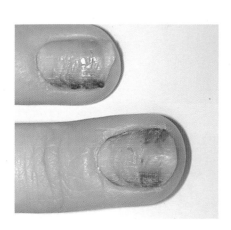

FIGURE 4.17 Chronic paronychia with secondary nail dystrophy and onycholysis

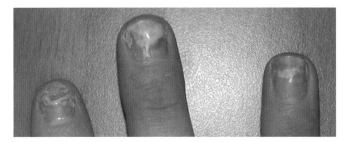

FIGURE 4.18 Onycholysis secondary to acrylates used to attach false nails

FIGURE 4.19 Onycholysis secondary to trauma

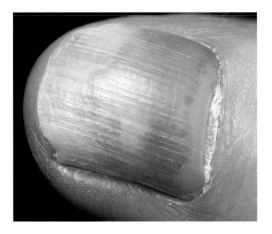

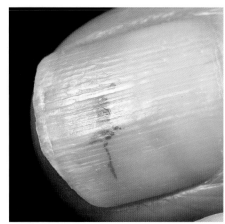

NAIL DYSTROPHY

Subungual hyperkeratosis

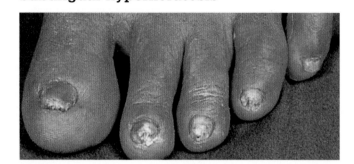

FIGURE 4.20 Subungual hyperkeratosis – fungal infection

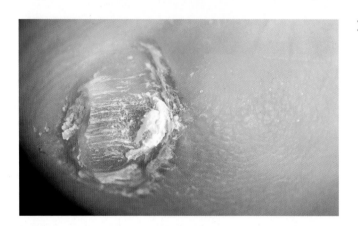

FIGURE 4.21 Subungual hyperkeratosis – trauma

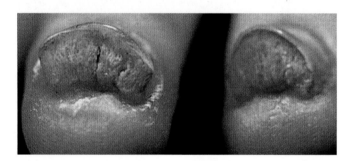

FIGURE 4.22 Pachyonychia congenita

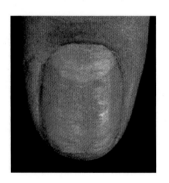 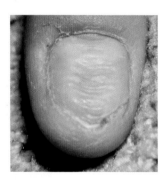

FIGURE 4.23 Habit tic – central nail dystrophy

NAIL DYSTROPHY

Central longitudinal

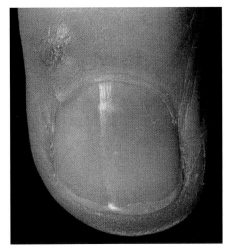 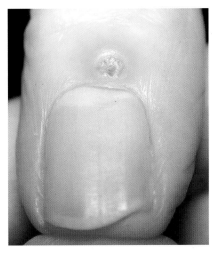 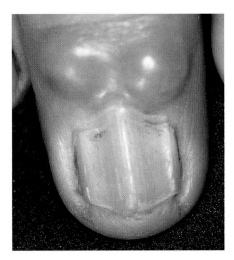

FIGURE 4.24 Central longitudinal ridge secondary to myxoid cyst

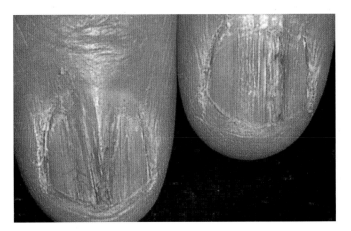

FIGURE 4.25 Lichen planus

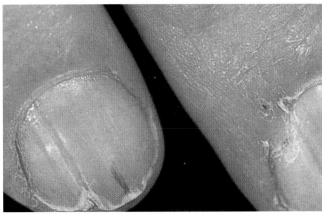

FIGURE 4.26 Darier's disease

NAIL DYSTROPHY

Transverse dystrophy

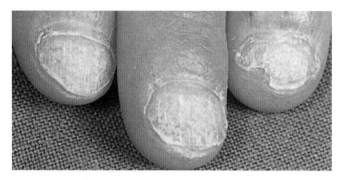
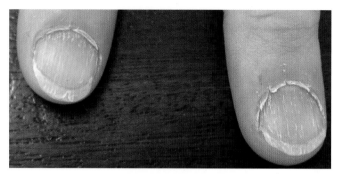

FIGURE 4.27 Twenty-nail dystrophy

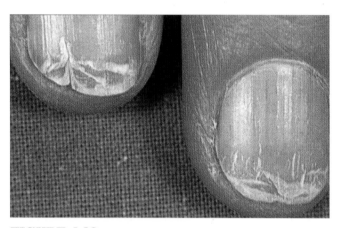

FIGURE 4.28 Lamellar dystrophy

NAIL DYSTROPHY

Other

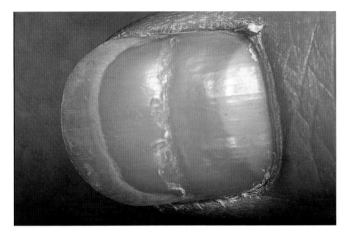

FIGURE 4.29 Beau's lines

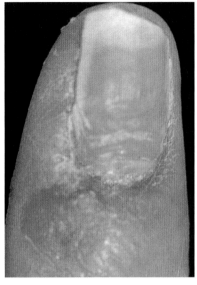

FIGURE 4.32 Dermatitis close to nail plate

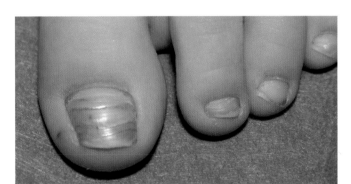

FIGURE 4.30 Nail ridging and separation due to repeated trauma

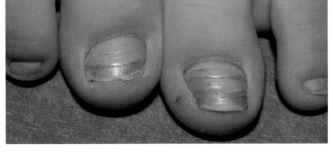

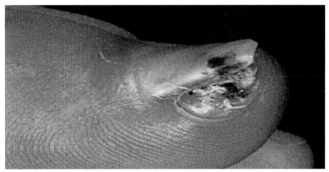

FIGURE 4.33 Subungual exostosis

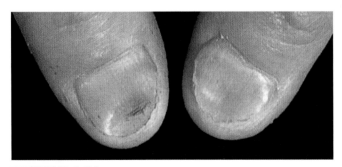

FIGURE 4.31 Koilonychia

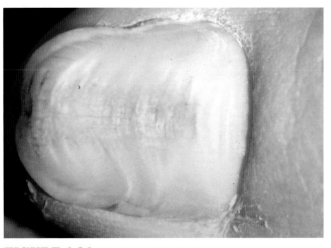

FIGURE 4.34 Median nail dystrophy

Chapter 5

Itch

Patients presenting with itch can be divided into two groups: those with a rash and those without. Patients with a rash should be approached as outlined in the rashes algorithm (Ch. 1). Patients without a rash or with merely manifestations of scratching (linear excoriations or excoriated papules) should first be investigated for underlying pathology. Full blood count, ESR, urea + electrolytes, bone biochemistry, liver function tests, thyroid function tests, serum iron and ferritin, fasting blood glucose and a chest X-ray will uncover most systemic causes of pruritus. The reader is directed to Chapter 12 in Section 2 for more detailed descriptions of these conditions.

Algorithm 5.1 Itch

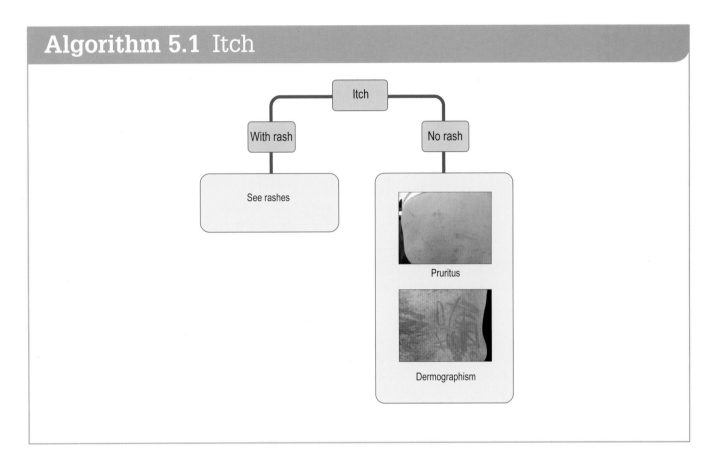

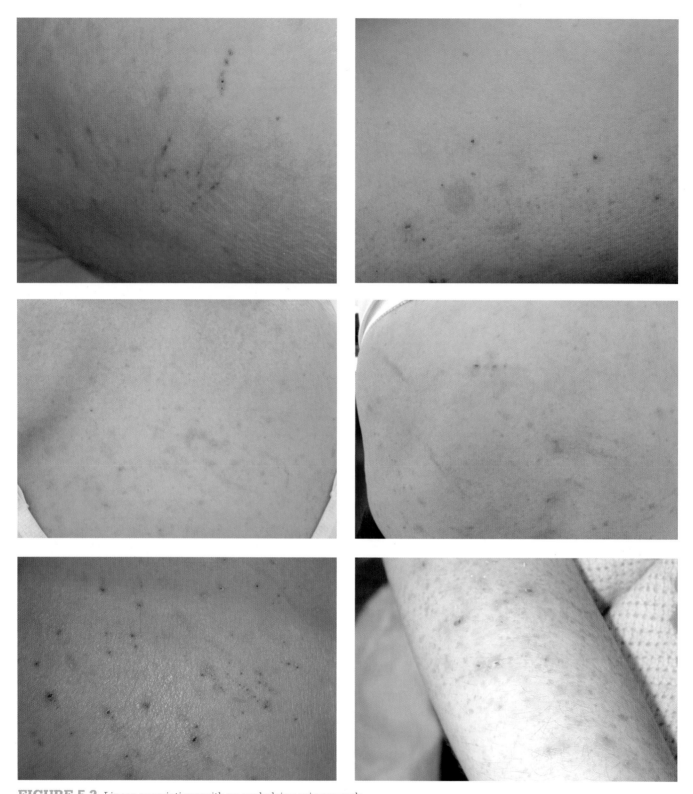

FIGURE 5.2 Linear excoriations with no underlying primary rash

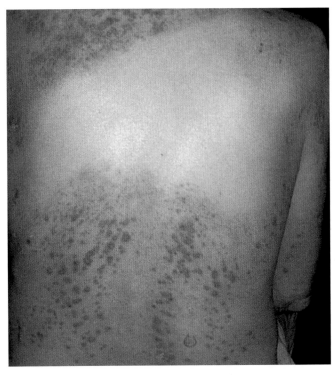

FIGURE 5.3 Central back spared in primary generalized pruritus

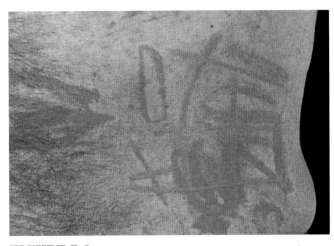

FIGURE 5.4 Dermographism is an important cause of generalized itch. No rash will be obvious until the patient scratches

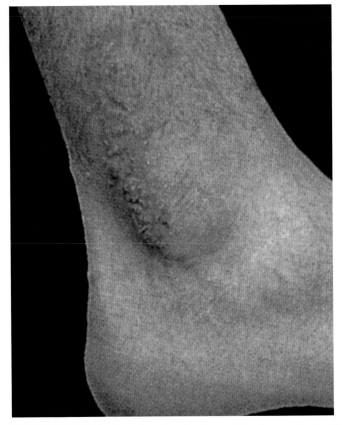

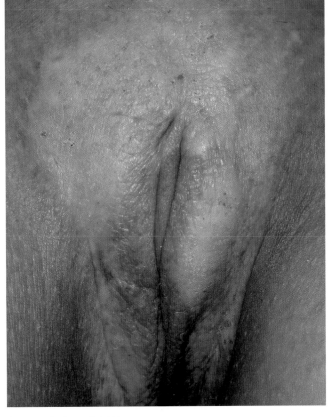

FIGURE 5.5 Lichen simplex chronicus of the leg and vulva due to repeated scratching

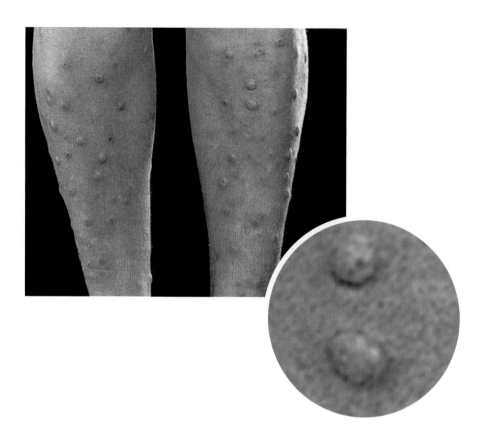

FIGURE 5.6 Chronic scratching may also result in extensive nodules – nodular prurigo

Chapter 6

Blisters

Summary

- ▇ Localized
- ▇ Generalized

Blisters can be divided into localized and generalized, with burns and insect bites being the most frequent cause of the former with infections and dermatitis also relatively common. Generalized blistering is relatively uncommon. Infections such as impetigo, varicella and drug reactions are the most common cause. Pemphigoid is a relatively uncommon but important diagnosis; pemphigus is fortunately very rare.

Algorithm 6.1

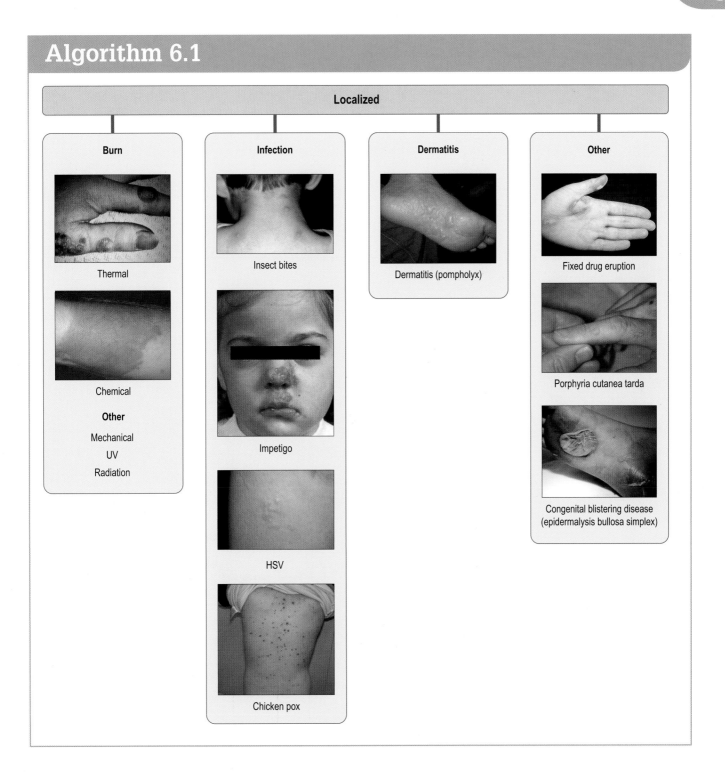

Localized

Burn

Thermal

Chemical

Other

Mechanical

UV

Radiation

Infection

Insect bites

Impetigo

HSV

Chicken pox

Dermatitis

Dermatitis (pompholyx)

Other

Fixed drug eruption

Porphyria cutanea tarda

Congenital blistering disease
(epidermalysis bullosa simplex)

Algorithm 6.2

Generalized

Small

Large

Viral infection

Varicella

Coxsackie
(hand, foot and mouth disease)

Acute dermatitis

Impetigo

Erythema multiforme/TEN

Bullous pemphigoid

Pemphigus

Congenital blistering disease
(dystrophic epidermolysis bullosa)

LOCALIZED

Burn

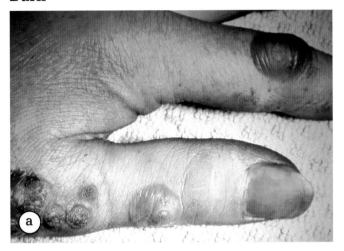

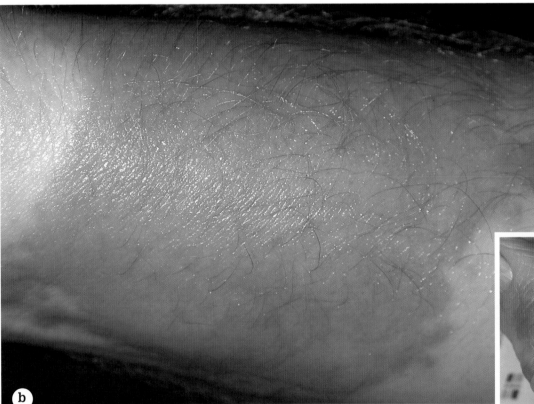

FIGURE 6.3 Burns from **(a)** liquid nitrogen, **(b,c)** chemicals

LOCALIZED Infection

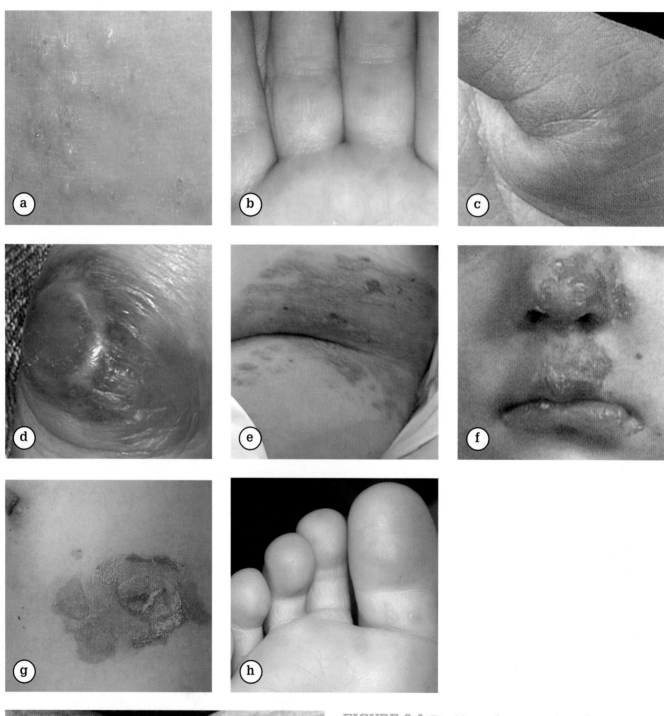

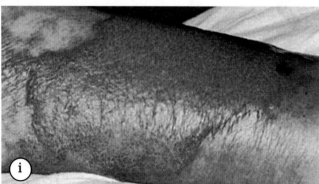

FIGURE 6.4 Tiny blisters from coxsackie infection (hand, foot and mouth disease) and HSV. Large blisters from staphylococcal impetigo, streptococcal cellulits, HZV and pox virus (orf). **(a)** HSV thigh, **(b)** hand, foot and mouth, **(c)** HSV thumb, **(d)** orf, **(e)** zoster, **(f,g)**, impetigo, **(h)** hand, foot and mouth, **(i)** cellulitis

LOCALIZED Dermatitis

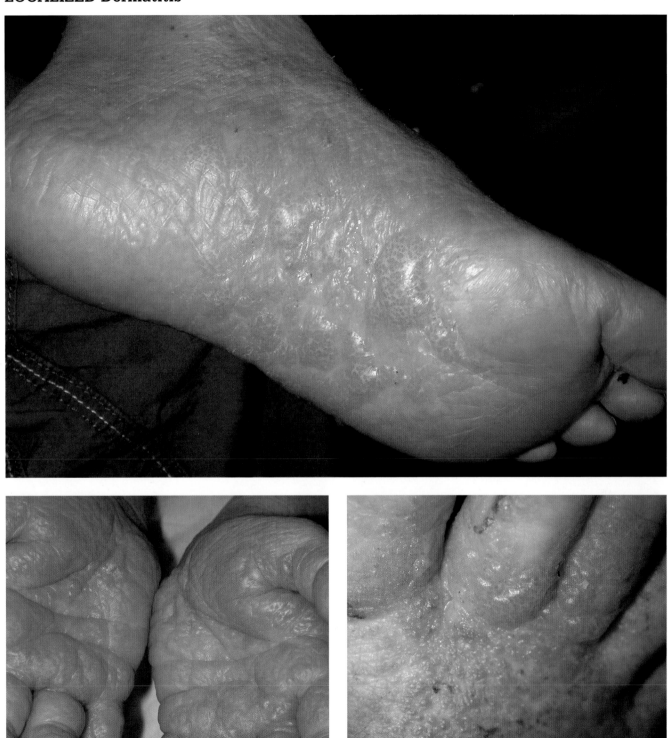

FIGURE 6.5 Dermatitis

LOCALIZED Other

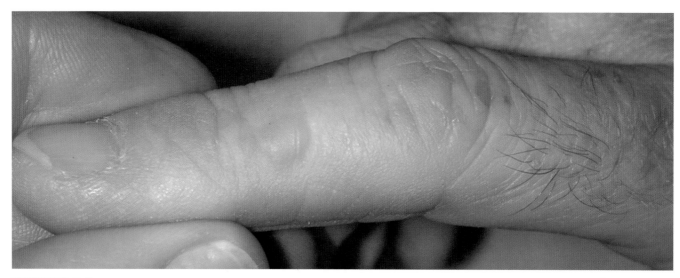

FIGURE 6.6 Porphyria cutanea tarda

GENERALIZED

Small blisters (vesicles)

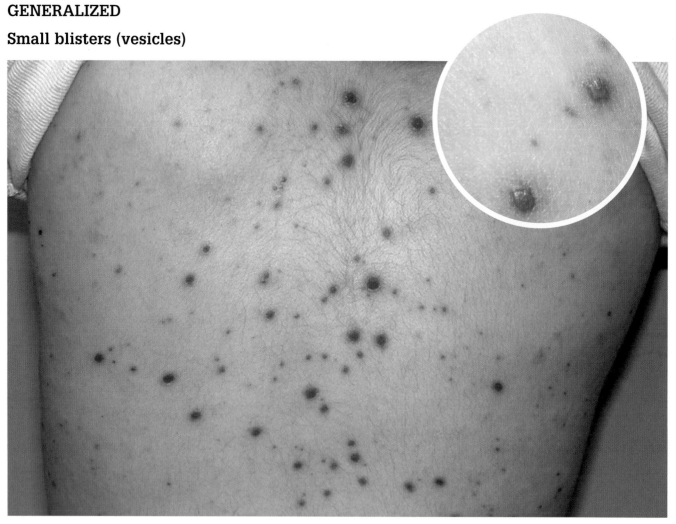

FIGURE 6.7 Chickenpox

GENERALIZED Small blisters (vesicles)

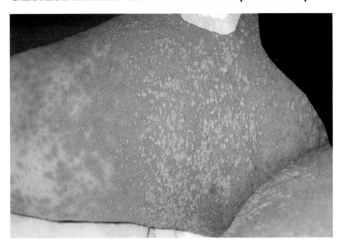

FIGURE 6.8 Acute pustular psoriasis

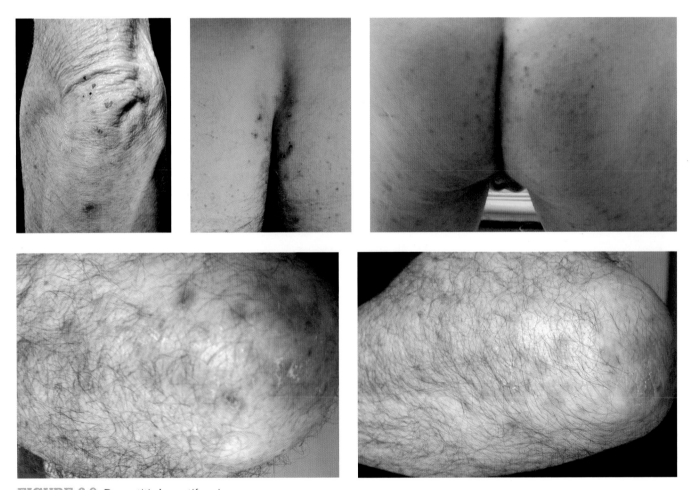

FIGURE 6.9 Dermatitis herpetiformis

GENERALIZED Large blisters

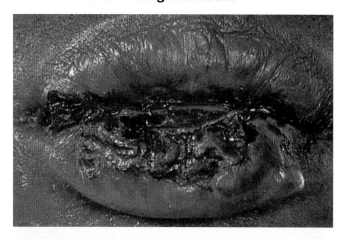

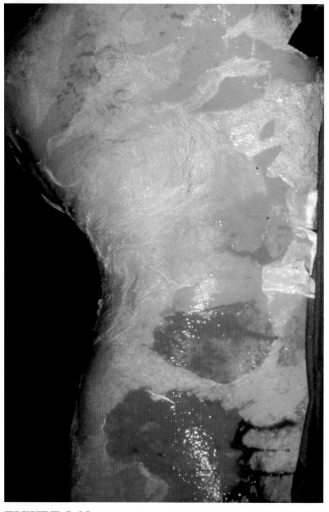

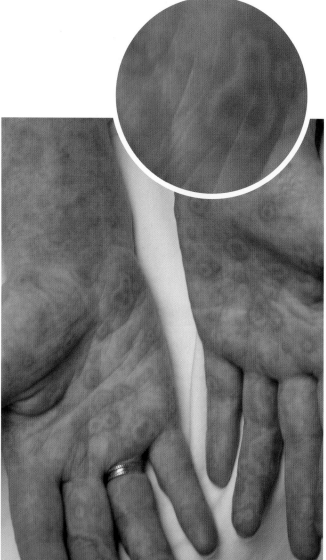

FIGURE 6.10 Erythema multiforme/TEN

GENERALIZED Large blisters

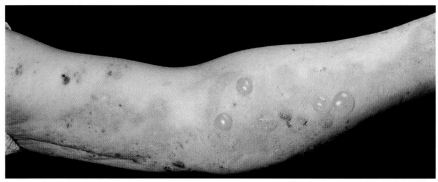

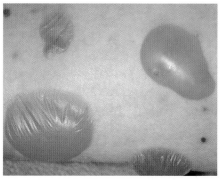

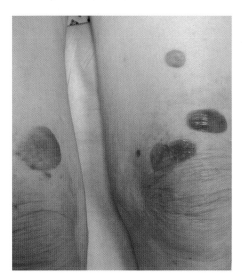

FIGURE 6.11 Tense and haemorrhagic blisters in bullous pemphigoid

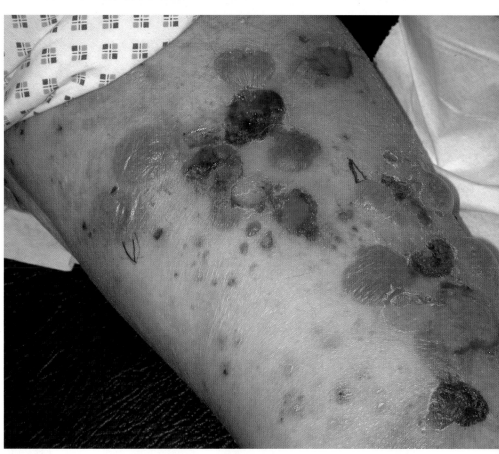

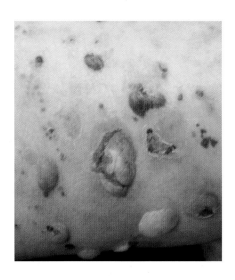

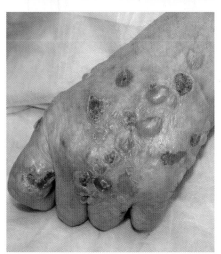

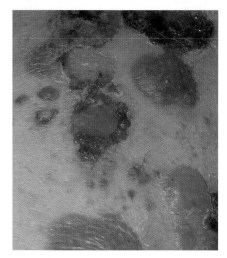

GENERALIZED Large blisters

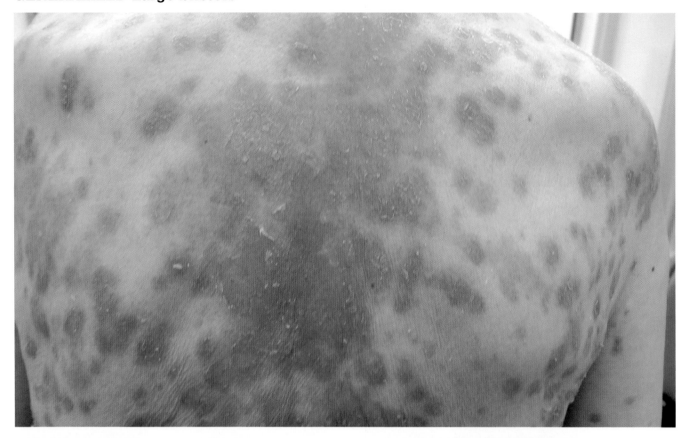

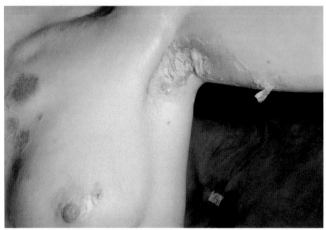

FIGURE 6.12 Fragile and superficial blisters in pemphigus vulgaris

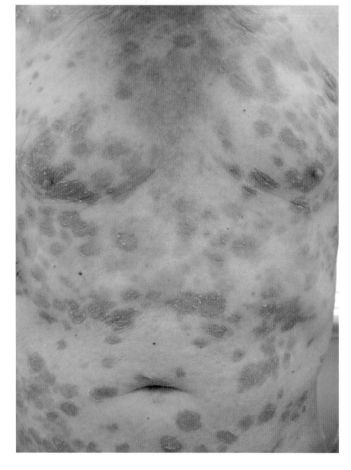

GENERALIZED Large blisters

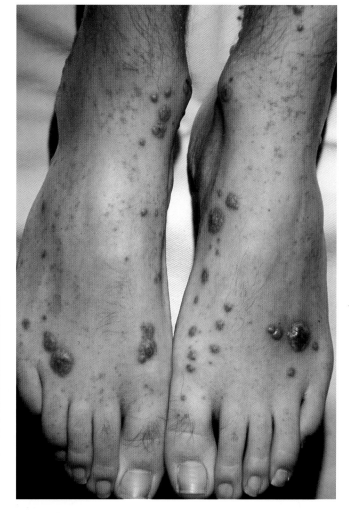

FIGURE 6.13 Vasculitis

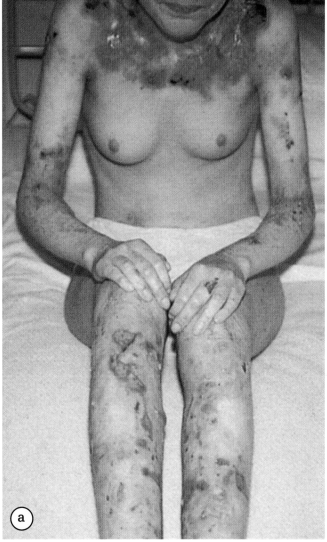

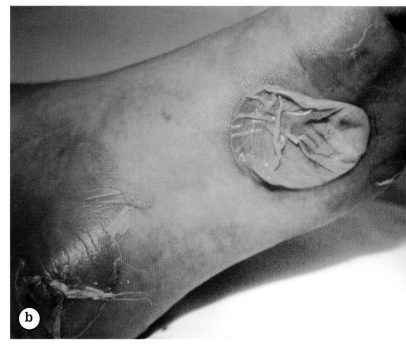

FIGURE 6.14 Congenital epidermolysis bullosa: **(a)** generalized dystrophic EB, **(b)** localized EB

Chapter 7

Pigmented Rashes

Summary

- Pigmented rash
- Depigmented rash

Pigmented rashes can be due to haemorrhage in the skin, as caused by venous hypertension, vasculitis and the related capillaritis. Post-inflammatory hyperpigmentation is caused by increased melanin production by melanocytes and can be seen after any intense inflammatory process in the skin. Phenotypically darker skin (skin type IV to VI) will be more prone to this problem. Photosensitivity particularly in females can cause hyperpigmentation as seen in chloasma and poikiloderma of Civatte and it is an occasional side effect of drugs such as minocycline and chlorpromazine. On the trunk tinea versicolor causes light-brown hyperpigmentation.

Hypopigmentation may be complete, as seen in vitiligo, or partial, as in post-inflammatory hypopigmentation. In tanned or darker skin tinea versicolor may cause hypopigmentation usually with a fine scale.

Algorithm 7.1

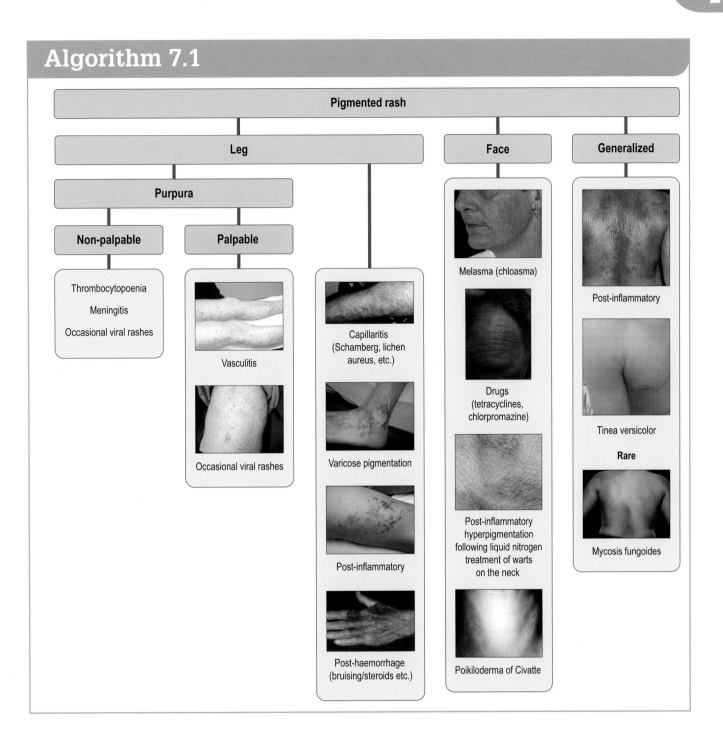

Pigmented rash

Leg

Face

Generalized

Purpura

Non-palpable

Thrombocytopoenia

Meningitis

Occasional viral rashes

Palpable

Vasculitis

Occasional viral rashes

Capillaritis
(Schamberg, lichen
aureus, etc.)

Varicose pigmentation

Post-inflammatory

Post-haemorrhage
(bruising/steroids etc.)

Melasma (chloasma)

Drugs
(tetracyclines,
chlorpromazine)

Post-inflammatory
hyperpigmentation
following liquid nitrogen
treatment of warts
on the neck

Poikiloderma of Civatte

Post-inflammatory

Tinea versicolor

Rare

Mycosis fungoides

Algorithm 7.2

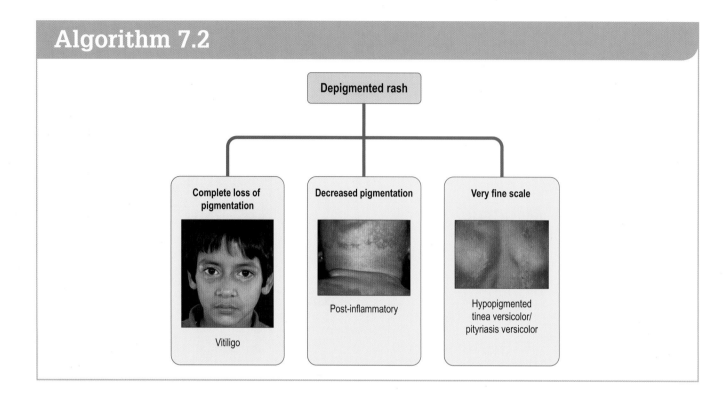

PIGMENTED RASH Legs, feet and hands

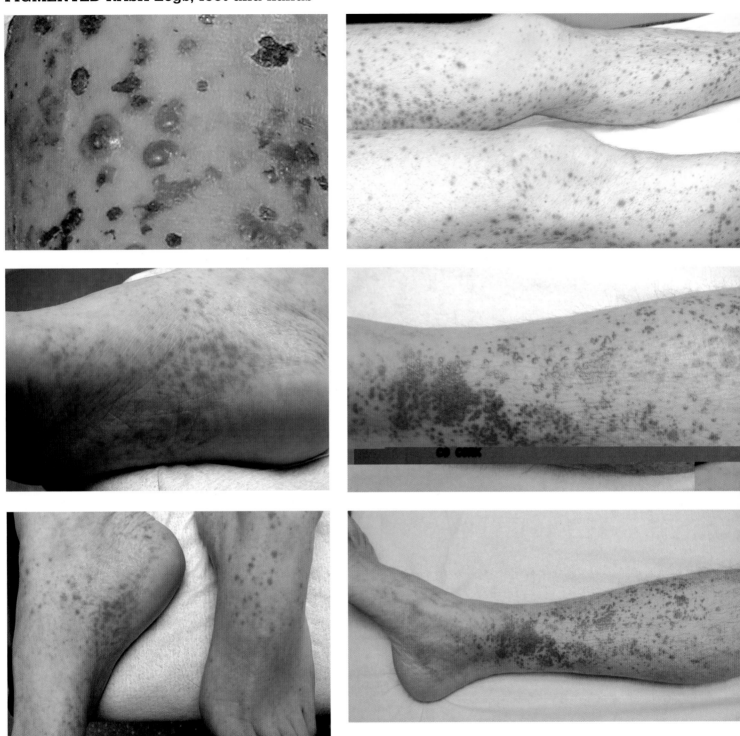

FIGURE 7.3 Vasculitis

PIGMENTED RASH Legs, feet and hands

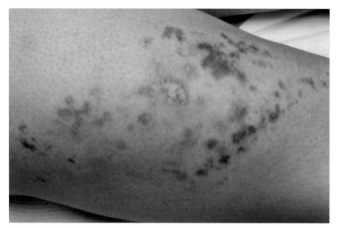

FIGURE 7.4 Post-inflammatory hyperpigmentation secondary to lichen planus

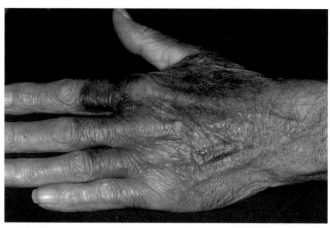

FIGURE 7.5 Senile purpura

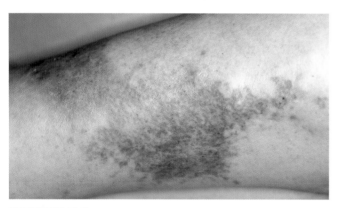

FIGURE 7.6 Venous stasis

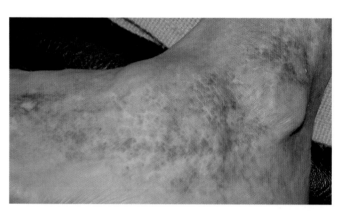

FIGURE 7.7 Varicose pigmentation

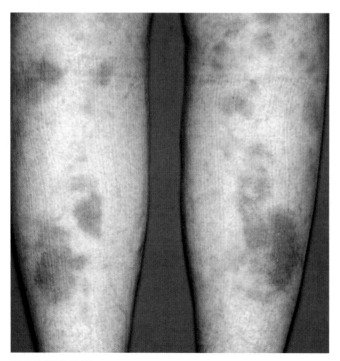

FIGURE 7.8 Minocycline pigmentation

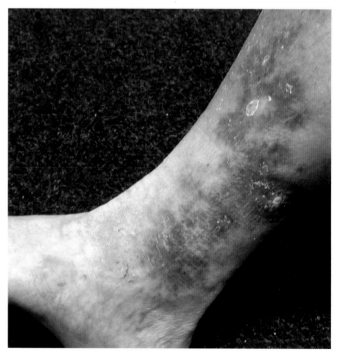

PIGMENTED RASH Legs, feet and hands

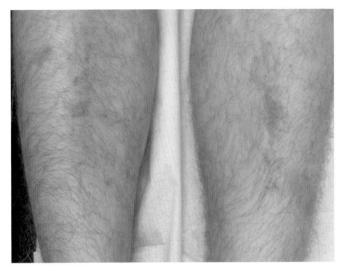

FIGURE 7.9 Capillaritis

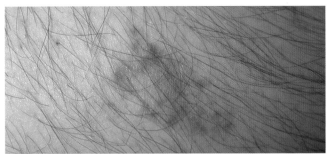

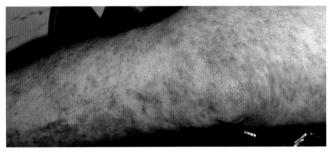

PIGMENTED RASH

Face

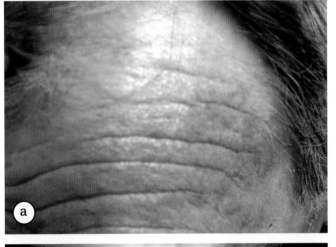
(a)

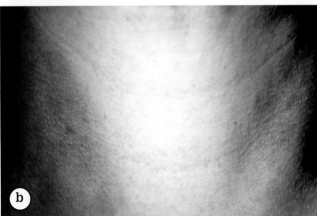
(b)

FIGURE 7.10 **(a)** Minocycline-induced pigmentation, **(b)** poikilodema of civatte

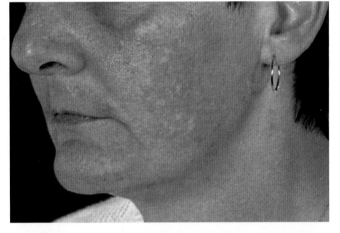

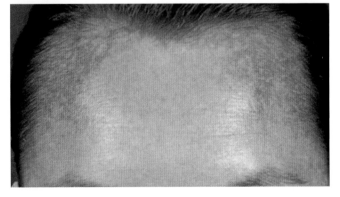

FIGURE 7.11 Chloasma

PIGMENTED RASH Generalized

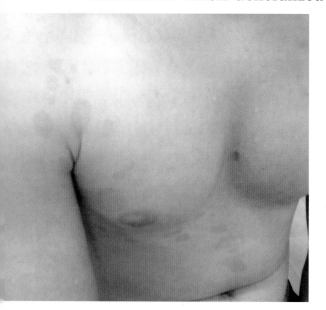

FIGURE 7.12 Pityriasis versicolor

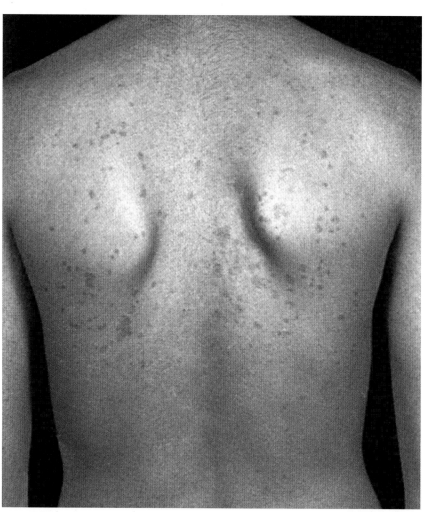

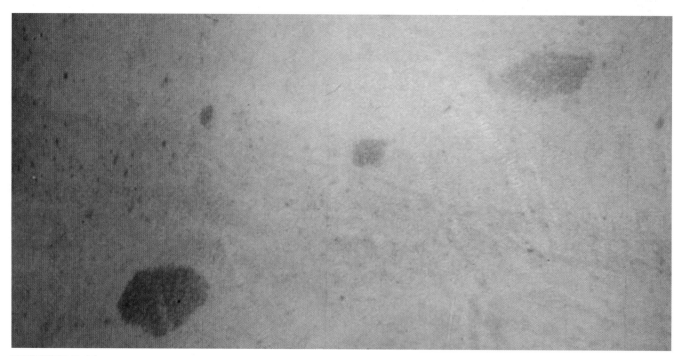

FIGURE 7.13 Café au lait patches

PIGMENTED RASH Generalized

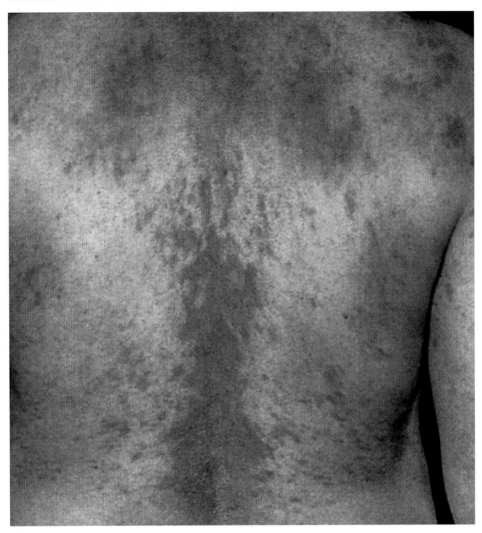

FIGURE 7.14 Post-inflammatory hyperpigmentation secondary to generalized dermatitis

DEPIGMENTED RASH

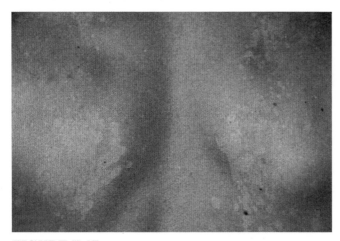
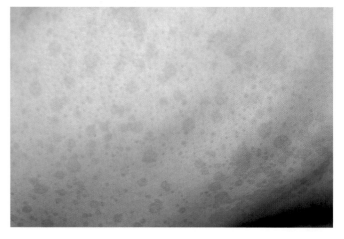

FIGURE 7.15 Pityriasis versicolor

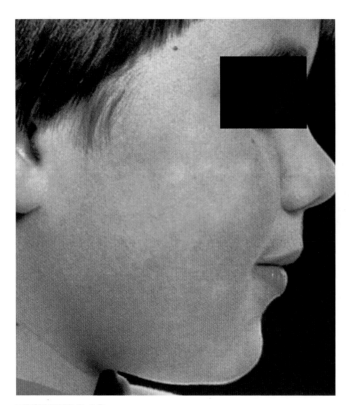
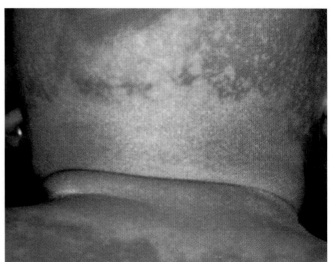
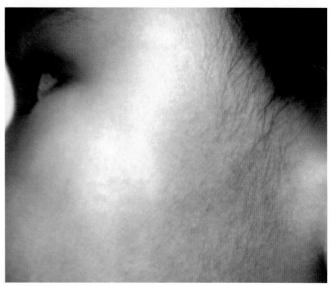

FIGURE 7.16 Post-inflammatory hypopigmentation from atopic dermatitis (pityriasis alba) and severe seborrhoeic dermatitis

DEPIGMENTED RASH

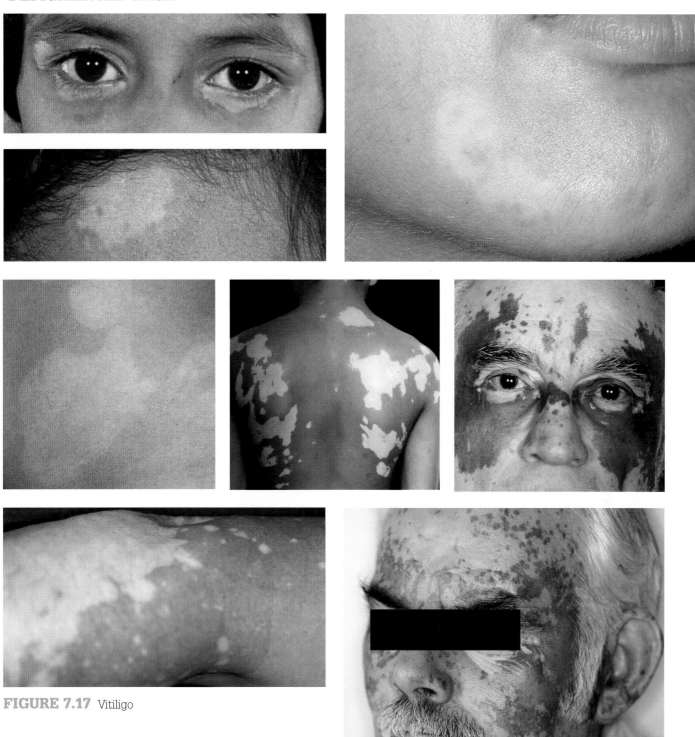

FIGURE 7.17 Vitiligo

Chapter 8

Pigmented Lesions

Summary

■ Congenital
■ Acquired

The importance of these lies in the differentiation between melanoma and benign lesions. Lesions which are present from birth or within the first year of life are usually congenital naevi. Only the larger ones carry a significant risk of melanoma. Dermal melanosis/Mongolian blue spot is mainly seen in Indo-Asian and Afro-Caribbean races. Café au lait patches may be present at birth but more commonly develop later and, if multiple, are a marker for neurofibromatosis. Acquired lesions can be divided into flat and raised. Freckles are the most common flat lesion and can occasionally be dark enough to simulate a naevus or even melanoma. Solar damage over time causes a benign proliferation of epidermal melanocytes in a linear fashion along the basement membrane, resulting in light-brown, generally uniformly pigmented lesions known as lentigo simplex or solar lentigo. The melanotic macule of the lip is similar although tends to be darker. Café au lait patches tend to develop in childhood on the trunk rather than sun-exposed areas. Darker flat lesions include junctional and atypical naevi, lentigo maligna and melanoma. Raised lesions are most commonly either waxy, warty seborrhoeic keratosis or rubbery, firm compound naevi, both of which need to be distinguished from melanoma. The reader is directed to Chapter 17 in Section 2 for more detailed descriptions of these conditions.

Algorithm 8.1

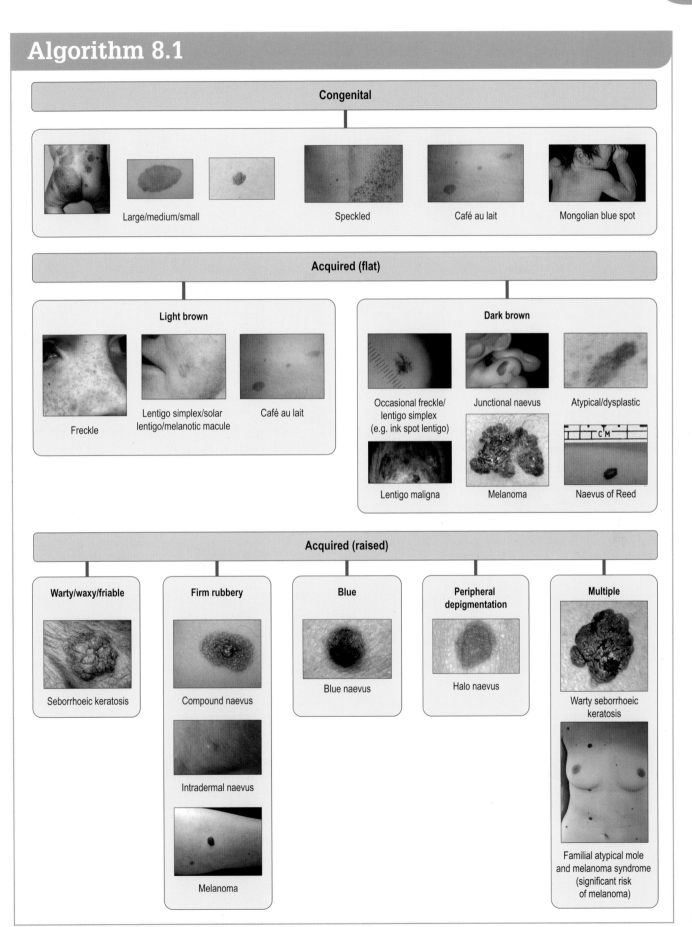

Congenital

Large/medium/small   Speckled   Café au lait   Mongolian blue spot

Acquired (flat)

Light brown

Freckle   Lentigo simplex/solar lentigo/melanotic macule   Café au lait

Dark brown

Occasional freckle/ lentigo simplex (e.g. ink spot lentigo)   Junctional naevus   Atypical/dysplastic

Lentigo maligna   Melanoma   Naevus of Reed

Acquired (raised)

Warty/waxy/friable

Seborrhoeic keratosis

Firm rubbery

Compound naevus

Intradermal naevus

Melanoma

Blue

Blue naevus

Peripheral depigmentation

Halo naevus

Multiple

Warty seborrhoeic keratosis

Familial atypical mole and melanoma syndrome (significant risk of melanoma)

CONGENITAL

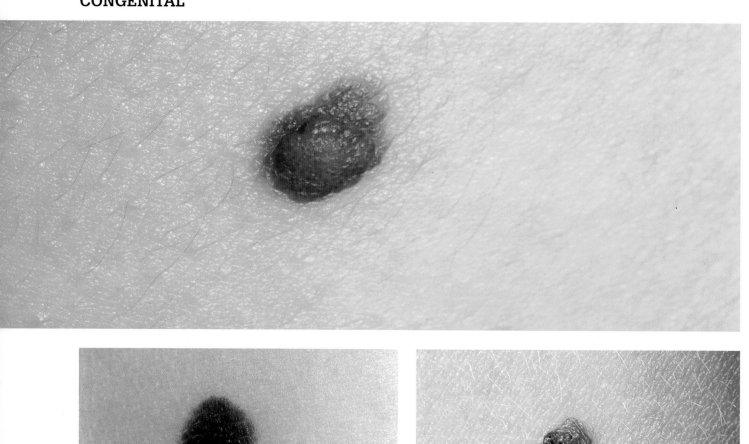

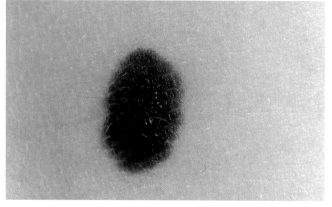

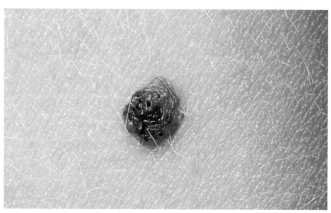

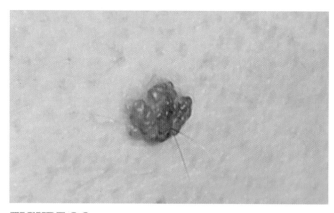

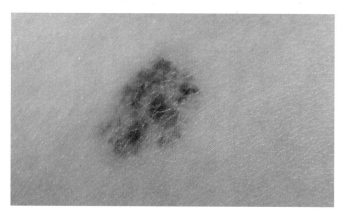

FIGURE 8.2 Small congenital naevi

CONGENITAL

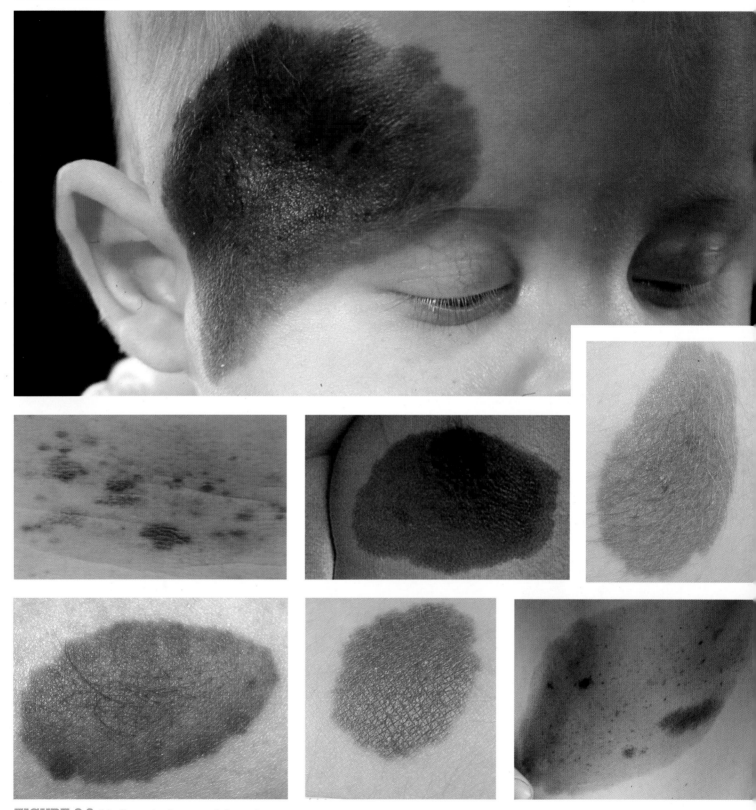

FIGURE 8.3 Medium-sized congenital naevi

CONGENITAL

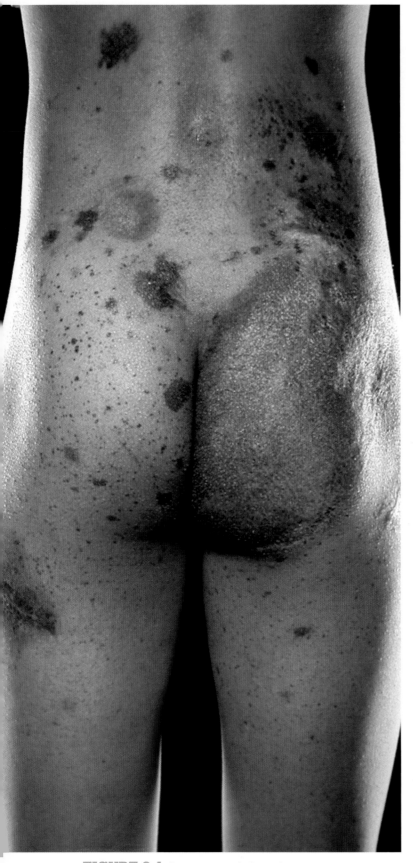

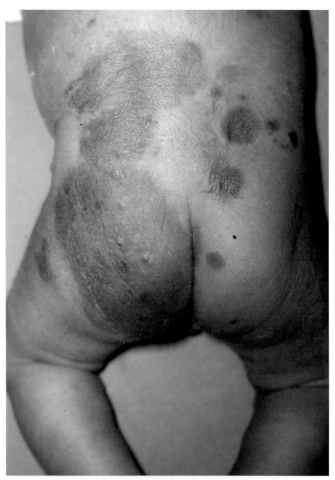

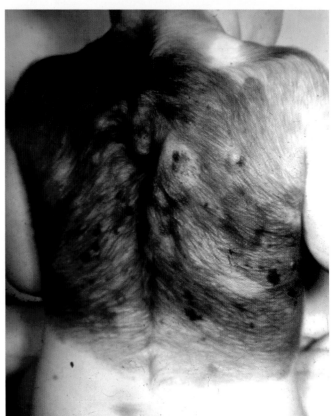

FIGURE 8.4 Large congenital naevi

CONGENITAL

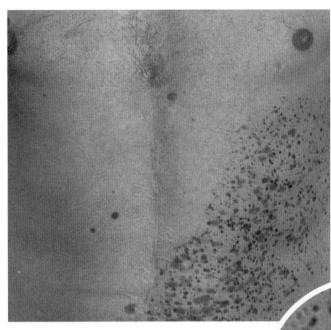

FIGURE 8.5 Speckled lentiginous congenital naevus

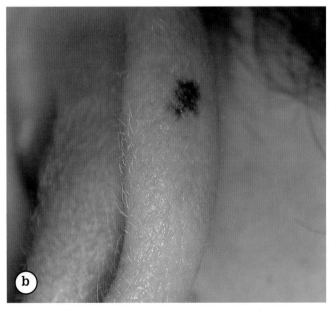

FIGURE 8.6 Mongolian blue spot

ACQUIRED

Flat

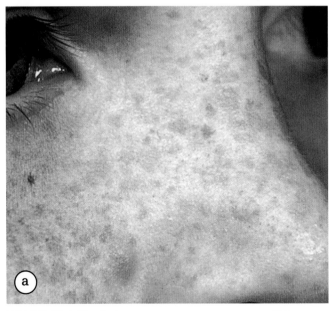

FIGURE 8.7 **(a)** Common freckles/ephelides **(b)** Common freckles/ephelides: occasionally freckles such as this one may be quite dark and require biopsy to exclude melanoma

ACQUIRED Flat

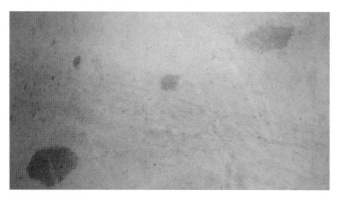

FIGURE 8.8 Café au lait patches

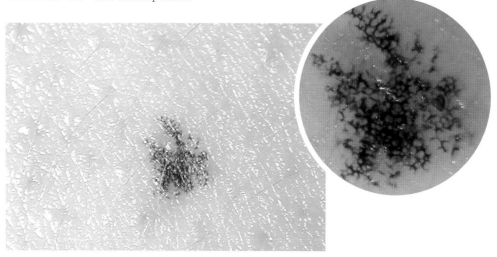

FIGURE 8.9 Ink spot lentigo with characteristic dermatoscopic appearance

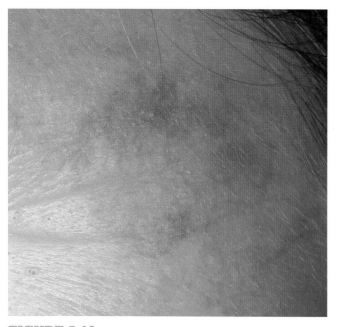

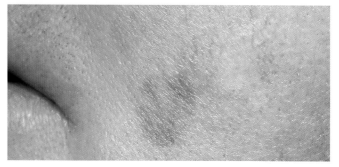

FIGURE 8.10 Solar lentigo/lentigo simplex

ACQUIRED Flat

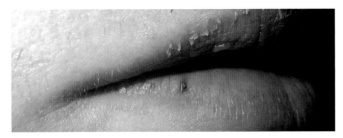

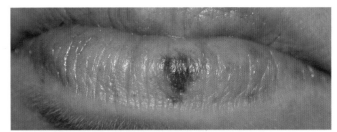

FIGURE 8.11 Labial melanotic macule

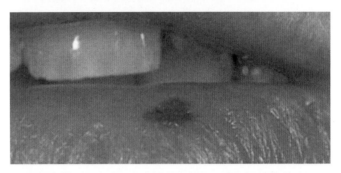

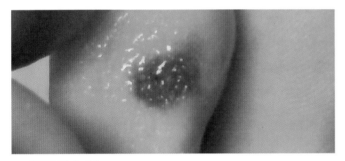

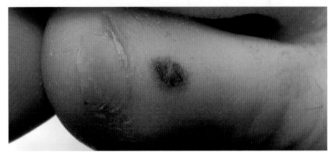

FIGURE 8.12 Junctional naevi

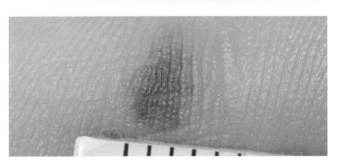

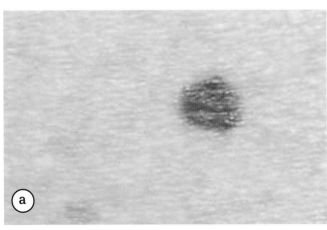

(a)

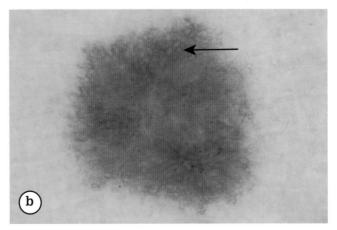

(b)

FIGURE 8.13 (a) Benign junctional melanocytic naevus. Lesion shows regular shape and even colour. **(b)** Dermoscopic view of **(a)** showing a regular pigment network (arrow) that fades to the edge

ACQUIRED Raised

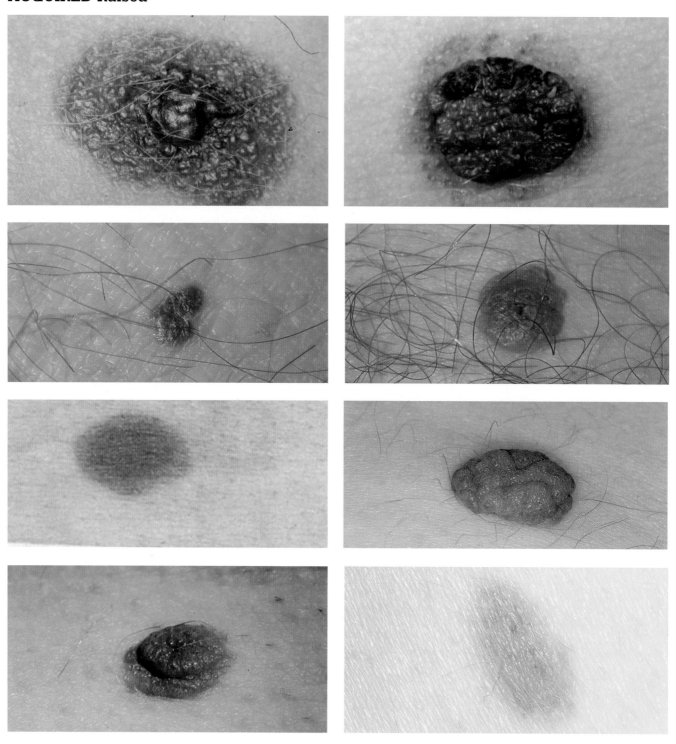

FIGURE 8.14 Compound naevi

ACQUIRED Raised

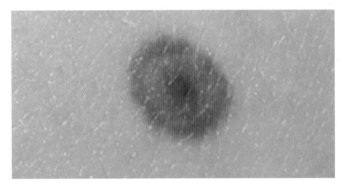

FIGURE 8.15 Naevus 'en cockarde'

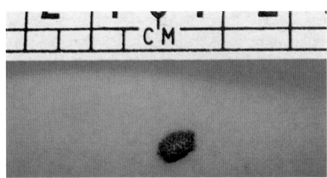

FIGURE 8.16 Naevus of Reed

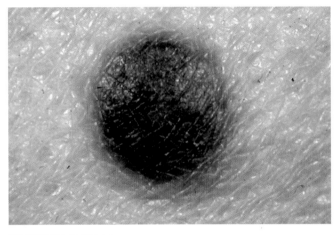

FIGURE 8.17 Blue naevus

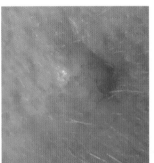 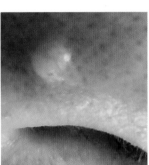

FIGURE 8.18 Intradermal naevus

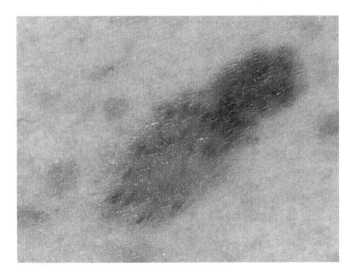

FIGURE 8.19 Irregular shape and pigmentation in dysplastic or atypical naevi

ACQUIRED Raised

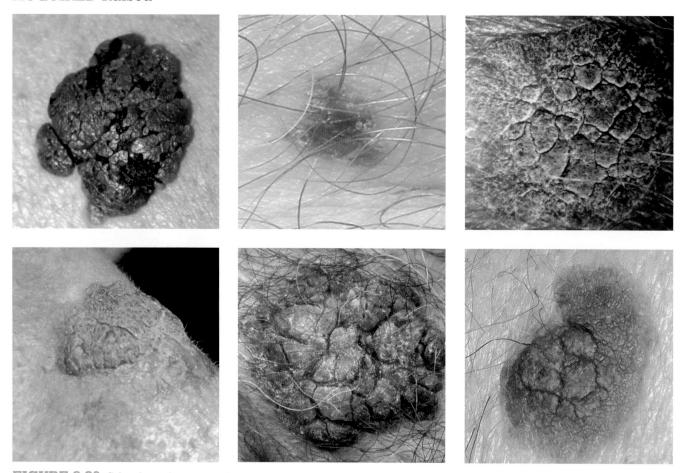

FIGURE 8.20 Seborrhoeic keratoses: characteristic warty lesions that may be single, often in or near hair-bearing areas or multiple, usually on the trunk

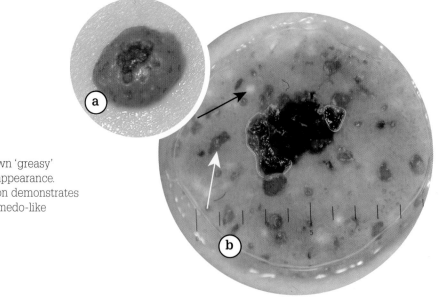

Fig 8.21 (a) Seborrheoic keratoses. A brown 'greasy' looking symmetrical lesion with a 'stuck-on' appearance. **(b)** Dermoscopic view of the above. The lesion demonstrates classical milia-like cysts (black arrow) and comedo-like openings (white arrow)

ACQUIRED Raised

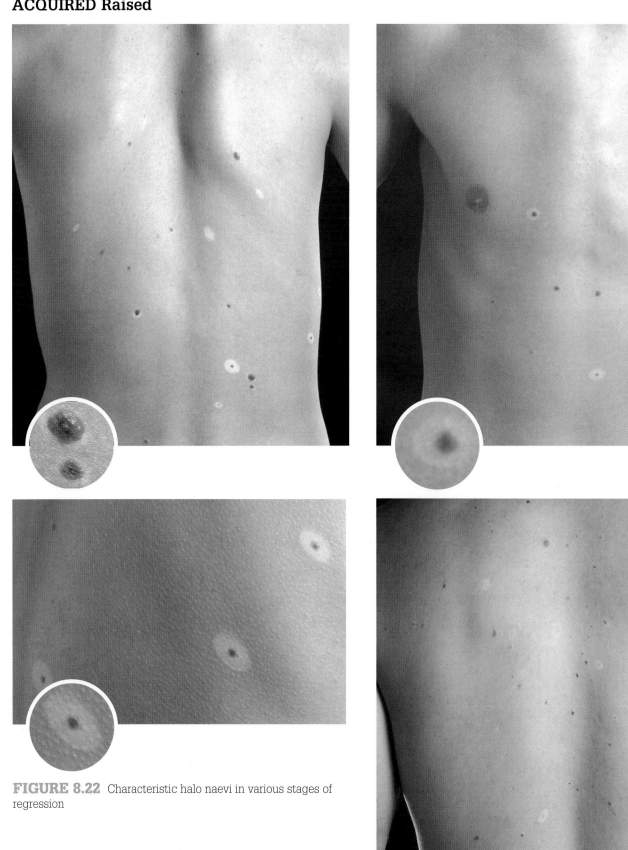

FIGURE 8.22 Characteristic halo naevi in various stages of regression

ACQUIRED Raised

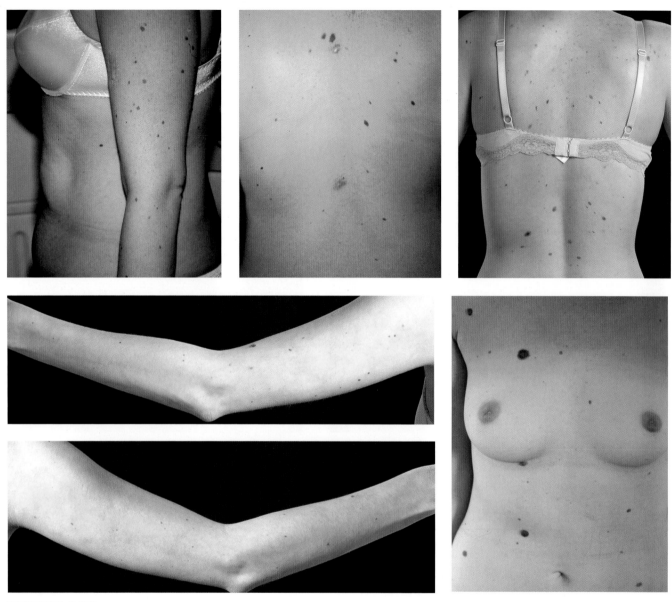

FIGURE 8.23 Familial atypical mole and melanoma syndrome: multiple atypical naevi with a family history of melanoma

ACQUIRED Melanomas

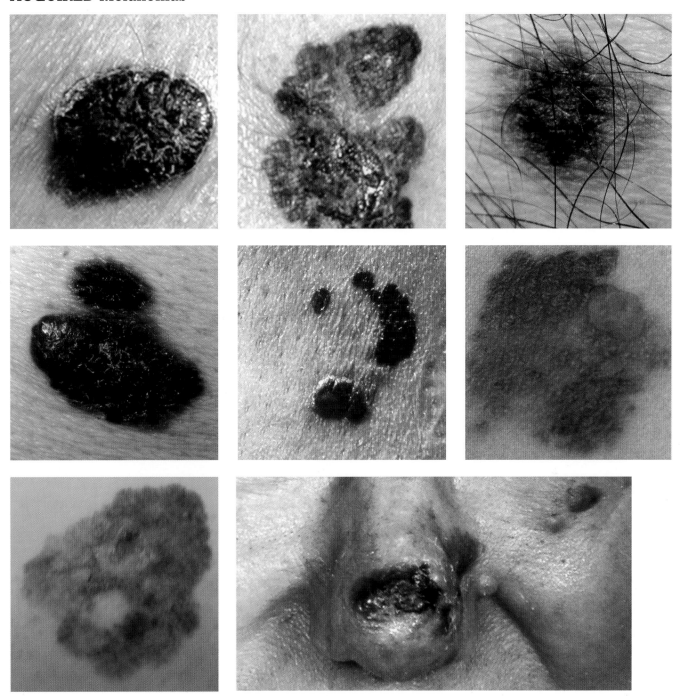

FIGURE 8.24 Characteristic irregularly shaped and pigmented melanomas

ACQUIRED Melanomas

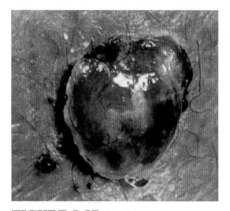
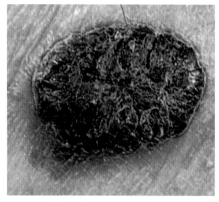
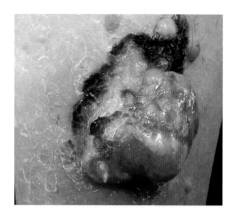

FIGURE 8.25 Nodular melanoma

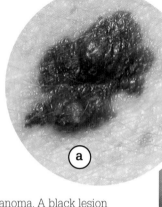

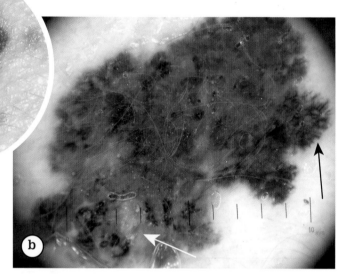

FIGURE 8.26 (a) Nodular melanoma. A black lesion with an irregular edge, and a 'bubbly' uneven surface. **(b)** Dermoscopic view of the above. Lesion shows a thickened irregular pigment network (black arrow) and a blue–white veil (white arrow)

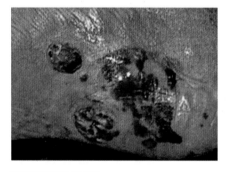
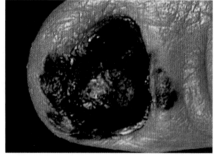
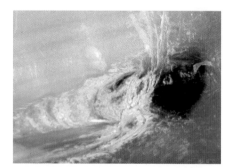

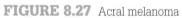

FIGURE 8.27 Acral melanoma

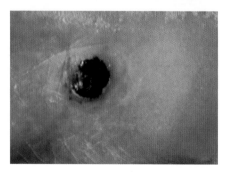

ACQUIRED Melanomas

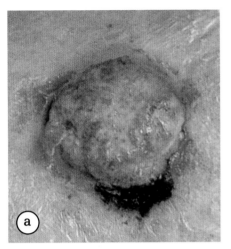
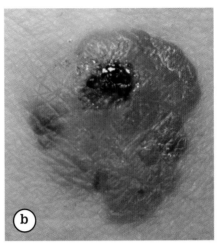
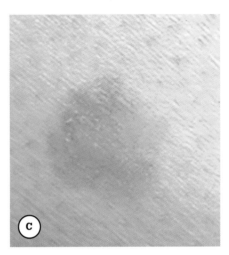

FIGURE 8.28 (a,b) Loss of pigmentation in late-stage melanoma. **(c)** Loss of pigmentation from the beginning – amelanotic melanoma

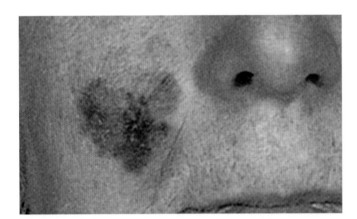

FIGURE 8.29 Lentigo maligna (*in situ*)

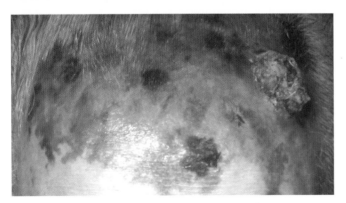

FIGURE 8.30 Lentigo maligna melanoma (invasive)

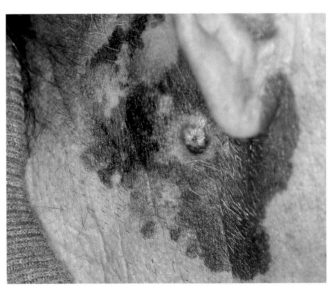

8

ACQUIRED Melanomas

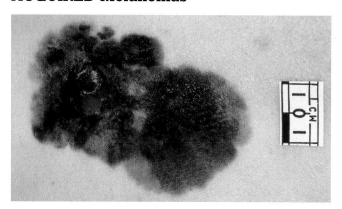

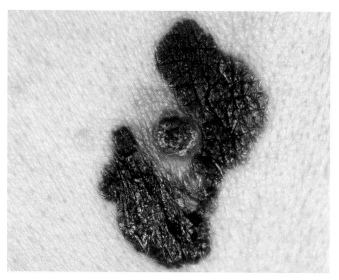

FIGURE 8.31 Superficial spreading melanoma

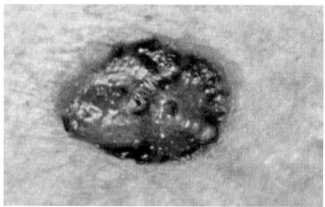

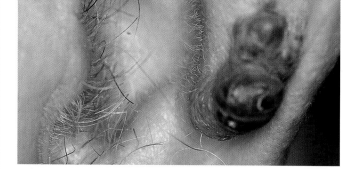

FIGURE 8.32 Melanoma

Chapter 9

Lumps and Bumps

Summary

- Vascular
- Non-pigmented

Lumps can be divided into vascular, pigmented and the rest. Pigmented lesions are dealt with in a previous chapter. Vascular lesions may be congenital of acquired. The most common congenital lesions are the flat port-wine stain and the raised haemangioma (strawberry naevus). The most common acquired lesions are spider naevi and Campbell de Morgan spots, which are essentially small haemangiomas. The remainder can be loosely divided into superficial smooth lesions such as milia, xanthelasma, dermatofibroma; and rough lesions such as solar keratoses, warts and squamous cell carcinomas. Deeper lesions such as lipomas and epidermoid cysts are relatively common and easily identified in most cases.

Algorithm 9.1

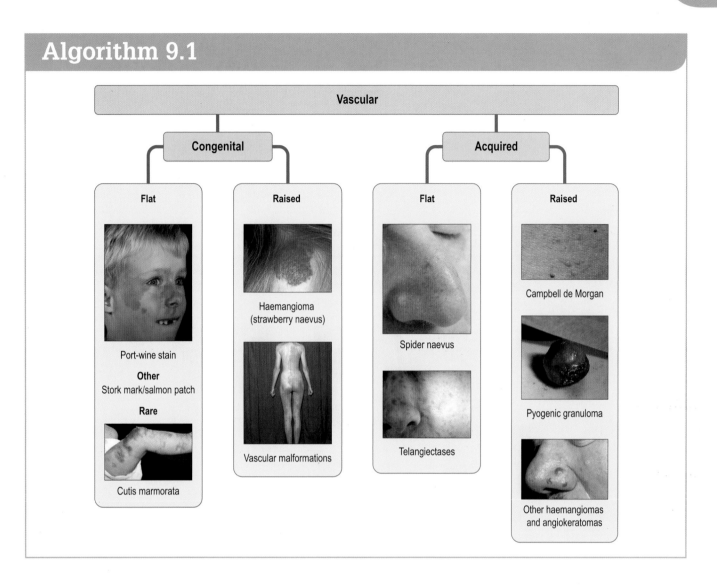

Algorithm 9.2

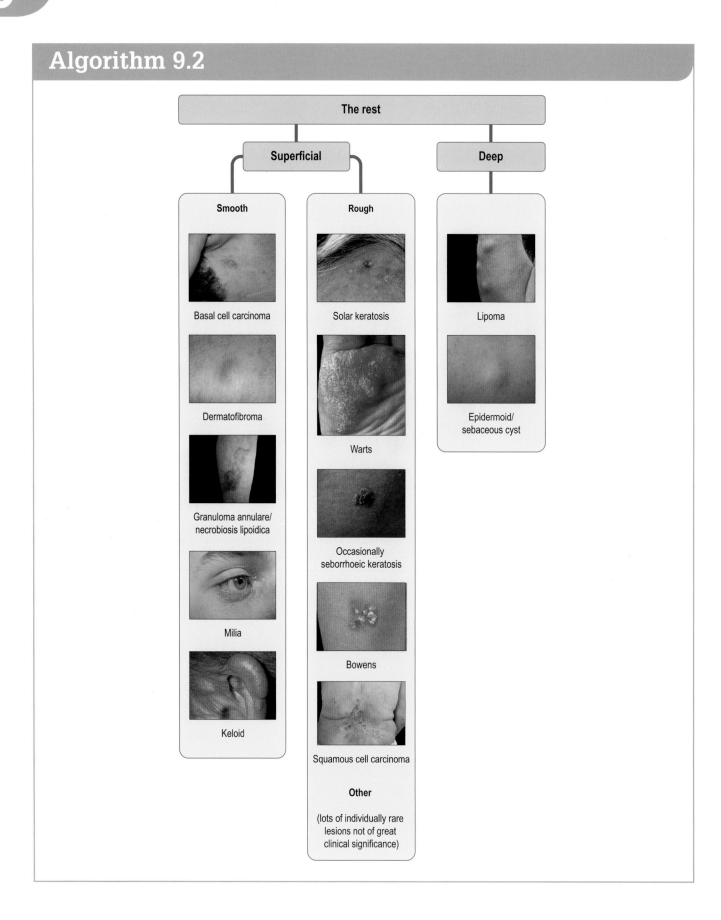

VASCULAR

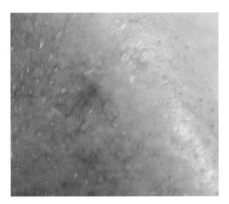 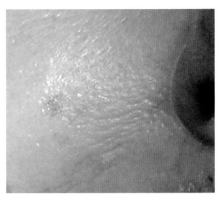 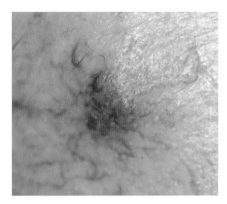

FIGURE 9.3 Spider naevi: note central darker arteriole

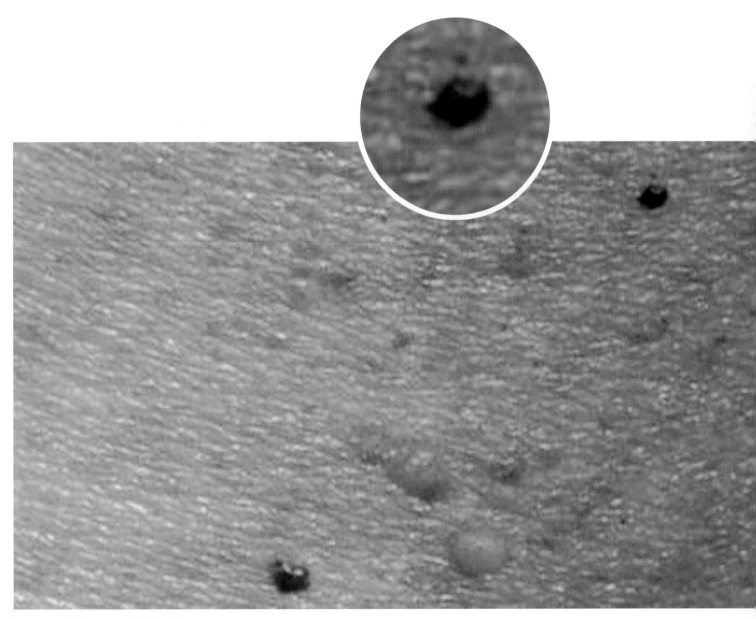

FIGURE 9.4 Campbell de Morgan spots

VASCULAR

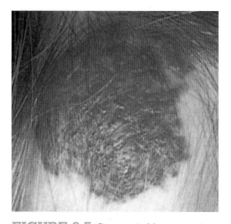
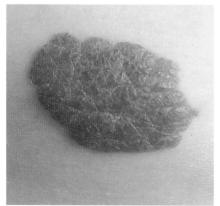
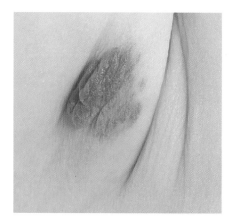

FIGURE 9.5 Congenital haemangioma

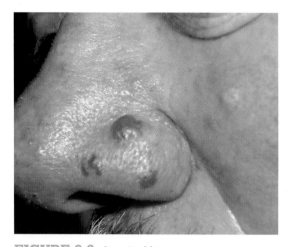

FIGURE 9.6 Acquired haemangioma

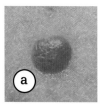
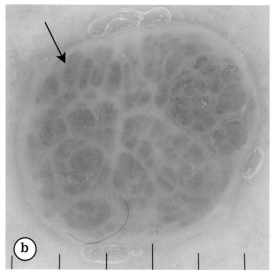

FIGURE 9.7 (a) Acquired angioma (haemangioma).
(b) Dermoscopic view of the lesion demonstrates red lagoons.

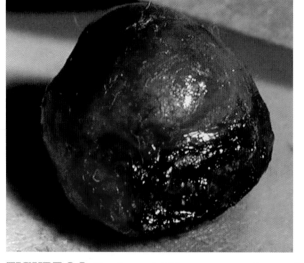
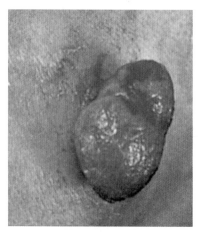

FIGURE 9.8 Bleeding painful lumps – pyogenic granuloma

VASCULAR

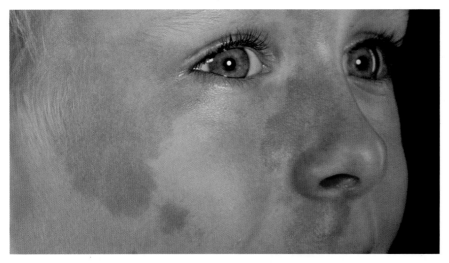

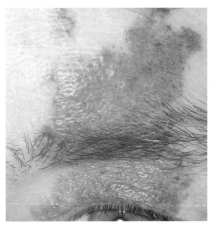

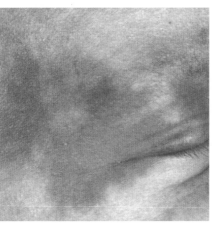

FIGURE 9.9 Port-wine stain: deeper congenital vascular malformations affecting the face and trunk – remember Sturge–Weber syndrome with lesions on the face and glaucoma with lesions near the eyes

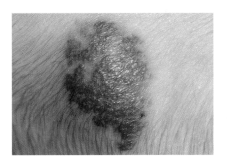

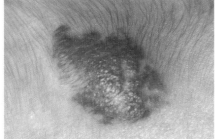

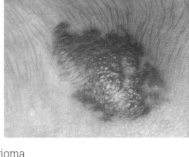

FIGURE 9.10 Small infantile haemangioma

NON-PIGMENTED Superficial *Smooth*

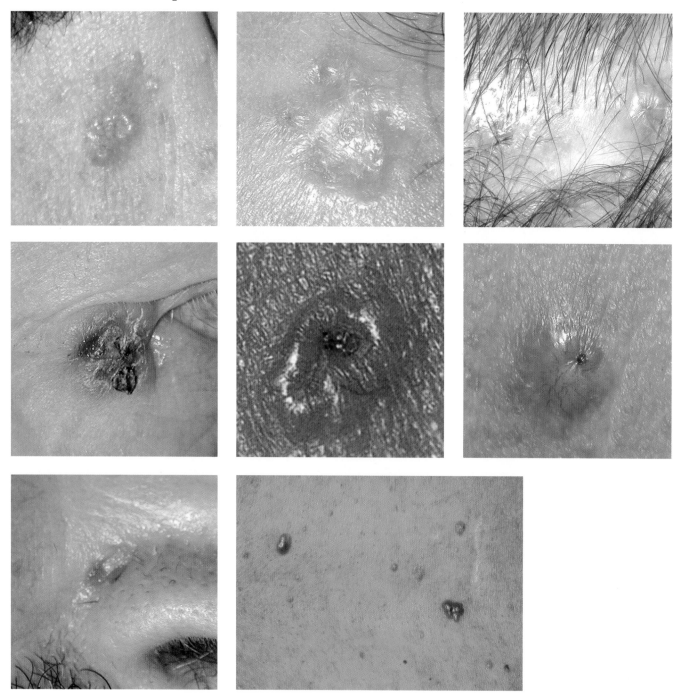

FIGURE 9.11 Typical basal cell carcinoma (BCC) with shiny pearly edge, telangiectasia ± ulceration

NON-PIGMENTED Superficial *Smooth*

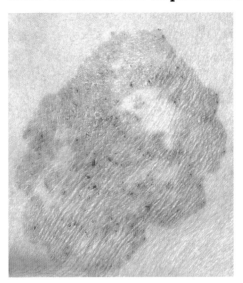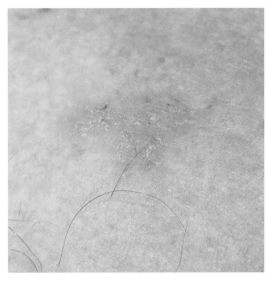

FIGURE 9.12 Superficial BCC on the trunk – may mimic plaques of psoriasis

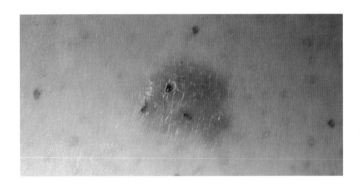

FIGURE 9.13 BCCs on the leg are often more erythematous, presenting as small smooth plaques approx. 1 cm in diameter

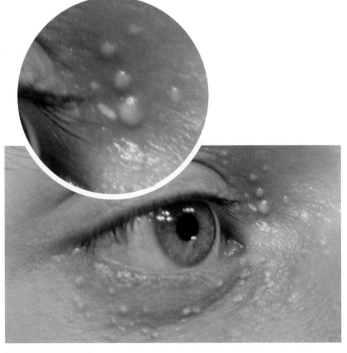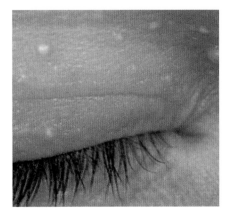

FIGURE 9.14 Milia around the eyes

NON-PIGMENTED Superficial *Smooth*

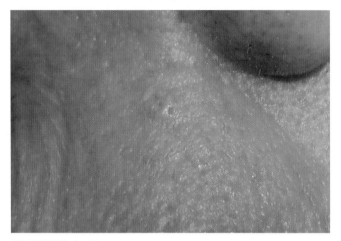

FIGURE 9.15 Sebaceous hyperplasia – may be single or multiple and mimic BCCs

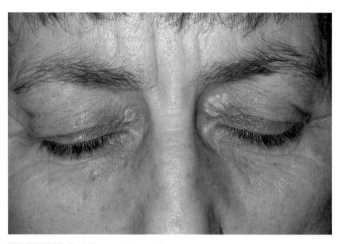

FIGURE 9.16 Xanthelasma

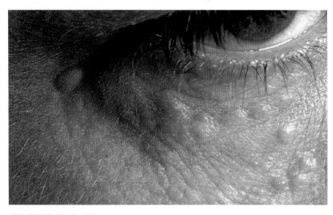

FIGURE 9.17 Syringomas

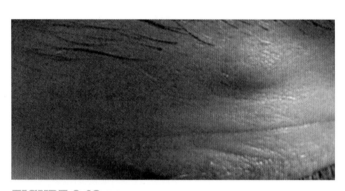

FIGURE 9.18 Pilomatricoma

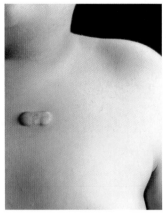 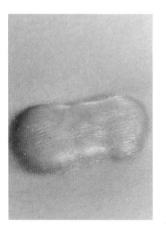 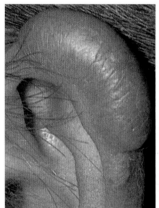 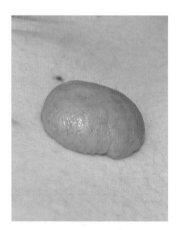

FIGURE 9.19 Keloids

NON-PIGMENTED Superficial *Smooth*

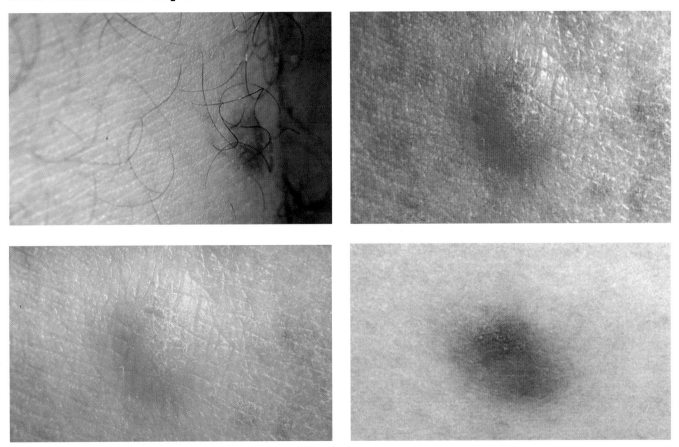

FIGURE 9.20 Dermatofibromas – firm, pea sized, varying in colour from pink to brown

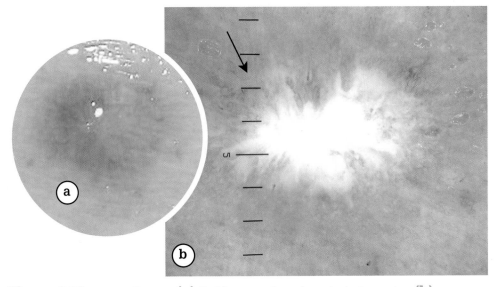

Figure 9.21 Dermatofibroma. **(a)** Red/brown–coloured regular lesion on leg. **(b)** Dermoscopic image of **(a)**. Lesion shows a pale white centre and a very fine peripheral pigment network (black arrow)

NON-PIGMENTED Superficial *Smooth*

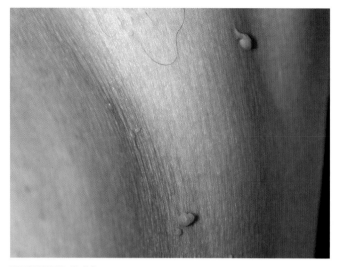

FIGURE 9.22 Skin tags

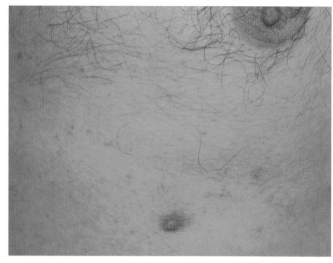

FIGURE 9.23 Accessory nipple

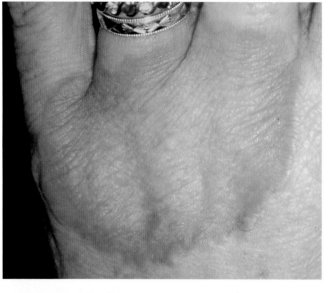

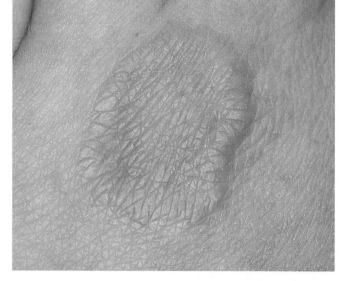

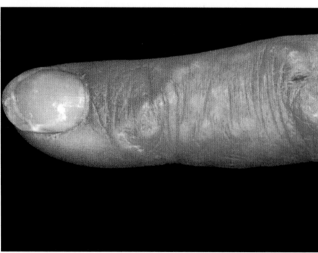

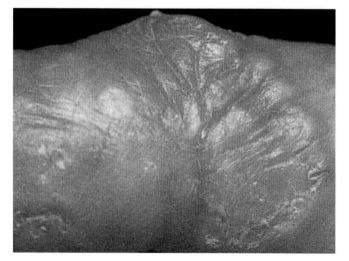

FIGURE 9.24 Annular slowly expanding lesions of granuloma annulare

NON-PIGMENTED Superficial *Smooth*

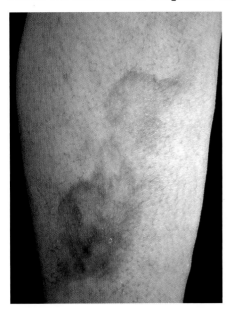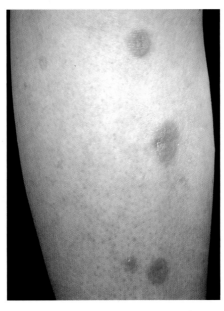

FIGURE 9.25 Annular slowly expanding lesions with central atrophy – necrobiosis lipoidica

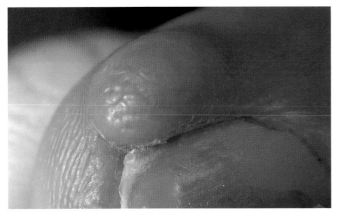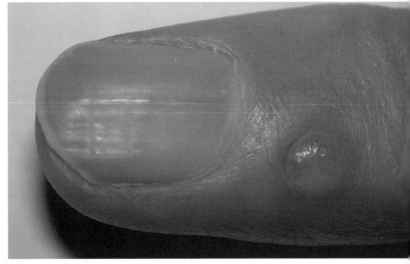

FIGURE 9.26 Translucent nodules close to a joint and often causing a linear depressed groove in the nail – myxoid cyst

NON-PIGMENTED Superficial *Rough*

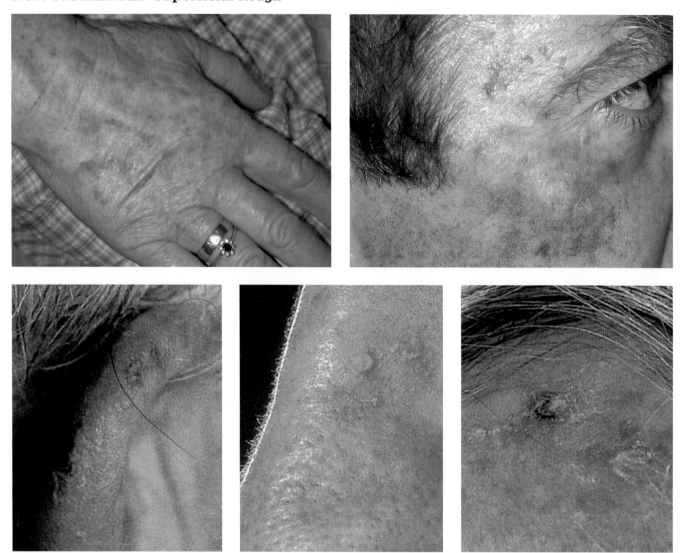

FIGURE 9.27 Typical crusted solar keratoses on the back of the hand, ear, nose and forehead

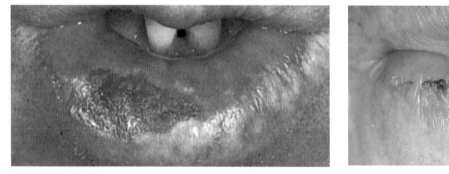

FIGURE 9.28 Similar lesions on the lips – also known as actinic cheilitis

NON-PIGMENTED Superficial *Rough*

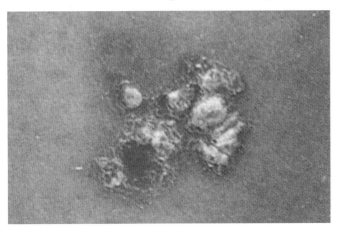

FIGURE 9.29 Typical psoriasiform plaque of Bowen's disease – SCC in situ

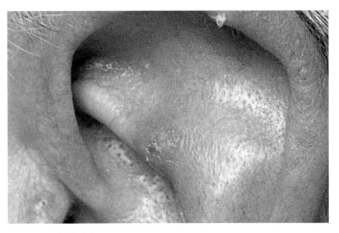

FIGURE 9.30 Painful lesion on the underside of the helical rim (nodularis helicis), often mistaken for SCC – chondrodermatitis

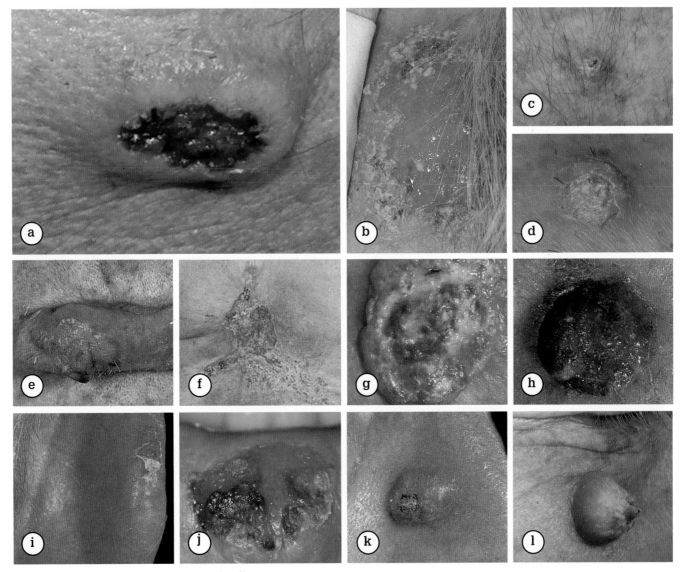

FIGURE 9.31 The spectrum of SCC **(a–j)** is considerable, varying from nondescript warty papules to fungating ulcerative masses. Raised firm edge may mimic BCC but grows more rapidly. **(k,l)** Show keratoacanthomas, rapidly growing self-healing varients of SCC with typical volcano-like appearance

NON-PIGMENTED Superficial *Rough*

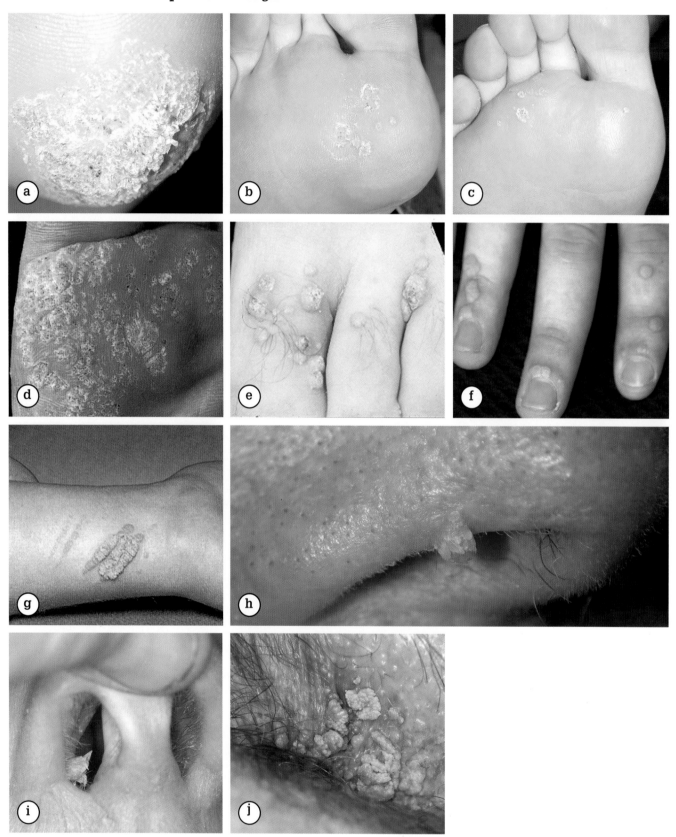

FIGURE 9.32 Typical warts on **(a–e)** the sole and dorsum of the foot, **(f)** fingers, **(g)** arm, **(h,i)** nose, **(j)** perianal

NON-PIGMENTED Superficial *Rough*

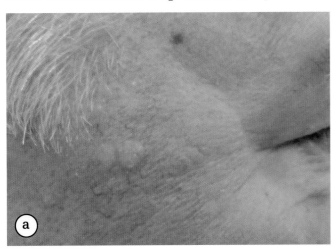

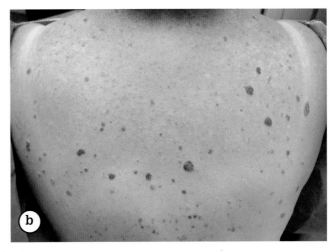

FIGURE 9.33 **(a)** Seborrhoeic keratosis on the face and **(b)** back

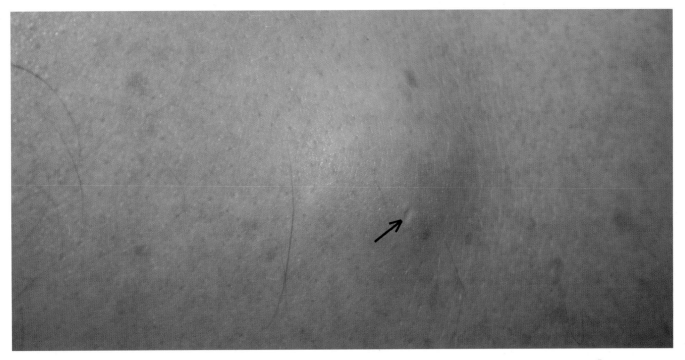

FIGURE 9.34 Fluctuant epidermoid 'sebaceous' cyst with punctum (arrow)

NON-PIGMENTED Deep lesions

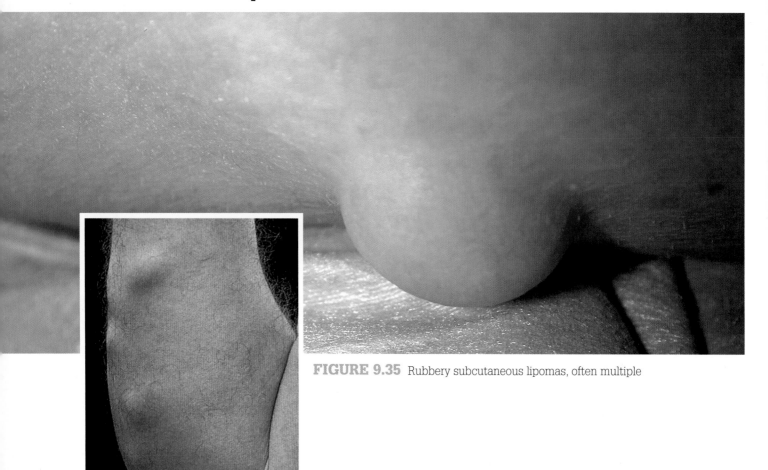

FIGURE 9.35 Rubbery subcutaneous lipomas, often multiple

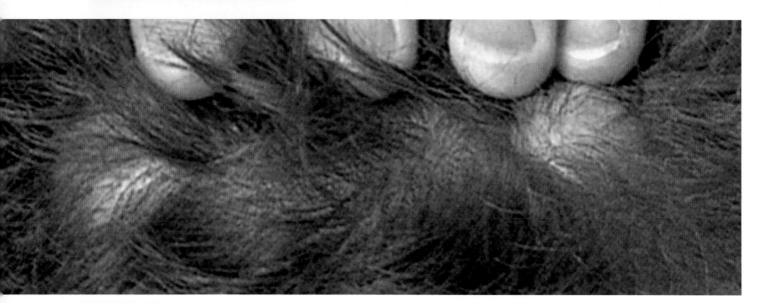

FIGURE 9.36 Multiple trichilemmomas

Common Conditions

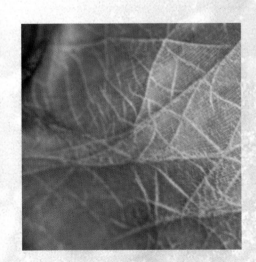

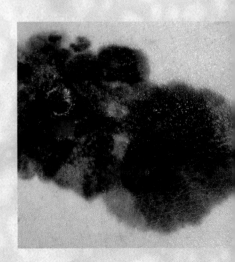

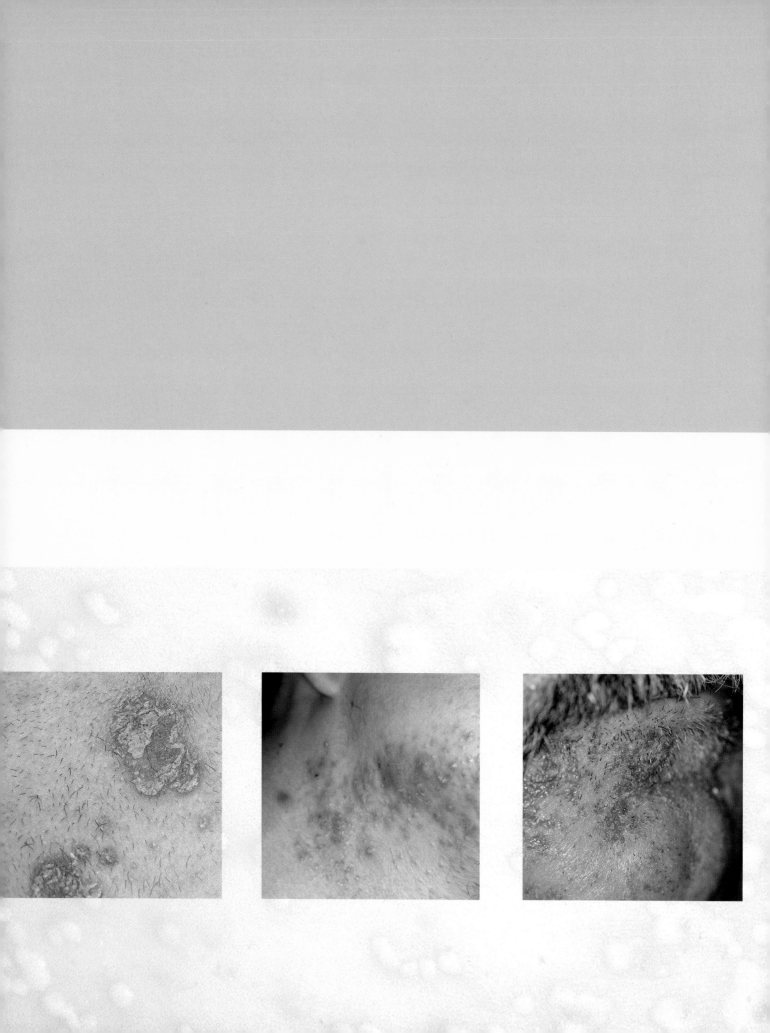

Chapter 10

Eczema

Summary

Clinical forms of eczema–dermatitis
- Primary irritant dermatitis
- Contact allergic dermatitis
- Atopic eczema (or atopic dermatitis; infantile eczema)
- Seborrhoeic eczema/dermatitis
- Discoid eczema (nummular eczema)
- Stasis dermatitis (varicose or gravitational eczema)
- Dermatitis of the hands and feet
- More unusual forms of eczema/dermatitis
- Eczema of special sites
- Infective eczema

Inflammation in the skin is one of the most important pathological processes and is a factor in a number of conditions. Psoriasis and lichen planus and, indeed, skin infections are invariably associated with a degree of inflammation. Some cutaneous inflammation is conventionally grouped together under the working title 'eczema' or 'dermatitis'. A working classification of this group of conditions is given in Box 10.1.

BOX 10.1 A classification of eczema–dermatitis

Exogenous

Primary irritant (Fig. 10.1)

Contact allergic (Figs 10.2, 10.3)

Secondary to pathogens (infective)

Endogenous

Atopic (Figs 10.4–10.6)

Seborrhoeic (Figs 10.7–10.9)

Discoid (Fig. 10.10)

Hand and foot:
    Hyperkeratotic/fissured (Figs 10.11–10.17)
    Vesicular (pompholyx) (Figs 10.18, 10.19)

Stasis (varicose) (Figs 10.20, 10.21)

Asteatotic (Fig. 10.22)

Superficial scaly dermatosis (xanthoerythrodermia perstans, digitate dermatosis) (Fig. 10.23)

Photo-provoked (Fig. 10.24)

Neurodermatitis (including lichen simplex chronicus and nodular prurigo) (Fig. 10.25)

However, at the outset it is important to stress that it may not be necessary, and indeed it may be unhelpful, to over-elaborate distinctions. For example, many people with an endogenous form of eczema will find that cutaneous irritation will trigger or exaggerate their problem, and contact allergic dermatitis may also be a complicating factor. In fact, nearly all eczema is caused by a combination of both endogenous (i.e. genetic) and exogenous factors. For example, atopic dermatitis clearly has a very significant genetic component (as shown by family involvement and the particularly high degree of concordance for the disease between identical twins). However, it seems highly likely that something in the environment needs to activate this genetic predisposition. The same is certainly true of irritant dermatitis, where the same exposure to irritants such as soaps or detergents will provoke a reaction much sooner in someone with a tendency to eczema than someone without.

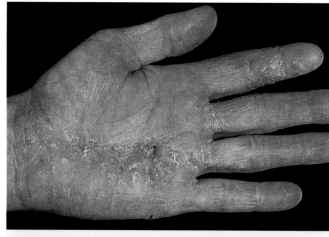

FIGURE 10.1 Irritant contact dermatitis of the hand

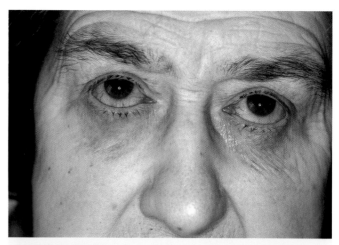

FIGURE 10.2 Contact allergic dermatitis to neomycin in eye drops

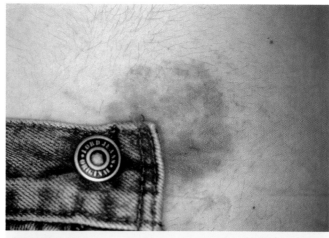

FIGURE 10.3 Contact allergic dermatitis to nickel in studs

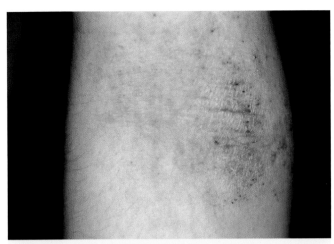

FIGURE 10.4 Atopic eczema: flexural changes

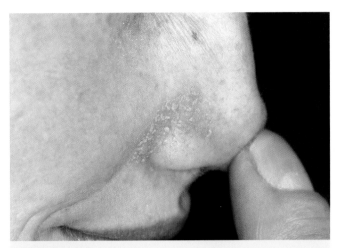

FIGURE 10.7 Seborrhoeic eczema: typical scale and erythema in the nasolabial fold

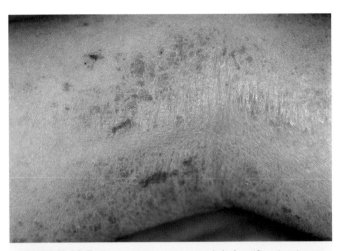

FIGURE 10.5 Flexural dermatitis with lichenification in atopic eczema

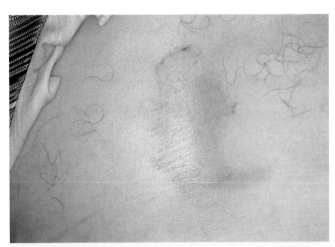

FIGURE 10.8 Seborrhoeic dermatitis

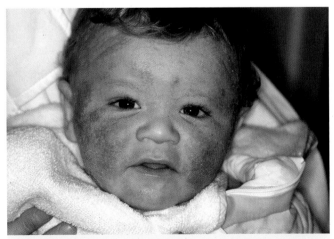

FIGURE 10.6 In children with atopic eczema, the face is prominently involved

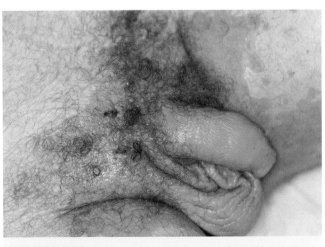

FIGURE 10.9 Seborrhoeic dermatitis: severe in the groin

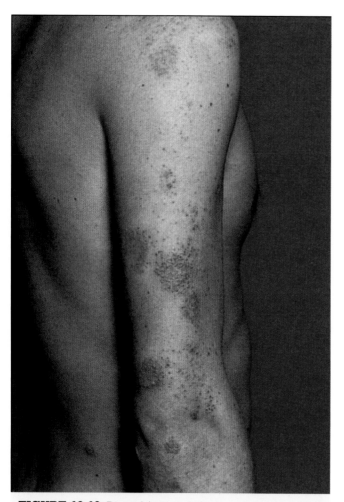

FIGURE 10.10 Discoid (nummular) eczema

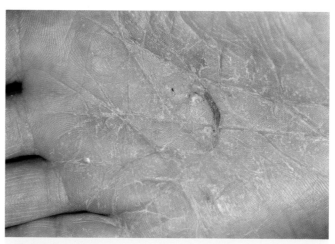

FIGURE 10.12 Hand eczema: hyperkeratotic

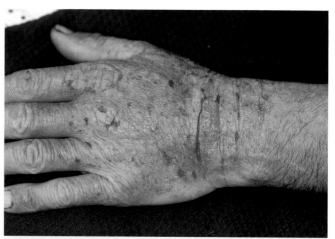

FIGURE 10.13 Hand dermatitis: irritant factors played a major role in this man

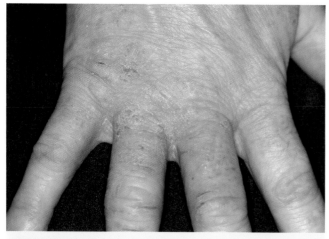

FIGURE 10.11 Hyperkeratotic/fissured hand dermatitis

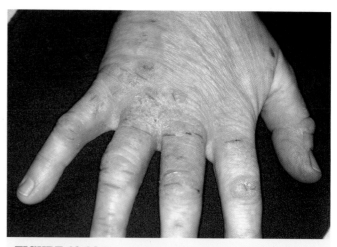

FIGURE 10.14 Hyperkeratotic/fissured hand dermatitis

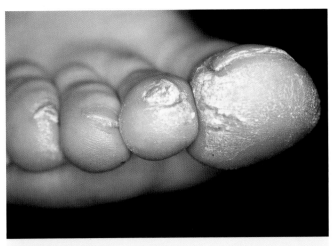

FIGURE 10.15 Foot eczema

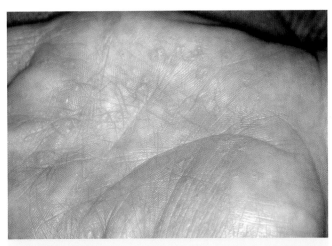

FIGURE 10.18 Tense blisters on the palm in pompholyx

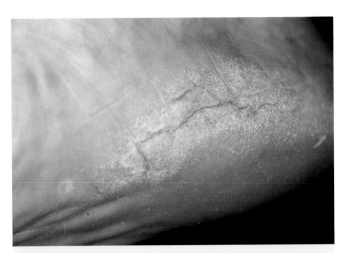

FIGURE 10.16 Foot dermatitis: hyperkeratotic areas on the heel

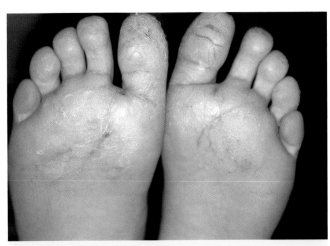

FIGURE 10.19 Glazed, fissured erythema of the forefoot in juvenile plantar dermatosis

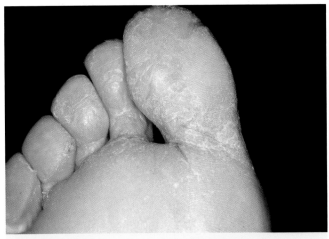

FIGURE 10.17 Foot eczema

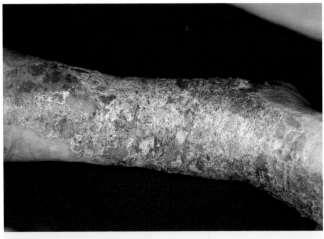

FIGURE 10.20 Severe stasis dermatitis

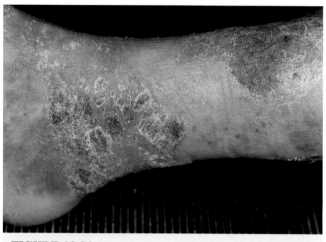

FIGURE 10.21 Localized areas of stasis dermatitis. Note also the hyperpigmentation

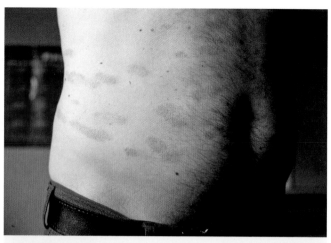

FIGURE 10.23 Finger-like patches of eczematous skin in 'digitate dermatosis'

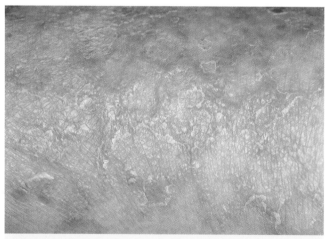

FIGURE 10.22 Eczema craquelé

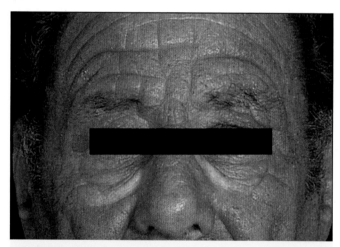

FIGURE 10.24 Photo-provoked

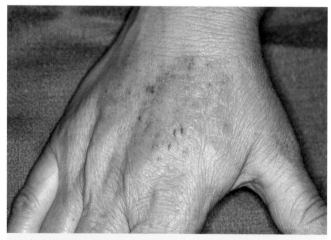

FIGURE 10.25 Lichen simplex

CLINICAL FORMS OF ECZEMA-DERMATITIS

PRIMARY IRRITANT DERMATITIS

Presentation

The skin is capable of withstanding a significant degree of chemical insult but, if such trauma is excessively prolonged or the materials involved are particularly harsh, an irritant dermatitis may develop. This occurs more quickly in some patients, often because of an endogenous eczematous tendency: irritant dermatitis is very much more troublesome in those with a previous history of atopic dermatitis. Common irritants include soaps and detergents, shampoos (especially in hairdressing), foodstuffs, water and cutting oils and so certain occupations predispose to the development of condition: hairdressers; cooks and caterers; machine-tool operators; washers-up; nurses; housewives/homemakers.

It often takes repeated injury over time for the reaction to develop but, once the process has begun, short remissions are followed by rapid deterioration. Occupational hand dermatitis will frequently improve over a period away from work, only to return on restarting.

Patient problems

The persistence of dermatitis may seriously interfere with the quality of life and may threaten the ability to carry out particular tasks.

Practical prescribing

The only permanent solution is the cessation of the provoking activity but if this is impossible (and it often is) some relief can be obtained by the judicious use of topical corticosteroids to suppress inflammation, the liberal use of emollients and non-soap cleansers, and avoidance measures such as gloves – plastic as opposed to rubber – and barrier creams.

CONTACT ALLERGIC DERMATITIS

This is the term used to describe type IV (delayed, cell-mediated) hypersensitivity to environmental allergens.

Presentation

Exposure induces dermatitis, predominantly at the site of contact. Often, only minute quantities of the offending agent are needed to cause reactions. A large number of agents can induce contact allergic dermatitis (Table 10.1).

Secondary spread from initial contact sites onto adjacent or even distant non-contact sites is common and may cause confusion: some sites are more prone to this, especially the eyelids, which are commonly inflamed in sensitivity to epoxy resins, plants, cosmetics and metal.

Materials that are volatile, or can be airborne in the form of dust, can give rise to *airborne allergic contact dermatitis*. This produces a diffuse dermatitis of the face, backs of hands and other exposed areas, simulating a light-sensitive eczema. However, the classical light-spared areas are usually involved.

Patient problems

The issues are essentially the same as in irritant dermatitis - the patient wants and needs to know what to avoid in order to stop the reaction occurring.

Practical prescribing

Investigation must begin with a careful history of exposure to potential sensitizers:

- Obtain a clear description of possible work and domestic sources.
- Establish all tasks carried out, hobbies and leisure pursuits.
- List cosmetics, toiletries and medicaments applied to the skin surface.

The key investigative technique is patch testing (see Ch. 23: 'Investigations').

Treat an acute attack with potent topical corticosteroids, together with soaking in potassium permanganate (1:10 000) solution if there is a vesicular or bullous component (see also 'Dermatitis of the hands and feet', below).

However, it is essential to remove the causative agent from the environment as far as possible.

ATOPIC ECZEMA (OR ATOPIC DERMATITIS; INFANTILE ECZEMA)

Atopic eczema (AE) is one of the commonest disorders in the Western world. At least 15% of UK children are affected by the age of 4 years.

AE is classically associated with the other common atopic diseases: asthma and allergic rhinitis–conjunctivitis (hay fever). Urticaria and urticarial reactions, especially after contact with foods and animal hair, are also common in AE.

Genetics are fundamentally important in atopic dermatitis but so are environmental factors.

Sadly not nearly enough is known about the complex interactions that must be taking place in AE. However, it is highly likely that disordered immunological function is fundamental in this host–environment interaction, as must be impairment of the skin barrier.

Table 10.1 Some common causes of contact dermatitis		
Antigen	**Common pattern/sites**	**Environmental source**
Nickel and cobalt	Eczema under jewellery, watches, fastenings	Non-precious metals
Chromates	Hands, feet, face (due to airborne contact)	Cement; tanned leather; industrial processes
Rubber chemicals	Hands, forearms, waist, feet	Gloves; shoes; elasticated materials
Colophony	Under sticking plasters	Sticking plasters
Epoxy resins	Face, hands	Domestic and industrial use
Phenylene diamines	Face, especially eyelids, which are often oedematous	Hair dyes
Formaldehyde, the 'parabens', ethylene diamine, and quaternium 15	Almost anywhere but often eyelids and face; may complicate varicose eczema and otitis externa	Preservatives in medicaments and toiletries – formaldehyde especially in shampoos
Lanolin	Anywhere; may complicate varicose eczema and otitis externa	Medicaments and toiletries
Aminoglycosides (especially neomycin)	Anywhere; may complicate varicose eczema and otitis externa	Medicaments
Corticosteroids	Anywhere	Medicaments
Plant antigens	Linear streaks at point of contact; face (due to airborne contact)	*Primula obconica* (UK); Rhus (poison ivy) (USA); Parthenium (India); Chrysanthemum and many others
Wood antigens	Hands, forearms, face (due to airborne contact)	Hardwoods, especially mahogany

Presentation

The diagnosis is a clinical one, but it is occasionally difficult to ascribe eczematous disease firmly to AE. Here a serum IgE may be helpful (it is often very high, but can be quite normal).

AE usually begins in childhood, often in the first year of life, but may appear at any age. In infancy the face is prominently involved, with red, inflamed skin. Similar changes appear over the trunk and limbs, more or less anywhere initially, but as time passes there is an increasing focus on flexural surfaces (antecubital and popliteal fossae; wrists and ankles). The skin may also become thickened and rough – a change known as lichenification (Fig. 10.26). A similar phenomenon occurs around the eyes, where the so-called 'Dennie–Morgan' infraorbital fold is common (Fig. 10.27).

Patients with AE have a generally 'dry' skin: the term *xerosis* is often used to describe this, although many children have changes amounting to a true ichthyosis.

There is usually abundant evidence of scratching because AE is always itchy.

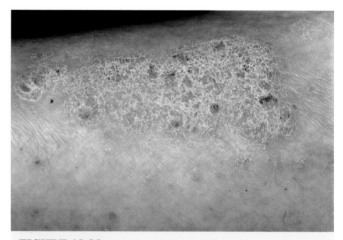

FIGURE 10.26 An area of lichenification

Weepy, yellow crusts caused by impetiginization (Fig. 10.28) are also common. However, distinguishing between true secondary infection and colonization by *Staphylococcus aureus* all the time is not straightforward.

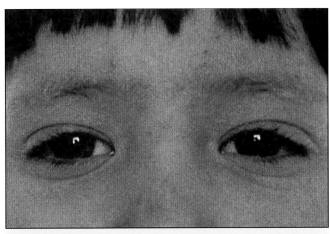

FIGURE 10.27 Arcuate skin creases of both lower eyelids ('Dennie–Morgan' folds) bilaterally

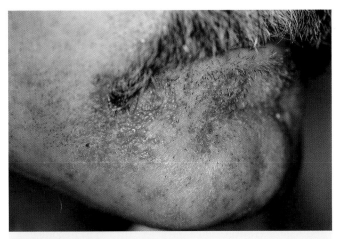

FIGURE 10.28 Impetiginization

Patient problems

The itch is probably the aspect of the disorder that causes the most distress. The symptom seems to become all-pervasive. Patients have feverish bouts of scratching, and some children seem never to stop rubbing and scratching at their skin. They may lie awake at night, keeping other family members from sleeping.

The other key management issue relates to the understanding that families and friends have about AE:

- There is a preconception that all (or even most) AE is 'due to an allergy', and that a search must be undertaken to find 'the cause'; to many it is obvious that this process should involve tests.
- There is far less knowledge about AE in some communities; in migrant families, for example, it may have been unheard of before the move to the West.

Outcome

AE spontaneously resolves in about 60% of children, but a significant number continue to have trouble into adolescence and adulthood. Furthermore, a large number of individuals with a past history of the disease develop primary irritant dermatitis from occupational or domestic exposure to chemicals.

Practical prescribing

There are few investigations that assist in the diagnosis or management of AE on a day-to-day basis. Swabs for bacterial culture may be valuable to determine antibiotic sensitivity. Samples for viral culture should be taken before commencing treatment if eczema herpeticum is suspected (see below). Allergy tests (prick tests and serum assays for total IgE and specific IgE) are usually unhelpful beyond confirming the atopic state, or in investigating acute, urticarial reactions, but are frequently requested.

Treatment is largely topical, relying on:
- The avoidance of irritants, such as soaps and harsh cleansers; cooler than average bath water and room temperatures; humidified air; cotton or man-made clothing (certainly not wool).
- The liberal use of emollients; these should be applied as often as is practical, especially at bath times.
- The judicious use of antiinflammatory agents; topical steroids work well, as long as agents of sufficient strength are employed; the key is to aim for effectiveness and intermittency; there are good studies showing that intermittent (twice weekly) potent steroids are safe; it is often possible, too, to commence with a stronger agent, gain control, and then serially reduce the strength. Occasionally it is justified to use very potent steroids on the face, but only in very short bursts.
- Topical calcineurin inhibitors (tacrolimus, pimecrolimus) have a role – especially on the face, and in allowing steroid-free windows.

In the event of failure, consideration should be given to:
- The use of sedative agents to aid sleep, i.e. sedating antihistamines.
- The introduction of antimicrobial therapy.
- A review of compliance.
- A check that allergic contact dermatitis related to medications is not a new complication.

Referral for:
- UVB phototherapy (in older patients who will tolerate the procedures involved, and in younger children where this will avoid the use of toxic systemic agents).
- Immunosuppressive drugs:
  - Systemic steroids, as long as there is an exit strategy.
  - Azathioprine in older patients.
  - Ciclosporin, preferably in short bursts.

171

Dietary manipulation is seldom effective, although one hears many tales of spectacular success. There may be intense pressure to assist with this, but uncontrolled dietary alterations are potentially dangerous. Any changes should be overseen by a qualified dietician.

Complications

In addition to secondary bacterial infection, patients with AE are more prone to invasion by viruses. Molluscum contagiosum is more prevalent and often more widespread in AE, but the main worry is superinfection by *Herpes simplex*: a state known as *eczema herpeticum* (or *Kaposi's varicelliform eruption*).

Viral lesions spread widely over the skin surface, creating an appearance resembling chickenpox (Fig. 10.29). This may be accompanied by a fever, particularly if this is the first exposure to the virus.

The condition can be life-threatening:

* The skin may cease to be an effective barrier to the retention of fluid and protein, leading to metabolic disturbances.
* The skin is susceptible to further invasion by bacteria that may cause septicaemia.
* Viraemia and viral encephalitis may occur.

If eczema herpeticum is suspected, and especially if the patient is febrile or unwell, intravenous therapy with acyclovir, or one of the newer alternative drugs, should be started immediately. Topical corticosteroids should also be suspended, and the patient should be kept under close observation.

SEBORRHOEIC ECZEMA/DERMATITIS

This is a very common clinical pattern of eczema seen in adults. There is also a condition known as *infantile seborrhoeic dermatitis*, which occurs (as the name implies) in infancy. The two are not directly related and must be considered separately.

Adult seborrhoeic eczema

Presentation

There are a number of unmistakeable features in a typical patient. In particular, the distribution is characteristic:

* Scalp – mild scaling (or dandruff) represents one end of the clinical spectrum, with marked scaling and erythema at the other.
* Nasolabial folds, spreading out on to the cheeks.
* Eyebrows.
* Behind the ears.
* Upper chest (both front and back) (Fig. 10.30).
* If the changes are very severe, check for HIV/other immunodeficiency.

The eruption consists of red, scaly, somewhat greasy-looking patches. Some patients also suffer from an inflammation of the eyelids (blepharitis). Others develop a more flexural (intertriginous) form in the axillae and groins, often producing a clinical appearance very similar to flexural psoriasis.

Adult seborrhoeic dermatitis usually presents in adolescence or early adulthood and, although the severity may fluctuate, the tendency often persists throughout life.

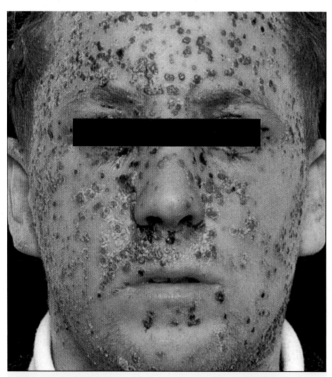

FIGURE 10.29 Extensive herpes simplex of the face in a patient with atopic dermatitis (eczema herpeticum/Kaposi's varicelliform eruption)

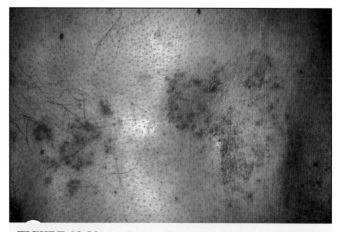

FIGURE 10.30 Adult seborrhoeic eczema: upper chest

Patient problems

Face and scalp disease is very upsetting. Flexural seborrhoeic eczema can be most uncomfortable. The skin changes can be seen in patients with HIV infection, especially when the CD4 count is falling.

Patients want to know why they have developed the condition. The generally accepted explanation is that a commensal yeast plays a major role in inducing and perpetuating the inflammation, but it is impossible to eradicate the organism permanently.

Practical prescribing

Patients may benefit from using a topical corticosteroid cream alone, or a topical antifungal agent such as miconazole, clotrimazole, or ketoconazole alone, but a combination of the two is generally superior.

Using the agents sequentially offers a chance to increase the intermittency of steroid application and reduce the potential for side effects. Occasionally, severe seborrhoeic dermatitis requires oral treatment with an agent such as itraconazole. Also, if persistent, low-dose systemic antibiotic with antiinflammatory activity, e.g. lymecycline 408 mg o.d., may be of additional benefit.

Scalp disease requires the use of an anti-yeast shampoo (zinc pyrithione, selenium sulfide and ketoconazole are all effective) and a topical steroid lotion.

Infantile seborrhoeic dermatitis

Some children develop a widespread eruption involving the nappy area, flexures and scalp (Fig. 10.31). *Infantile seborrhoeic dermatitis* is much less common than it once was (reason unknown), but it generally appears in the

first 3 months of life. The rash appears not to be itchy, although the nappy area may be sore and weepy. The skin lesions respond well to mild topical corticosteroids (often combined with an antifungal agent because of a fear of superadded candidal infection). The scalp changes (known as cradle cap) do well with oils and gentle shampooing but may require more aggressive therapy with salicylic acid.

DISCOID ECZEMA (NUMMULAR ECZEMA)

Presentation

Patients (both children and adults) present with round or oval patches of eczema. These are exquisitely itchy and may arise almost anywhere (though they are fortunately rare on the face). They can be distinguished from psoriasis because they are itchy, lighter in colour and lack classical scale, Auspitz's sign is negative and there is a rapid response to topical steroids. Untreated lesions either settle over a few days or may grumble on, sometimes merging with adjacent patches. The cause is unknown.

Practical prescribing

The treatment of discoid eczema relies on topical corticosteroids used early enough to prevent lesions from developing into large plaques, but the condition often continues to erupt, causing trouble over many months or years. The lesions in some patients are secondarily infected with *S. aureus*, and oral antibiotics may be helpful.

STASIS DERMATITIS (VARICOSE OR GRAVITATIONAL ECZEMA)

Alongside the other changes associated with venous incompetence (see Ch. 16: 'Leg ulcers and lymphoedema'), patients frequently develop eczematous areas on the lower legs. These may be diffuse, involving the whole 'gaiter area', or more localized. Occasionally, the changes appear directly over varicose veins. Secondary spread to more distant sites is common and may indicate the development of an allergic contact dermatitis to some of the topical medication, a situation which is particularly common in stasis dermatitis. The lesions may also be purpuric, especially around the ankles and on the foot.

Practical prescribing

Emollients – if the skin is very dry, use of ointment such as Epaderm at night might also be needed. If itch continues despite this, symptomatic relief can be obtained with minimum intermittent dose of topical corticosteroids,

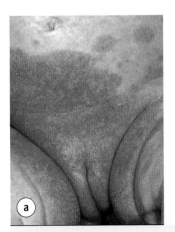
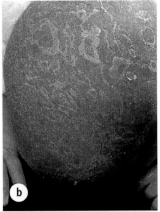

FIGURE 10.31 **(a)** Infantile seborrhoeic dermatitis: widespread eruption involving the nappy area and flexures. **(b)** Infantile seborrhoeic dermatitis affecting the scalp

173

but watch out for skin thinning and for sensitivity to constituents of any treatment that is applied to this condition. It is essential to promote active treatment of the underlying venous condition: compression or surgery, as judged appropriate.

DERMATITIS OF THE HANDS AND FEET

Hand and foot dermatitis is one of the commonest patterns of eczematous inflammation encountered in clinical practice. Either hands or feet may be involved alone but it is common to see both affected simultaneously. Hand and foot dermatitis may also be part of a more generalized eczema (e.g. atopic dermatitis). The hands are frequently involved in primary irritant dermatitis, and both hands and feet may be affected by contact allergic dermatitis. It is a simple, but reasonably useful, rule of thumb that *exogenous* dermatitis mostly involves the dorsa of the hands and feet, and the finger and toe web spaces, while changes predominantly on the palmar and plantar surfaces probably represent a largely major *endogenous* process.

Patch testing is a normal part of the investigation of any patient with hand or foot dermatitis. However, common as these problems are, many patients present with dermatitis of the hands and feet for which no obvious external cause can be found, or in whom exogenous factors are only part of the picture.

Presentation

There are several changes that reflect dermatitis on the hands and feet. These are not mutually exclusive. Three main patterns can be distinguished:

- *Hyperkeratotic/fissuring*. There may only be one or two plaques present, or the whole palmar and plantar surfaces may be involved; lesions may be localized to specific sites, such as the fingertips and the base of two adjacent fingers and part of the palm (the so-called apron pattern). Hyperkeratosis may be indistinguishable from palmar or plantar psoriasis. Symptoms arise from the cracking and splitting that occurs; the tenderness can be so severe as to render patients effectively disabled. Physical stiffness is a nuisance, especially if fine manual manipulation is important to the patient.
- *Pompholyx*. The predominant feature is blistering: deep-seated vesicles appear in crops on the palms and soles or along the sides of the digits. Occasionally the lesions may become very large and frankly bullous. Symptoms are very variable, but patients often use words such as 'pricking' and 'tingling' to describe the early phases. As lesions progress, the skin may become more inflamed and some splitting and fissuring may follow.
- *Juvenile plantar dermatosis*. Some children go through a phase when the forefoot becomes permanently glazed,

red and cracked. The cause is unknown but there may be a link with atopic eczema.

Practical prescribing

Hyperkeratotic/fissuring

Treatment is difficult. Avoiding external irritants and the use of emollients and potent topical steroids (under occlusion if necessary) may keep some patients comfortable. Others require more aggressive treatment: PUVA (psoralen plus ultraviolet A), particularly using local soaks with psoralen solutions, may be helpful. A few patients need systemic treatment with low-dose systemic steroids or acetretin and immunosuppressants simply to be able to lead a normal life.

Pompholyx

Treatment with potent topical corticosteroids may help to some degree, but the most effective remedy for an acute attack of pompholyx is potassium permanganate, diluted 1:10000 and used as a soak. Oral antibiotics may be required if secondary infection supervenes. Some patients have such severe pompholyx that the use of systemic steroids may be justified, at least in short bursts.

Juvenile plantar dermatosis

This disorder is generally unresponsive to steroids. The liberal use of heavy-duty emollients may help. Some authorities recommend a switch from trainers to more 'open' footwear – but is this practical? The condition tends to clear at puberty. What about cork insoles?

MORE UNUSUAL FORMS OF ECZEMA/ DERMATITIS

Asteatotic eczema (eczema craquelé, xerotic eczema)

This term is applied to skin changes generally attributed to defatting of the skin. An appearance resembling 'crazy paving' is seen, often on the lower legs in elderly patients. It may occur more readily in the winter, and may be seen in patients admitted to care facilities and in whom washing arrangements are radically altered. The treatment of choice is the liberal use of emollients – ointments may be needed.

Chronic superficial scaly dermatosis (xanthoerythrodermia perstans, digitate dermatosis)

This is a highly characteristic eruption, most commonly seen in older males. Round, oval, or elongated lesions appear on the trunk and limbs, giving a finger-like appearance. The surface is slightly scaly; itching is seldom significant. The lesions tend to persist and increase in number over the years. Phototherapy can be helpful.

Similar changes are seen in the very early stages of cutaneous T-cell lymphoma (mycosis fungoides). It is therefore sensible to obtain some histology and keep a special eye on these patients; histology may miss early cases of mycosis fungoides.

Photo-provoked eczema and chronic actinic dermatitis

Some patients develop dermatitis in response to light of various wavelengths.

Presentation

Eczematous changes appear on light-exposed sites (see Fig. 10.24), with characteristic sparing of shaded areas such as the eyelids and under the chin. Occasionally the skin of the face, scalp and neck becomes grossly thickened.

Patient problems

Affected patients have a miserable life. Sunscreens do not help much and active treatment is required.

Practical prescribing

Patch testing should always be considered because some of these patients have complex photoallergies, particularly to flowers of the chrysanthemum family. Topical steroids may help. In severely affected patients, systemic azathioprine is effective, as is ciclosporin.

Neurodermatitis (including lichen simplex chronicus and nodular prurigo)

Some patients develop eczematous changes, either over widespread areas of the body or in localized patches, a significant component in the initiation and perpetuation of the lesions appearing to be the development of an 'itch–scratch' cycle. Lesions are very excoriated (scratched and abraded) and may become heavily thickened (or lichenified – a term used to describe the rather flat-topped nature of the lesions). Classical sites for the localized form of this disorder (lichen simplex chronicus) (Fig. 10.32) are the shins, forearms, palms, perianal and vulval skin, and the back of the neck.

Nodular prurigo is generally considered to be a variant, and presents a striking clinical picture. Dome-shaped lesions develop, varying in size from a few millimetres to 1–2 cm in diameter (Fig. 10.33). There may be a few lesions or many. Patients complain of an insatiable and uncontrollable desire to scratch, often coming in intense bursts.

Treating these forms of skin inflammation, where itching is the major problem, and scratching is probably part of the pathogenesis of individual lesions, is extremely challenging. Simple topical therapy with corticosteroids, together with occlusion under medicated bandages impregnated with tar, ichthammol or zinc paste, is the usual starting point, but is often ineffective in the long term, especially with nodular prurigo. Some authorities recommend the use of tranquillizers and other psychotropic agents. Ultraviolet B phototherapy and PUVA may help some patients, and there are reports of success with powerful immunosuppressant drugs.

ECZEMA OF SPECIAL SITES

There are a number of sites on the body where eczematous inflammation presents particular problems and for which a few additional notes are worthwhile.

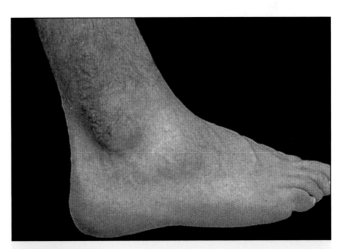

FIGURE 10.32 Lichenified plaque of dermatitis on the lateral aspect of the ankle in lichen simplex chronicus (neurodermatitis)

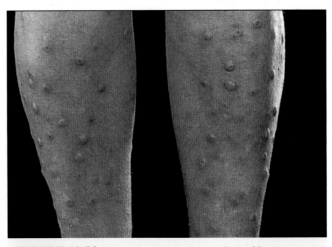

FIGURE 10.33 Nodular prurigo: dome-shaped lesions

Otitis externa

Eczema of the outer ear is common and extremely annoying. There may be subtle features of seborrhoeic eczema, but often no obvious cause. Contact allergic dermatitis, especially due to medicaments, is a very common complicating feature. All patients with otitis externa should undergo patch testing. Treatment involves the use of various topical steroids. Aminoglycosides and other sensitizing agents (which are commonly present in preparations used in the ears) should be avoided as far as possible.

Eyelid dermatitis

Eyelids may be involved as a primary dermatitis, as part of a more generalized endogenous eczema (e.g. atopic dermatitis, seborrhoeic dermatitis) or be caused by contact allergy (Fig. 10.34), especially to hair dyes, nail varnish and medicaments. Contact eyelid allergy is often accompanied by oedema. Treatment requires careful moderation of topical steroids, because eyelid skin is very prone to atrophy and there is the risk of inducing glaucoma. Tacrolimus and pimecrolimus may be useful. Patch testing should be considered.

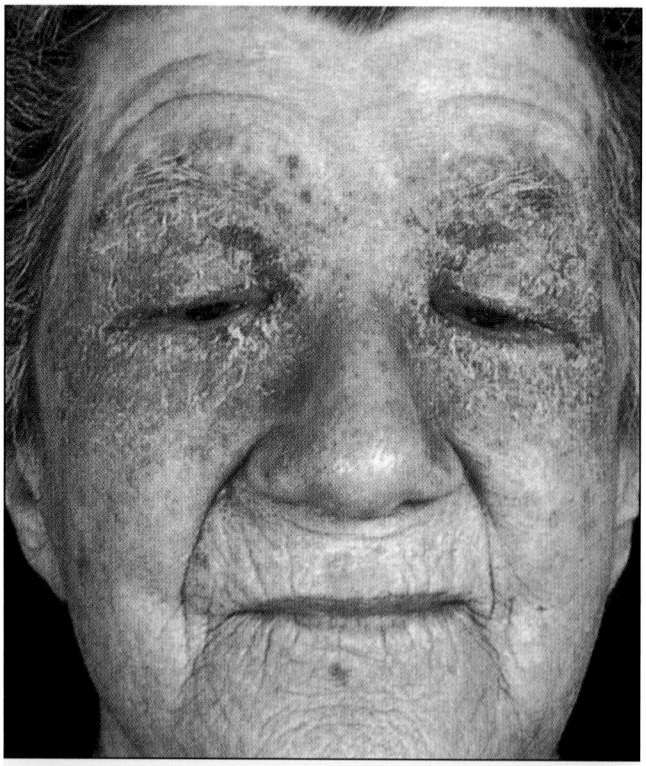

Paronychial dermatitis

When eczema involves the dorsa of the ends of the fingers and toes, a marked nail dystrophy is commonly seen (Fig. 10.35).

Perineal and genital dermatitis

The skin of the vulva, penis and anus is frequently involved in eczematous dermatitis of various kinds. The intertriginous groin folds may be affected by seborrhoeic dermatitis, and the vulva and perianal skin are common sites for lichen simplex chronicus.

The anal skin is subject to irritation for obvious reasons and this may be exacerbated by haemorrhoids or other anal conditions. Anogenital epithelium seems, like the ears, eyelids and lower legs, to be particularly susceptible to contact allergic sensitization by medicaments (Fig. 10.36).

The glans penis may also become inflamed (balanitis). In older, usually uncircumcised males, a non-specific balanitis is common. This usually responds to mild topical steroids. More troublesome is the florid inflammatory condition known as Zoon's erythroplasia/balanitis, in which moist, shiny, deep-red patches appear on the glans and foreskin (Fig. 10.37). Histology is benign, but the condition responds only partially to topical corticosteroids and circumcision may need to be considered.

INFECTIVE ECZEMA

Eczematous changes can be induced by invading organisms, and the concept of an 'infective' eczema is useful.

FIGURE 10.34 Eyelid dermatitis due to contact sensitivity to neomycin in eye drops

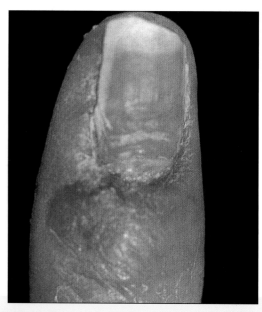

FIGURE 10.35 Paronychial dermatitis: nail dystrophy

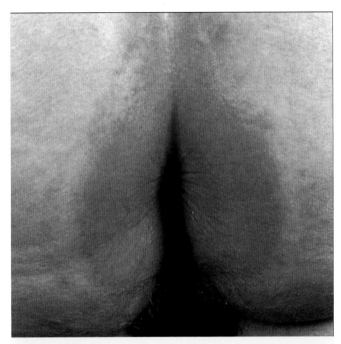

FIGURE 10.36 Perianal dermatitis due to ethylenediamine in Triadcortyl cream

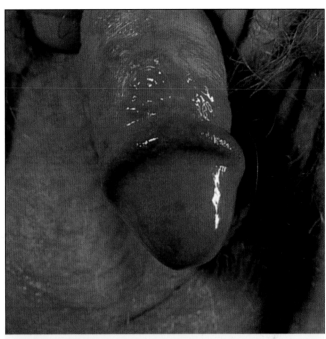

FIGURE 10.37 Zoon's erythroplasia/balanitis, in which moist, shiny, deep-red patches appear on the glans and foreskin

The red, itchy rash of ringworm (tinea) is actually nothing more than an inflammatory response to the presence of fungal organisms in the skin. Typical eczematous dermatitis also occurs commonly around areas of molluscum contagiosum, especially in children with an underlying tendency to atopic eczema. Bacterial infections may occasionally produce similar changes.

Psoriasis

Presentation

Psoriasis affects around 3% of most of the ethnic groups that live in the UK and, since it tends to be pretty persistent once it has appeared, a GP is bound to see patients with the disease. Because it is so common, it is important to remember that more 'unusual' forms will be encountered from time to time, and that these can be difficult to diagnose; a one-off specialist referral for a definitive diagnosis may therefore be necessary in addition to seeking advice on treatment of recalcitrant disease.

In addition to the discomfort of having psoriasis, joint involvement is a well-recognized complication and is said to affect 5–10% of patients.

Psoriasis does not usually affect the patient's general health, apart from with the very rare acute pustular psoriasis or widespread 'brittle' disease, both of which can be life-threatening, especially in the elderly. The psychological effects, though, can be profound and there is also evidence that patients with severe psoriasis may severely abuse alcohol. This may have implications for the choice of therapy and, of course, for the patient's general health and well-being.

Box (cont)

Nail changes (Figs 11.7, 11.8)

Nail changes are very common and are said to be universal in psoriatic arthropathy

Pits are very common (BUT BEWARE: nail pits are not always due to psoriasis)

Onycholysis is also common

Arthritis (Figs 11.9, 11.10)

Distal interphalangeal joints

Resembling rheumatoid arthritis

Large joint

Spondylitis

Arthritis mutilans

Pustular (Fig. 11.11)

Widespread pustules, often with fever and malaise

Localized to palms and soles (Figs 11.12, 11.13)

BOX 11.1 Presentations of psoriasis

Plaques (Fig. 11.1)

Classically occur on knees, elbows, base of spine

Isolated plaques may appear anywhere at all

Plaques are red, well demarcated and surmounted by very typical (silvery) scale

Facial lesions may show very little scale

Dandruff/scaling of the scalp (Figs 11.2, 11.3)

Psoriasis affects the scalp very frequently

Palpable scaling in the scalp in an adult is almost certainly psoriasis; there are usually areas of normal scalp

Extends a few millimetres from the hairline, with a well-defined edge

Multiple lesions

Psoriasis may present with many lesions all at once

The lesions may be small and drop-like: 'guttate' psoriasis (Fig. 11.4)

Lesions may be of various shapes and sizes

Flexural changes (Figs 11.5, 11.6)

Psoriasis affects the axillae, groins and natal cleft more often than you might think

---

Patient problems

There are a number of reasons why someone with psoriasis will seek medical advice.

BOX 11.2 Reasons for psoriasis patients seeking medical advice

Diagnosis

Counselling on what is likely to happen to the patient and/or their relatives

First-line treatment

Modification of first-line regimens: combination or 'try-again' treatments

Second-line treatments

Seeking referral for specialist treatment and/or advice

Diagnosis

When anyone first develops skin lesions they want to know what it is. The diagnosis of psoriasis is often very obvious: it usually presents with at least some of the 'classical' features. However, there are some useful tips on what to look for specifically if psoriasis is in your differential diagnosis.

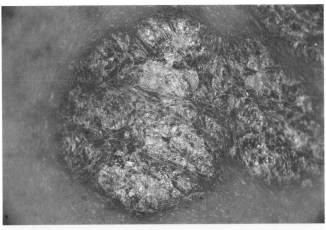

FIGURE 11.1 A typical plaque of psoriasis demonstrating the 'silvery' scale

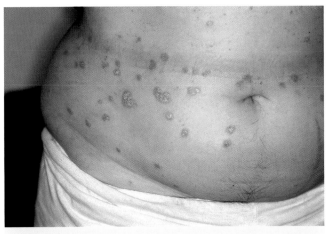

FIGURE 11.4 Small 'drop-like' plaques in guttate psoriasis

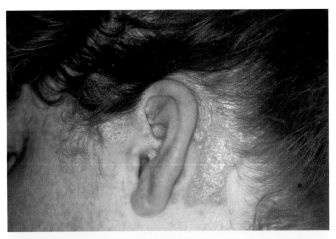

FIGURE 11.2 Classic sites for psoriasis: the scalp, scalp margin and behind the ear

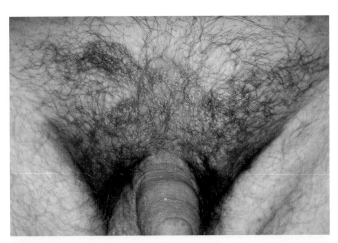

FIGURE 11.5 Flexural changes

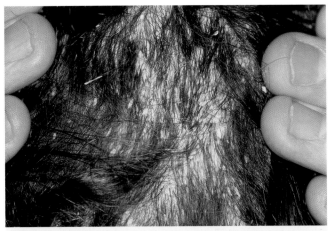

FIGURE 11.3 Extensive, adherent hyperkeratosis in pityriasis amiantacea

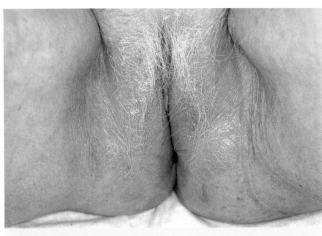

FIGURE 11.6 Psoriasis affects the genital area more often than is sometimes appreciated

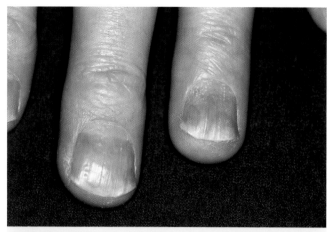

FIGURE 11.7 Pits and onycholysis of the nails in psoriasis

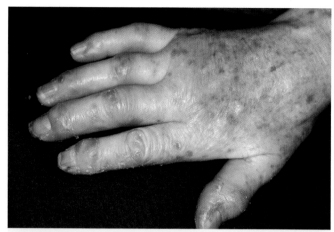

FIGURE 11.10 Painful arthropathic changes in a patient with psoriasis

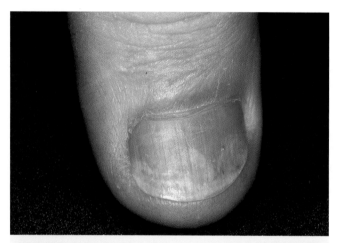

FIGURE 11.8 Nail changes

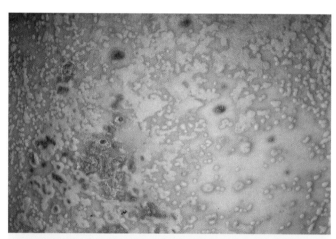

FIGURE 11.11 Acute pustular psoriasis: a dermatological emergency

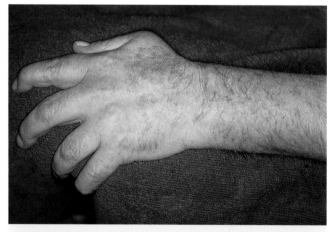

FIGURE 11.9 Arthritis

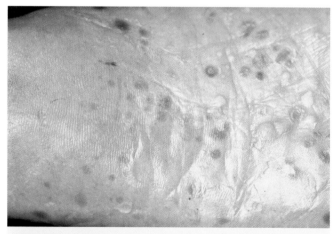

FIGURE 11.12 Pustular psoriasis localized to palms and soles

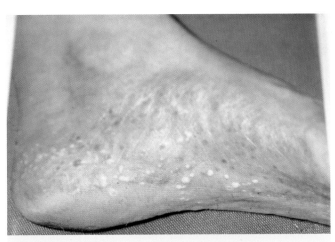

FIGURE 11.13 Chronic palmoplantar psoriasis

BOX 11.3 Diagnostic tips if you are thinking of psoriasis

Look out for:
> Any sign of pinkness or scaling on the knees or elbows
> Scalp involvement
> Umbilical involvement
> Nail changes (see Figs 11.7, 11.8)

Counselling on what is likely to happen to the patient and/or their relatives

Developing psoriasis must surely have an adverse effect on self-esteem and self-image. Most people find coping mechanisms, but in some patients the psychological effects of psoriasis are profound. This may be amplified by the dawning realization of the chronicity of psoriasis: that they may have to live with irritable, scaly, red patches for the rest of their life. The more visible and exposed they are, the worse it is and, of course, for anyone in a close personal relationship, 'exposed ' can be anywhere.

Furthermore, genes play a major role in psoriasis – especially in those with a young age of onset – and a number of patients will already be aware of this because of other affected family members. For some, however, it is a new experience and it may take some time for the news that others close to them may yet develop the disease, to sink in. This is particularly unwelcome to most patients in relation to their children.

First-line treatment

Patients presenting for the first time will expect immediate treatment and, most often, will expect success. One key piece of advice in dealing with psoriasis is to try (without sounding too negative) to create a sense of realism about what can be achieved – better that than have to explain why the first (or second, or third ...) attempts at treatment have not eliminated the problem for good.

Suggestions about how to start treating a psoriatic patient are given below.

Modification of first-line regimens: combination and "try-again" treatments

Often, when treatment doesn't work straight away, the temptation is immediately to switch to a new modality or class of agent. This is often a mistake, because modifications and reinforcement of the use of first-line agents may be enough. For example, the enhanced use of emollients may increase the effectiveness of other modalities, such as topical steroids or vitamin D analogues. Using topical steroids as part of a rotation with a vitamin D analogue will often produce a much greater level of improvement than either alone.

Dermatologists have used mixtures of different agents for years. Some are rather outdated and difficult to obtain (e.g. steroid + tar + salicylic acid) but there are some proprietary combinations that are definitely worth exploring if one alone is unsuccessful (e.g. steroid + salicylic acid, steroid + calcipotriol).

Second-line treatments

There may come a point when the use of conventional, topical treatments is either just not good enough, or has itself become so laborious as to interfere significantly with life. Consideration of second-line therapies is then justified and there is no reason why, with the right support and monitoring, some of these could not be initiated and/or managed wholly or partly in primary care.

Nothing short of second-line systemic therapy will work in psoriatic nail disease.

Chronic palmoplantar pustulosis/pustular psoriasis of palms and soles

A particular problem may be encountered in the diagnosis, and subsequent successful management, of this chronic disorder. Waves of pustules develop on an erythematous background. It is important to consider both pompholyx and tinea pedis in the differential diagnosis. Treatment is often unrewarding, but would usually begin with topical vitamin D analogues ± topical corticosteroids. Many units recommend psoralen plus ultraviolet A (PUVA), while systemic therapy can be justified because of the disabling nature of the problem in some patients.

Seeking referral for specialist treatment and/or advice

Patients come to recognize that there are certain things that will probably only be available in larger, specialist centres: phototherapy; photochemotherapy (PUVA); dithranol day therapy; second-line drugs in the majority of instances; biologicals.

They may therefore take the initiative and request a referral for consideration of further management approaches. At present, specialist advice is generally available only in larger, acute-based or acute-base linked centres.

Practical prescribing

BOX 11.4 Effective therapies for psoriasis

First-line therapies

Emollients

Vitamin D analogues

Topical steroids

Salicylic acid

Tar

Dithranol

Calcineurin inhibitors

Topical vitamin A derivatives

Specialist and second-line therapies

Variations of topical regimens

UVB

PUVA

Systemic therapy:
    Methotrexate
    Acitretin
    Ciclosporin
    Biologicals
    Fumarates

Treatment for arthropathy

The fact that there are such a large number of treatments for psoriasis sends a powerful message: none of them work perfectly for everyone. In many ways, all of them represent a compromise between effectiveness, safety and convenience.

Emollients

The liberal use of emollients will often keep psoriasis plaques smoother and more comfortable, but they are messy and adult patients can find their use too difficult and time-consuming, especially in the morning.

In general, the heavier the agent is the better it will work, but that has to be balanced with what is practical and cosmetically acceptable.

Vitamin D analogues

Calcipotriol, calcitriol and tacalcitol have assumed enormous importance in the management of psoriasis in the past few years. Generally safe, they may bring quite extensive disease under control if used regularly. They may also usefully be combined with topical steroids (see below), either in combination and simultaneously, or as part of an alternating regimen. The advantages of the latter approach are that the local side effects of steroids may be reduced.

They are not so useful on the scalp, nor are they always tolerated on the face (and for which they are not licensed) or flexures. There are also a number of patients in whom they simply don't work well.

Topical steroids

Despite what some accounts say, topical steroids have a definite role in managing psoriasis. They really do work in suppressing plaques. There is no point in using anything other than a potent steroid on lesions of trunk, limbs and scalp. Very potent steroids may be valuable in very short bursts. The use of mild- to moderate-potency agents on the face and flexures, however, is one of only a few topical options, and should be rotated with other agents (e.g. vitamin D analogues). Whatever agent is being used, its application must be made sufficiently intermittent to avoid skin thinning.

Salicylic acid

A 'keratolytic' agent, salicylic acid has been used for decades in combination with other topical therapies, especially for patients presenting with very scaly psoriatic plaques. 2% salicylic acid in yellow soft paraffin for the first 1–2 weeks will remove much of the scale and allow other agents to penetrate better.

Salicylic acid is included in a useful proprietary scalp application and ointment combination with betamethasone (Diprosalic).

Tar

Tar is the essential ingredient in Cocois, a scalp preparation that is undoubtedly the most effective treatment for scalp psoriasis – if used properly. It has to be massaged in and left on for 6 hours (usually overnight). It is important to warn patients that it smells and will make a mess on bed linen.

Dithranol

Once the mainstay of psoriasis treatment, dithranol has rather fallen from grace. This is largely because it is messy (it stains everything it touches) and it can cause burns. Patients should also be warned that it will leave the skin discoloured for some time. It requires a disciplined approach which may take an hour or more each day. However, if used properly, it can be very successful, and may keep the psoriasis at bay longer than any other topical treatment.

It should be applied carefully to plaques while protecting normal skin, starting with lower concentrations and gradually increasing to tolerance, left on for about an hour and then removed.

Calcineurin inhibitors

Tacrolimus and pimecrolimus are not licensed for psoriasis, but can be useful on facial lesions and in the flexures.

Topical vitamin A derivatives

Some authorities find tazoratene (which is a gel formulation) useful. In general it has only a modest effect, but does allow patients to avoid continuous use of topical steroids.

Variations of topical regimens

As indicated above, a combination of these topical agents and/or simultaneous use with systemic drugs or physical therapies may be worth considering. Much will depend on the specific response and responsiveness of the individual patient.

UVB and PUVA

These are generally only available through specialist centres. Exposure to sunlight has been known to help psoriasis for many years, although it does not benefit everyone. The effective 'rays' have been shown to be in the mid-UV range (UVB). It is now most common to use a very narrow band or peak in the middle of the spectrum (hence the term 'narrow band'). Courses usually involve increasing periods of exposure to UVB two to three times a week over 6–8 weeks. There are risks, notably sunburn and the premature induction of skin cancer, and most units limit lifetime doses.

Very occasionally patients may acquire a set of lamps for home use. While this can be managed by a very well-educated and motivated individual, it is expensive.

PUVA is another modality that has secured a place in the therapy of chronic psoriasis. It is even more likely to induce skin cancer than UVB and is reserved for severe, chronic and extensive disease. Its use is even more restricted than UVB.

Both forms of treatment can be (and usually are) used in combination with other modalities, both topical and systemic

Systemic therapy

Specialists may well offer patients with severe, resistant disease one or other of a range of agents.

Methotrexate is the oldest and remains one of the best options, especially in middle-aged or elderly patients who have completed their families. It has a reputation for toxicity that far outstrips reality. Excessive dosing is highly dangerous (it should absolutely NEVER be given more often than once weekly), but lower, standard doses are usually safe as long as monitoring is careful and rigorous. One key addition to routine haematology, biochemistry and liver function is a procollagen III peptide assay that 'predicts' liver fibrosis. This will normally be offered three times a year through secondary centres. Methotrexate is teratogenic and also affects spermatogenesis.

Acitretin is a close relative of isotretinoin, the great acne drug. It is generally not as effective as methotrexatre, but is a useful alternative, especially in younger patients. It also causes a troublesome cheilitis, disturbances of liver function and elevation of triglycerides and cholesterol. Like isotretinoin, it is teratogenic.

Ciclosporin is nephrotoxic, and causes hypertension and a long list of less 'serious' side effects. It can be tremendously effective in controlling psoriasis, although close monitoring of renal function and blood pressure is essential and patients often have to come off it after a year or two.

Biologicals are new, exciting and horrendously expensive. Although NICE has approved the introduction and use of some in restricted circumstances, their place in the gamut of treatments is unknown at this stage. Long-term safety remains to be established.

Fumarates are widely used in northern Europe and occasionally in the UK. They are unlicensed, expensive and may be poorly tolerated because of flushing and diarrhoea. They do work well sometimes, though.

Treatment for arthropathy

Dermatologists and rheumatologists often share the care of patients with psoriatic joint disease. Biologicals such as adalimumab, infliximab and etanercept have revolutionized the treatment of these patients and may replace older regimens.

Chapter 12

Generalized Pruritus

Presentation

By definition, the presenting symptom is itch, usually all over or moving around from one site to another in a seemingly random fashion. The problem most commonly presents in older people and the temptation in the elderly is to attribute the itching to so-called *senile* pruritus. While this may, indeed, be the final diagnosis, it is important to exclude treatable conditions at any age.

A very careful examination of the skin is essential. The key signs that need to be sought are excoriations (scratch marks; Figs 12.1 and 12.2), which confirm the history, and anything that might suggest a primary cutaneous or systemic cause of the problem (Fig. 12.3). In particular, look out for subtle changes of dryness (xerosis) and even eczema craquelé (Fig. 12.4). Check, too, for dermographism (Fig. 12.5).

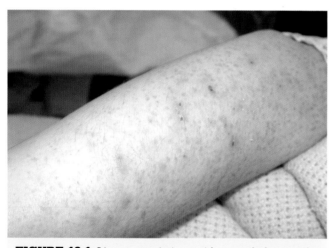

FIGURE 12.1 Linear excoriations with no underlying rash

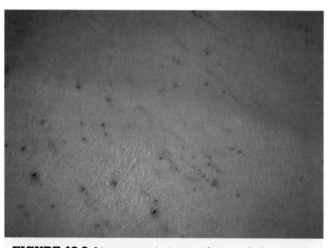

FIGURE 12.2 Linear excoriations with no underlying rash

BOX 12.1 Important signs in a patient with generalized pruritus

Excoriations

Confirmation that the patient is suffering from significant irritation

Signs of primary skin disease

Eczema	Eczematous changes
Scabies	Burrows; sparing of head and neck
Dermatitis herpetiformis	Blisters or papules on extensor surfaces

Signs of systemic disease

Liver disease	Icterus; clubbing; hyperpigmentation
Renal disease	Muddy complexion; nail changes
Malignancy	Weight loss; anaemia; lymphadenopathy
Iron deficiency	Anaemia; dry, lacklustre hair and skin; nail changes
Polycythaemia	Ruddy complexion; splenomegaly
	NB: history of triggering by water contact
Thyrotoxicosis	Tachycardia; atrial fibrillation; sweating; weight loss; exophthalmos; pre-tibial myxoedema
Myxoedema	Bradycardia; dry skin; loss of outer eyebrows
Pregnancy	Should be obvious!
Coeliac disease	A rare presentation of a rare disorder
Diabetes	May rarely be a feature

Patient problems

There are very few symptoms that are as intrusive as persistent, severe itching. Although scratching is, in its way, a pleasurable exercise, the effect of chronic irritation can be truly miserable. The problem is never far from the patient's mind (nor, often, from the mind of their close friends, relatives and carers). Sleep is frequently disturbed, so tiredness may further compound the problem. And – unless a treatable cause can be found – there is the very real prospect of the misery continuing indefinitely.

Sadly, there is much less often an easy solution than one would like.

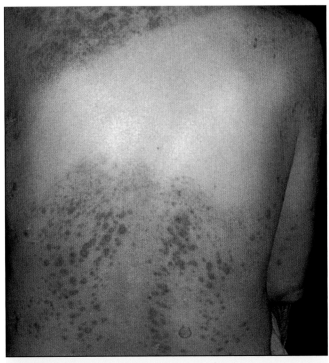

FIGURE 12.3 Central back spared in primary generalized pruritus

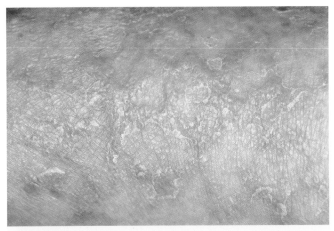

FIGURE 12.4 Eczema craquelé

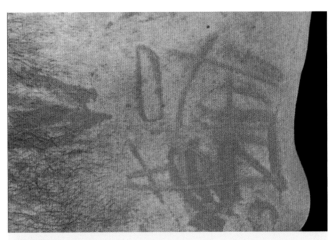

FIGURE 12.5 Dermographism is an important cause of generalized pruritus. No rash will be obvious until the patient scratches

Occasionally, though, an investigative screen will throw up something really important. We have seen several cases of lymphoma present in this way – a few with no overt lymphadenopathy or other signs – and of haematological disorders, notably iron deficiency. Primary biliary cirrhosis is another disorder for which unexplained generalized itch is a classical presentation.

Investigations need, therefore, to be aimed at eliminating as many of these putative aetiologies as possible – or of course finding one and treating it.

> **BOX 12.2** Test for generalized pruritus
>
> FBC; iron/ferritin; U&E; LFTs; TFT; bone screen; glucose; CXR
>
> Immunoglobulins/plasma electrophoresis in older patients
>
> Appropriate investigations (e.g. endoscopy, imaging, including CT) if weight loss or other significant symptoms

Investigation

Most undergraduates can, at the time of finals at least, rattle off a list of causes of generalized pruritus, and any good textbook of dermatology will contain one with more or less the same range of conditions to consider. In practice it is relatively uncommon to find one of these diseases by test alone. If the itch is due to liver or kidney disease, for example, the underlying condition has usually already been established or there will be clear signs that something else is afoot: jaundice, for example, in a patient with obstructive jaundice.

Practical prescribing

Let us assume that no cause has been established for the patient's itch. There are generally two scenarios. In the first, there is a degree of cutaneous dryness or *xerosis*, and in the second, the skin is texturally normal.

Scenario one: dry skin

Conventional wisdom suggests the use of liberal emollients, 1% menthol in aqueous cream as a cooling agent and, perhaps, some dilute topical steroid, at least for a short while to assess response. This can be helpful but there are three key problems:

BOX 12.3 Systemic causes of generalized pruritus

Liver disease	Hepatitis; obstruction, including physical
Renal disease	Chronic renal failure
Haematological disorders	Iron deficiency
	Polycythaemia vera
Thyroid disease	Thyrotoxicosis
	Hypothyroidism
Malignancy	Lymphoma, including Hodgkin's disease
	Carcinomas
Pregnancy	Associated with cholestasis

- Many older people are physically limited; applying creams and ointments to some parts of the body is difficult enough for the young and fit; it is a real challenge to an older person with arthritis.
- Many older people live alone, compounding the problem of achieving successful application.
- Creams and ointments may increase the hazards associated with old age – notably falls – by making the skin and the surfaces on which the skin seeks to operate slippery.

Scenario two: skin of normal texture, or where emollients alone are ineffective

This is a much more difficult situation to manage. Potent topical steroids may help in the short term, but there are obvious hazards with their long-term application.

Sedative agents, such as hydroxyzine, may reduce itching – especially at night – but they can often result in excessive drowsiness and confusion.

UVB phototherapy may work, but is often impractical in the elderly frail.

A number of psychotropic agents may be helpful: doxepin (10–50 mg at night), amitriptyline (25–75 mg, again at night), and gabapentin up to 2 g daily in divided doses.

Scenario three

Pruritus associated with hepatic or renal disease, or malignancy, can be especially difficult to treat. The agents used in idiopathic pruritus may be helpful, particularly UVB. Two other agents reported to be helpful, especially in renal failure, are naltrexone and rifampicin. The latter is relatively contraindicated in hepatic disease and should only be used with care.

Scenario four

As a diagnosis of exclusion, one should consider the possibility of psychological causes. Many patients are anxious or depressed by their skin complaint, and disentangling this from underlying primary disturbances can be a challenge. However, if identified, appropriate treatment can be very rewarding.

A rare but very distressing and difficult condition is *delusional parasitosis*, in which patients develop an unshakeable belief that they are infected with some kind of creature – usually an insect. Psychotropic drugs are said to work but patients rarely agree to take them.

Chapter 13

Urticaria and Vasculitis

Summary

- Urticaria (and angioedema)
- Vasculitis

URTICARIA (AND ANGIOEDEMA)

Presentation

Urticaria is a disorder that can be diagnosed from the history alone, but lesions may, of course, be present at the patient's first visit too. The condition is characterized by the appearance of multiple cutaneous wheals (Figs 13.1–13.4). These raised swellings of the skin are caused by leakage of fluid from vascular spaces into the dermis. Angioedema (Fig. 13.5) is the same process, but involving the subcutaneous tissues.

Individual wheals arise and disappear within a short period of time (from about 30 minutes to 3–4 hours) and leave no visible mark. The only exception to this is seen with *delayed pressure urticaria*, where wheals may take up to 24 hours to develop. Crops of wheals generally continue to appear anywhere on the body surface. Otherwise, if lesions last beyond the expected time, a diagnosis of *urticarial vasculitis* should be considered (see below).

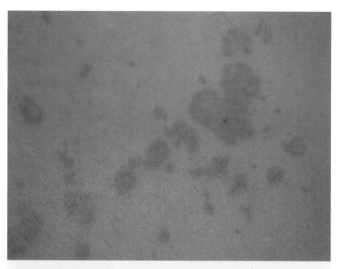

FIGURE 13.3 Generalized idiopathic urticaria

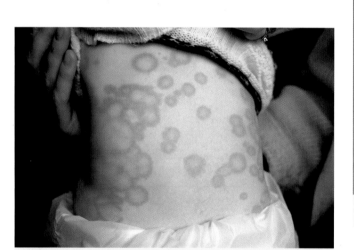

FIGURE 13.1 Urticaria

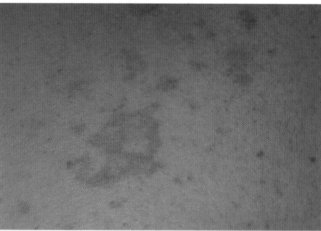

FIGURE 13.4 Generalized idiopathic urticaria

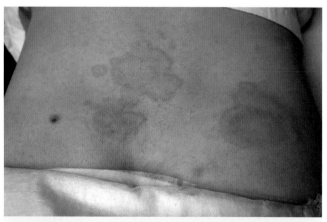

FIGURE 13.2 Generalized idiopathic urticaria

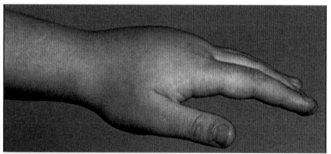

FIGURE 13.5 Angioedema

Patient problems

The overwhelming problem in urticaria is itch, whatever the cause. This may be intolerable, interfering with sleep, work and all other aspects of life.

Acute urticaria

In many patients, the problem lasts for a few days at most, in which case it is worth searching hard for a trigger. Indeed, after two or three attacks of this acute form of urticaria (Fig. 13.6), most patients will work out what the likely cause is for themselves (see Box 13.1).

Physical urticarias

Another important set of triggers are physical – hence the term *physical urticarias* (see Box 13.2).

Chronic idiopathic urticaria

In other patients, the process can continue for months or years, although there may be days free of whealing and others where the problem is much more intense. Here the problem is probably an autoimmune process, and it is usually impossible to identify a trigger, although patients are told that they have an 'allergy' by many well-meaning people, both lay and professional. In consequence they continue to search hopelessly for a cause, and may end up exploring all sorts of 'alternative health solutions'.

Angioedema

Swelling of the soft tissues around the face (lips, tongue and eyelids) or other areas (e.g. genitals) can be frightening, especially if there seems to be any obstruction to the airway.

In the very rare *hereditary angioedema*, there are never any urticarial wheals. Abdominal pain is a common symptom, and there is often a family history.

Anaphylaxis

Rarely, urticaria is part of a more generalized systemic reaction to injected, ingested or inhaled proteins. This situation, known as anaphylaxis, may be associated with profound lowering of blood pressure and even death from hypovolaemic shock.

Practical prescribing

Once a diagnosis of urticaria has been firmly established, two things should follow: appropriate investigation and symptomatic treatment.

Investigations

It is important to take a good history, which will help to reveal potential triggers. It is usually prudent to perform simple haematological and biochemical screening, especially if the condition is associated with malaise or there are other general symptoms: urticarial rashes are sometimes seen with hepatitis and other infections, including dental abscesses. Some clinicians routinely perform a range of IgE-based tests, including skin-prick tests, although these can be difficult to interpret if the patient is continuing to have spontaneous wheals. An alternative is serum antibody screening (RASTs), but these seldom reveal a clear trigger.

BOX 13.1 Triggers of acute urticaria

Drugs: aspirin, NSAIDs, antibiotics

Foods: many, including nuts, fish, shellfish, milk, strawberries, eggs

Contact with: grass, animal hair/fur, milk, eggs, latex

BOX 13.2 Physical urticarias

Cold	Patients complain of whealing in cold air/wind
Heat	Whealing occurs with hot drinks or contact with warm objects
Water	Any temperature of water may be responsible
Sunlight	Take care to distinguish from polymorphic light eruption, sunburn or other causes of acute photosensitivity
Sweating	*Cholinergic* urticaria usually occurs on the trunk
Dermographism	Everyone is familiar with the tendency to wheal on scratching
Delayed pressure	Wheals occur up to 24 hours after sustained pressure

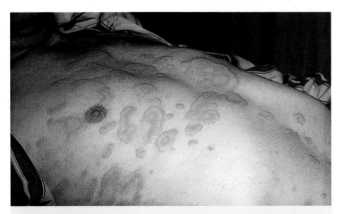

FIGURE 13.6 Widespread acute urticaria. In this case urticaria was due to penicillin allergy

If it is suspected that the urticaria has a physical basis, a challenge test is appropriate: ice applied to the skin for cold urticaria; hot water in a container for heat-induced urticaria; ultraviolet radiation for solar urticaria; water for aquagenic urticaria. To test for delayed-pressure urticaria, a heavy weight should be left in contact with the skin, and any response over 12–24 hours noted.

If hereditary angioedema is a possibility, the level of C1 esterase inhibitor should be measured.

Treatment

Any evident triggers should be avoided. In cold-induced urticaria, swimming in cold water can cause a massive urticarial reaction resulting in shock. Aspirin and NSAIDs should be discouraged as far as possible.

The drug treatment of choice for most forms of urticaria begins with an H_1 antihistamine. Early H_1 antihistamines produced marked sedation in most individuals but there are now a number of agents in which this side effect is much less troublesome (e.g. fexofenadine, desloratidine, levocetirizine); these would normally be used as first-line therapies. Be sure to give an adequate dose! This is often higher than would be used for hay fever. For example, we frequently prescribe fexofenadine 180 mg twice daily. Some authors advocate the addition of H_2 receptor antagonists (there are also H_2 receptors in the skin) when the urticaria is not easily controlled by monotherapy, e.g. ranitidine 150 mg twice daily. Some forms, especially the physical urticarias, are largely unresponsive to antihistamines of either class. A more aggressive approach involving systemic steroids or even ciclosporin may be required in a few patients, especially those in whom the urticaria is part of a major systemic allergic response.

Treatment of anaphylaxis

Patients in a state of anaphylaxis succumb to anoxic brain damage and die. The most immediate requirement is adrenaline (epinephrine) to improve circulatory performance. Patients may also need systemic steroids, antihistamines and intensive-care support. It is crucial that potential triggers are identified and avoided as far as possible.

VASCULITIS

Cutaneous blood vessels are prominently involved in many situations. When the superficial vessels are inflamed and damaged, become leaky and allow red cells (and other blood constituents) into the surrounding dermis, the term *cutaneous vasculitis* is applied. This is often qualified by adjectives such as 'allergic', 'leukocytoclastic', 'small vessel' or 'necrotizing', but these are of limited value in the general setting in which most clinicians first meet cutaneous vasculitis.

Patient problems

The first, and obvious, issue is the appearance of an unexplained rash. Vasculitis in the skin causes *palpable* petechiae/purpura (Fig. 13.7), although very new lesions are often pink.

When accompanied by joint pains, fever, abdominal discomfort and renal damage, the condition is often termed *Henoch–Schönlein syndrome*. The same skin changes occur, though, alone or in other contexts (e.g. following drug ingestion, lupus erythematosus and rheumatoid arthritis).

Sometimes the vascular damage is severe, leading to necrosis, blisters and ulcers. If larger vessels are involved (as, for example, in polyarteritis nodosa) tissue damage may be extensive.

Urticarial vasculitis

A particular clinical pattern is sometimes seen in which what at first appear to be typical urticarial lesions last much longer than normal and fade to leave purplish staining. This is known as *urticarial vasculitis* and is seen in a number of systemic disorders, including systemic lupus erythematosus.

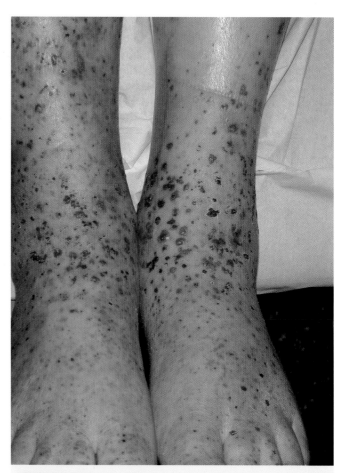

FIGURE 13.7 Vasculitis

Erythema multiforme

The term erythema multiforme is given to a highly characteristic disorder in which vasculitis is a fundamental component. The lesions are round and are therefore called 'iris' or 'target' lesions (Fig. 13.8). They can appear anywhere, but involvement of the extensor surfaces of the limbs, and of the palms and soles, is often prominent. If the process is severe enough, bullae may form (Fig.13.9): a situation called *Stevens–Johnson syndrome*.

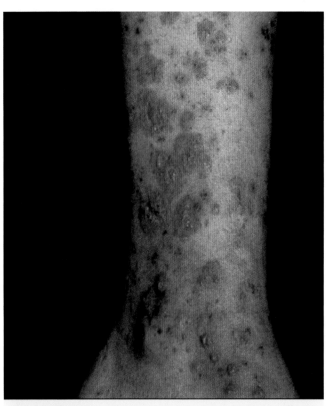

FIGURE 13.9 Stevens–Johnson syndrome: multiple lesions with superficial blistering in severe disease

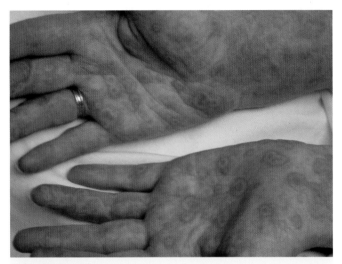

FIGURE 13.8 Erythema multiforme

Practical prescribing

The most important initial step is to confirm the diagnosis (which requires a skin biopsy). A careful history is important, focusing on possible drug or infective triggers. Following this, a full haematological, biochemical and immunological screen should be performed; check the ASO (anti-streptolysin O) titre, as streptococcal infection is a common trigger. A CXR should be performed. It is particularly important to keep a close watch on renal function: regular urinalysis and biochemistry are mandatory while the process is active.

In severe vasculitis, strict bedrest is valuable and may result in complete clearance on its own. However, the lesions often recur on remobilization. Drug treatment may therefore be necessary. Dapsone is usually the first-line drug (some clinicians use alternative sulfones such as sulfapyridine and sulfamethoxypyridazine). Systemic corticosteroids may be required, at least initially.

Urticarial vasculitis may be suppressed by dapsone, but systemic corticosteroids are more effective.

Erythema multiforme seldom needs specific treatment because the reaction settles over 10–21 days. Occasionally, in the more severe forms with blistering, patients need extra nursing and medical support. Systemic steroids, while tempting, are contraindicated.

Chapter 14

Acne and Rosacea

Summary

- Acne
- Rosacea

ACNE

Presentation

A degree of acne is said to affect up to 80% of the population at some point. The typical presentation is of a teenager, often with early signs of pubertal change, with a variety of lesions, cropping and settling. A number of types of skin change may be seen.

Acne may be seen outside the typical age range.

BOX 14.1 Skin changes in acne

A combination of some or all of:

    Greasiness

    Closed comedones ('whiteheads') (Fig. 14.1)

    Open comedones ('blackheads') (Fig. 14.2)

    Papules (Fig. 14.3)

    Pustules (Fig. 14.4)

    Small scars

would justify a diagnosis of *acne vulgaris* (Figs 14.5–14.8).

The addition of:

    Multi-headed comedones (macrocomedones)

    Nodules (Fig. 14.9)

    Cysts (Fig. 14.10)

    Abscesses

    Large scars, including keloids (Fig. 14.11)

would indicate *nodulocystic* or *conglobate* acne (Fig. 14.12)

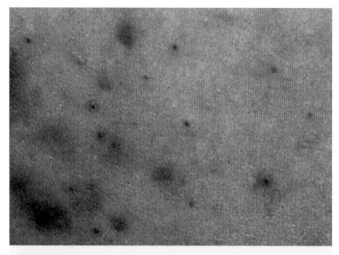

FIGURE 14.2 Open comedones (blackheads)

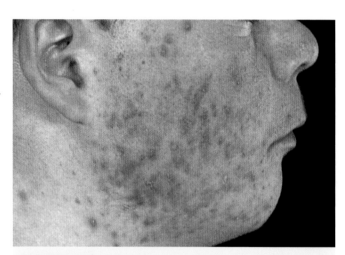

FIGURE 14.3 Erythematous papules on the cheeks of an adolescent male with greasy skin in acne vulgaris

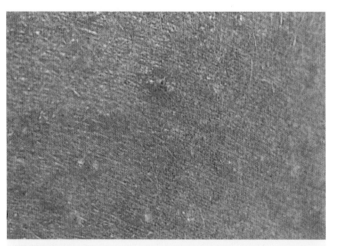

FIGURE 14.1 Closed comedones (whiteheads)

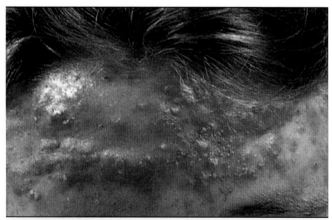

FIGURE 14.4 Papules and pustules on the forehead in acne vulgaris

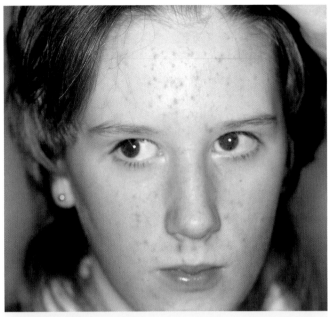

FIGURE 14.5 Mild papulopustular acne

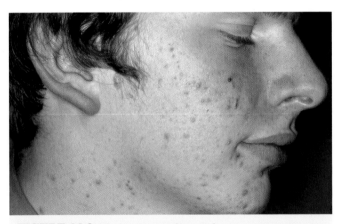

FIGURE 14.6 Moderate papulopustular acne

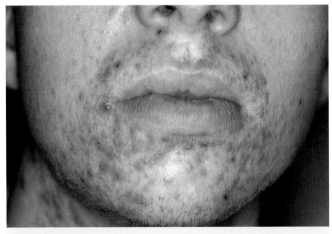

FIGURE 14.7 Extensive inflammatory papules and pustules

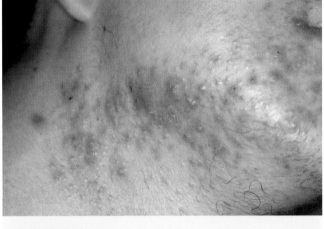

FIGURE 14.8 Extensive inflammatory papules and pustules

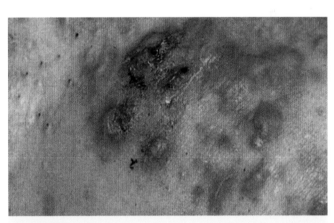

FIGURE 14.9 Nodulocystic acne

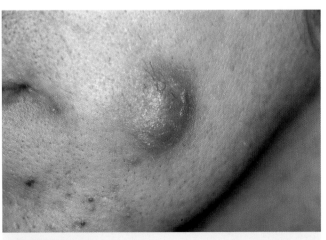

FIGURE 14.10 A typical acne cyst

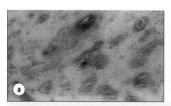
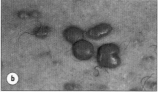

FIGURE 14.11 **(a)** Atrophic, **(b)** hypertrophic scars (keloids) in severe acne

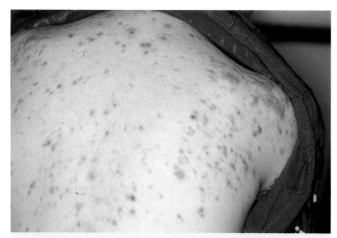

FIGURE 14.12 Extensive acne of the back leading to scars, some of which are hypertrophic

Infantile/juvenile

Identical changes are also occasionally seen in infants and children and, although it usually settles with treatment, it may be followed by a severe recrudescence in adolescence(Fig. 14.13).

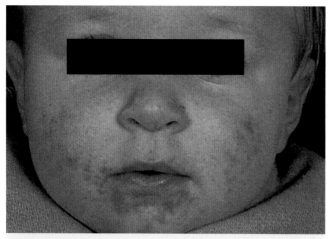

FIGURE 14.13 Infantile/juvenile acne

Persistent and mature onset

Acne usually reaches a peak during adolescence, and subsides over the following 3–4 years, but some patients continue to have significant lesions well into their thirties and beyond. Some, particularly women, develop acne for the first time in their late twenties or thirties.

Patient problems

The lesions of acne are often painful or itchy – and in severe, nodulocystic disease they always are – and symptoms can be the main reason for seeking advice.

For most patients, however, the key issue is the psychological upset that results from having recurrent lesions on the face and upper trunk. Acne of any severity is capable of producing a very significant alteration in the individual's sense of well-being, and their ability to interact satisfactorily with those around them.

As the disease is predominantly one of the formative, adolescent years, its impact is magnified by peer pressure to conform to a societal 'appearance norm' and by the increasing drive to appear attractive to a partner as Desmond Morris's 'pair-bonding' gets underway. Personal appearance is central to our feelings of self-worth and acne strikes at an age when the way one looks is particularly critical. We instinctively know that people like us less if we have imperfections, and there is evidence to support this in that employers are inclined to favour those with clear complexions when making job offers. People with facial blemishes are never totally at ease with them, and teenagers can become completely obsessed with their acne, even if there are not all that many active lesions. It is all too common to hear that a young person simply will not go out in the evenings but, instead, sits alone in his or her room nurturing feelings of despair and rejection. Suicides have been reported.

Another common reason for patients seeking attention is the fear, or the reality, of scarring and the desire to avoid these wherever possible or to deal with established lesions. Sadly, the tendency to scar is not as predictable as one would like. Furthermore, the system in both the UK NHS and the private sector tends to obstruct early, aggressive intervention to prevent scarring, and is poor at arranging funding for scars, once they have developed, deeming such treatment to be 'cosmetic'.

Practical prescribing

Conventional wisdom indicates a stepwise approach to the management of acne, with treatment being tailored to the severity of the condition, but there is an argument for looking more holistically at the situation and offering more potent, and potentially more permanent, therapy earlier rather than later. The psychological impact of acne is only very loosely related to the number or size of lesions, and if the goal is the prevention of scarring then early, aggressive treatment ought to be the order of the day.

Current licensing of acne therapies and the "gate-keeper" system in place in the UK, though, do not encourage such an approach.

BOX 14.2 Therapy of acne

Topical

Comedolytics	Benzoyl peroxide
	Retinoids (retinoic acid; adapalene)
Antimicrobial	Oxytetracycline
	Erythromycin
	Clindamycin
Intermediate	Intralesional steroid

Systemic

Frontline	Antibiotics
	Anti-androgens*
	13-*cis*-Retinoic acid (isotretinoin)
Back-up/specialist	Systemic steroids
	Dapsone

Physical

Hyfrecation

Laser; dermabrasion

Initiating treatment therefore depends on a judgement of severity and on the circumstances of each patient. This includes a consideration of age: tetracyclines should *not* be used in a child under the age of 12, or in a pregnant or breast-feeding woman. Trimethoprim should be avoided in pregnancy.

In mild disease, topical therapy alone may suffice.

Benzoyl peroxide should be applied to the whole area daily – not just to spots; begin with low strength, then increase.

Retinoic acid, isotretinoin and adapalene are all derived from vitamin A. They should be applied to the whole area daily – not just to spots.

Although topical retinoids are safe to use by any age group they must be avoided in pregnancy.

If the severity is greater, topical antibiotics (tetracyclines, erythromycin, clindamycin) should be applied to the whole area daily. In patients with a lot of comedones a combination of retinoic acid and topical antibiotics may be helpful.

In more severely affected patients, with moderately severe disease, the addition of systemic therapy to the topical agents listed above is indicated. There are several choices:

- Oxytetracycline or erythromycin 500 mg b.d.
- Lymecycline 408 mg daily.

Both oxytetracycline and lymecycline should be taken on an empty stomach.

- Minocycline 100 mg daily (either in one or two doses); there have been some reports of serious side effects with minocycline; while these are extremely rare in practice, it is as well to perform regular liver function tests and autoantibody screens (especially for antinuclear antibodies (ANA) and anti-neutrophil cytoplasmic antibodies (ANCA)).
- Doxycycline 100 mg daily; in summer months or on sunny holidays, patients should be advised to use additional sun protection with this drug.
- Trimethoprim 300 mg b.d; research evidence is only available for this dose of trimethoprim; in practice, 200 mg b.d. is reasonable.

These should all be given for 3 months initially, or for longer if successful.

In females only, the anti-androgen *cyproterone acetate* can be very helpful. It is taken in combination with oestrogen as Dianette™. The Committee on Safety of Medicines (CSM) warns about the increased risk of thromboembolism, about which it is essential to warn the patient. The drug should be used for the shortest period possible.

In severe disease or in milder forms where the treatments above are unsuccessful, the next step is *isotretinoin*. A 4- to 6-month course at a dose 0.5–1 mg/kg per day is the recommended approach. It is important to explain very carefully about side effects, to check liver function and lipids regularly, and to follow the approved pregnancy prevention programme in all female patients – the drug is highly teratogenic.

In very inflamed acne, the addition of *systemic steroids* may provide more rapid control, but this should not be a routine approach. *Dapsone* has been advocated by some for resistant acne, especially where isotretinoin is contraindicated, or where the patient is unwilling to take the drug.

Injections of triamcinolone directly into cysts will often speed up resolution dramatically.

BOX 14.3 Key side effects of isotretinoin

Dry lips and skin

Muscle aches and pains

Hyperlipidaemia (especially triglycerides)

Liver function test abnormalities

Teratogenicity

Depression*

*This is controversial, but there are several case reports of suicide in patients taking isotretinoin.

Unusual complications of acne

Gram-negative folliculitis

Very occasionally, a patient with acne appears to become resistant to antibiotic therapy. The morphology of the eruption may become rather more uniform, with masses of small follicular pustules being seen. Swabs reveal not the normal skin commensals but any one of a number of Gram-negative organisms. This condition may be becoming less common as a consequence of earlier retinoid therapy.

The likelihood of antibiotic resistance developing may be reduced by the use of zinc, and by avoiding different combinations of systemic and topical antibiotics.

Benzoyl peroxide for 2–4 weeks may also help if resistance is an issue.

Acne fulminans

Very occasionally severe, usually nodulocystic, acne is accompanied by a fever, malaise and joint pains. Most patients require a combination of antibiotics and systemic steroids, with isotretinoin being introduced later, when the generalized disturbance has settled. Such patients often have a long and uncomfortable journey, with severe scarring being a major risk.

Physical treatments

Patients with large numbers of macrocomedones may benefit from light cautery/hyfrecation.

For individuals with significant scarring, a range of techniques has been developed, including dermabrasion and the use of carbon dioxide and erbium YAG lasers. These are routinely available in many parts of the world and work well in relatively superficial scars, although the skin never returns entirely to normal. Deeper scars, especially the 'ice-pick' type, keloids and lesions on the trunk, do not do well. Pigmented skin needs to be handled with care.

ROSACEA

Presentation

Rosacea most commonly presents as symmetrical facial erythema and papulopustulation (Figs 14.14 and 14.15), frequently resulting in a 'cruciform' distribution: forehead, both cheeks, nose and chin. Many patients also complain of facial flushing, or may admit to it on questioning. The absence of comedones distinguishes the eruption from acne.

Rarely, these changes are accompanied by fluctuant or permanent swelling of the cheeks due to lymphoedema, and some patients develop ocular irritation and soreness due to a keratitis (Fig. 14.16).

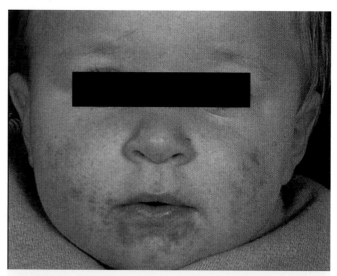

FIGURE 14.14 Rosacea, particularly affecting the cheeks

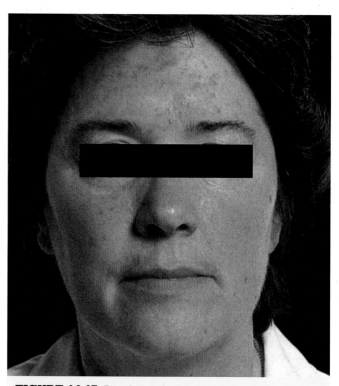

FIGURE 14.15 Papules and telangiectasia on the cheeks and forehead in acne rosacea

Also very uncommon is the development of *granulomatous rosacea*, in which the papules are much firmer and more persistent (Fig. 14.17).

Patient problems

The main issue, as any other facial eruption, is the patient's perceived disfigurement, although the degree of flushing can be severe and this, too, may cause distress.

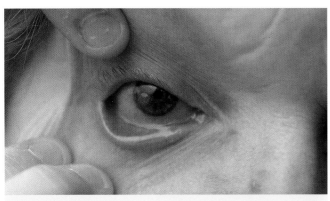

FIGURE 14.16 This woman with rosacea also developed persistent redness and discomfort; this is rosaceous keratitis

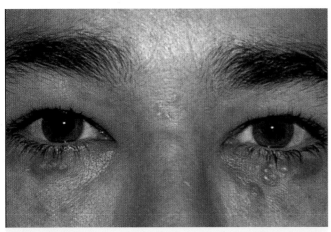

FIGURE 14.17 Granulomatous papules on the eyelids in acne agminata

Practical prescribing

There are only two treatments that are generally accepted as being supported by hard evidence of success: antibiotics of the classes used in acne and topical metronidazole. Many dermatologists will try isotretinoin if the patient has had an adequate course of conventional therapy, but the results are variable. Facial flushing has been managed with β-blockers and clonidine, but with varying success.

The most effective agents by far are oral tetracyclines or erythromycin. The criteria by which the prescriber would choose which drug are essentially the same as for acne – as is the dosage.

Sadly, for many patients, while the papulopustular lesions respond well, the redness and telangiectasia are much less responsive. Here there may be a role for laser therapy, although results are variable and treatment is seldom funded through the NHS.

Rhinophyma (Fig. 14.18) is another important complication of rosacea. Once fully established, any attempt to improve the situation will need to be either by laser or surgery, but very early rhinophyma may respond to oral isotretinoin in similar doses to those used in acne, due to its ability to reduce sebaceous gland proliferation.

Key pitfall

It is very tempting to apply topical corticosteroids to rosacea. The involved areas are red, irritable and will settle (often very significantly) following a few days of hydrocortisone. However, there is always a relapse and usually a degree of rebound which leads slowly but surely to a worsening of the underlying condition. So-called *steroid rosacea* is much less common than it was, but we still see it.

Perioral (periorificial) dermatitis (Fig. 14.19)

The appearance of multiple small, red, follicular papules in the area around the mouth and the nasolabial fold (and occasionally around the eyes) is classically associated with the prior and repeated application of creams and ointments, especially topical steroids.

Treatment with one of the antibiotics used for acne or rosacea is usually curative as long as the 'responsible' topical applications cease.

Hidradenitis suppurativa (Fig. 14.20–14.22)

Hidradenitis is an unpleasant condition characterized by chronic, relapsing suppuration in the axillae, groins and, in women, around the breasts. It requires a combined approach using antibiotics, retinoids and surgery.

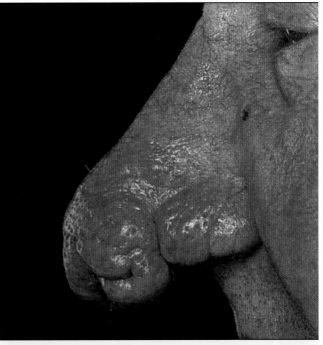

FIGURE 14.18 Bulbous nose in chronic rosacea (rhinophyma)

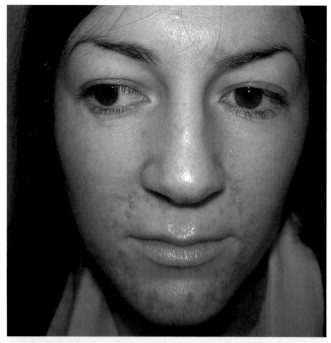

FIGURE 14.19 Perioral (periorificial) dermatitis

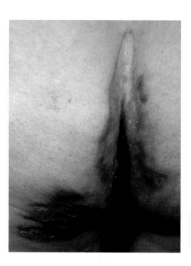

FIGURE 14.20
Hidradenitis suppurativa

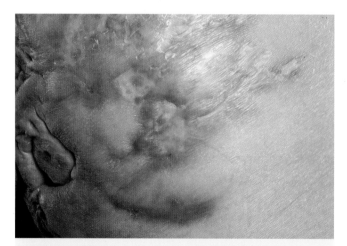

FIGURE 14.21 Hidradenitis suppurativa

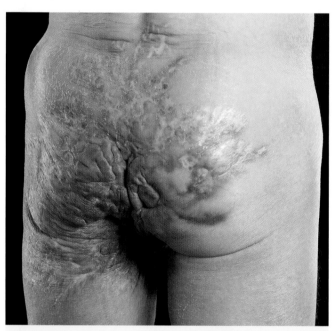

FIGURE 14.22 Hidradenitis suppurativa

Chapter 15

Infections and Infestations

Summary

- Bacterial infections
- Viral infections
- Fungal infections
- Ectoparasite infections

STAPHYLOCOCCAL INFECTIONS

Staphylococcal infections include folliculitis, impetigo, boils (furuncles), carbuncles and staphylococcal scalded skin syndrome.

Staphylococcal organisms are ever-present on human skin. *Staphylococcus epidermidis* is a normal commensal. While this bacterium can cause minor infective problems (see below), the most troublesome member of the family is its much more pathogenic cousin *Staph. aureus*.

Staph. aureus too is carried as a harmless passenger by many healthy people. However, this only involves certain sites, such as the nasal passages. An exception to this is the skin of patients with atopic eczema, where *Staph. aureus* multiplies and survives on the skin surface.

A special mention should be given at this point to MRSA (methicillin-resistant *Staph. aureus*). This organism has become a major problem for all health professionals in recent years. It has been an important addition to the complexity of the assessment and management of superficial skin infections. For example, it is increasingly common to have to confront MRSA when dealing with secondarily infected atopic eczema.

Folliculitis

Presentation

Small aggregations of organisms can create a pustular reaction in the superficial part of the hair follicle (Fig. 15.1). This is particularly common on the buttocks and thighs, and on the lower legs, often as a result of depilatory activities.

Patient problems

The individual spots are unsightly and may be uncomfortable. Post-inflammatory pigmentary disturbances are also a common cause of complaint.

Practical prescribing

Treatment is not always required, but it is sensible to avoid tight-fitting clothes as far as possible. Shaving and other depilatory techniques may need to be suspended. Antibiotics, such as tetracyclines or erythromycin, and the regular use of topical antiseptic washes are sometimes useful.

Furuncles (boils)

Presentation

Furuncles comprise a deeper and much more substantial involvement of a hair follicle than that seen in folliculitis.

Lesions are initially red and tender, but begin to 'point' after a day or so (Fig. 15.2). The content of the pustule discharges and the area heals, sometimes leaving a small scar.

Patient problems

While an individual boil is a nuisance, the main difficulties arise in those who develop multiple, and recurrent, boils.

Practical prescribing

Single lesions

Treatment depends on the frequency and severity the patient is experiencing. Most lesions will settle with simple oral antibiotics and local antisepsis, but large boils may benefit from lancing.

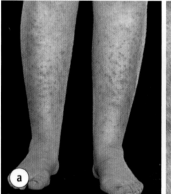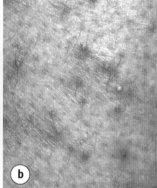

FIGURE 15.1 (a) Folliculitis: follicular pustules on the legs of a woman. **(b)** Close-up of the same patient

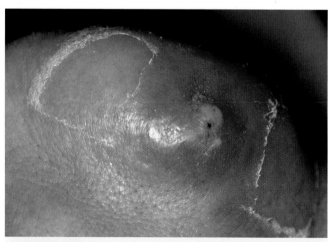

FIGURE 15.2 The typical appearance of a staphylococcal furuncle or boil

Recurrent boils

Some individuals develop crops of boils that recur over months and years; occasionally, this may be a presenting feature of diabetes, but patients are usually entirely well, and investigation of immune status is also generally unrewarding; in most patients, however, it would appear that the skin simply seems receptive to a strain of *Staph. aureus* that is pathogenic to the individual concerned. Empirically, these patients are probably best managed by a long-term course of antibiotics together with an antiseptic skin scrub; the tendency normally disappears in time.

Carbuncles

Carbuncles represent an even deeper and more extensive infection of hair follicles than boils. Carbuncles generally only occur in the elderly, the ill, in patients with diabetes and in patients on systemic steroids.

Presentation

Several adjacent pilosebaceous units are involved and a large, indurated, red mass develops. After a few days, multiple 'heads' appear, discharging pus, and the centre may break down.

Patient problems

Carbuncles are very painful and can take weeks to heal. Scarring is common.

Practical prescribing

Systemic antibiotics are essential, as is good nursing care, often including the need for regular dressings and debridement.

A search for underlying systemic problems should be undertaken.

Impetigo

Impetigo is a very superficial infection, the organism remaining within the outer layers of the epidermis. It is more common in children than in adults, particularly in temperate climates.

Presentation

Impetigo is most common on the head and neck, although any area of the body may be affected. Lesions are classically round or oval, beginning as small pustular areas which rapidly extend. Superficial bullae may remain intact, but usually rupture, leaving an oozy surface covered in honey-coloured crusts (Figs 15.3 and 15.4).

Patient problems

Impetigo is highly contagious and is spread easily from site to site, and from person to person. Very rarely, an outbreak may occur in neonates in intensive care facilities. This situation (*pemphigus neonatorum*) can be devastating, with a high mortality rate.

Practical prescribing

Topical treatment may be adequate for very limited disease, but a 5- to 7-day course of systemic anti-staphylococcal antibiotics is indicated in most cases. Some attempt at isolation, or a reduction in direct contact, for a few days is also a good idea, to avoid the infection spreading. Impetigo heals without scars, but may leave temporary discoloration.

In recurrent staphylococcal infections, it is worth taking swabs from the patient and relatives (including nasal), to determine the presence of carriage. If present, the use of nasal mupiricin is valuable.

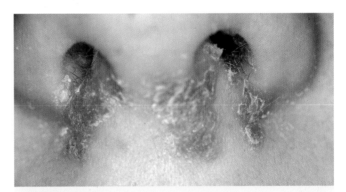

FIGURE 15.3 Impetigo: superficial bulla

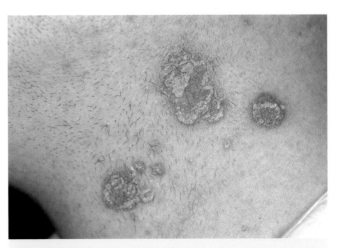

FIGURE 15.4 Impetigo: annular erythematous lesions with honey-coloured crusts; there may be preceding blistering

207

Secondary impetiginization

Secondary staphylococcal infection (impetiginization) is also very common, particularly in association with the eczemas (see Fig. 10.28), superimposed on viral infections (e.g. herpes simplex), and in cutaneous ectoparasite infections such as scabies and head lice.

'Staphylococcal scalded-skin syndrome'

The 'staphylococcal scalded-skin syndrome' is extremely rare. Some staphylococci produce a toxin that causes the epidermis to disintegrate. Sheets of skin peel away, producing an appearance resembling a severe burn from boiling water (Fig. 15.5). Adequate treatment with antibiotics, probably parenterally, is required. As important is good general nursing and metabolic support, without which the outcome is not nearly as successful.

STREPTOCOCCAL INFECTIONS

Streptococci are very important cutaneous pathogens. They may complicate impetigo, but their main importance is as the causative organism of scarlet fever (scarlatina), erysipelas/cellulitis, necrotizing fasciitis, erythema nodosum, glomerulonephritis, rheumatic fever and in their ability to trigger immunological reactions: Henoch–Schönlein purpura and guttate psoriasis.

Scarlet fever/scarlatina

Some streptococci produce toxins that induce a widespread erythema. The illness caused by these organisms is generally less severe nowadays, perhaps because a different strain is now responsible.

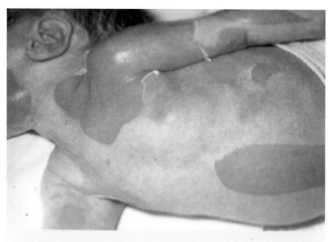

FIGURE 15.5 Staphylococcal scalded skin syndrome: the changes are very dramatic and children can be extremely unwell

Presentation

Accompanying, following, or independent of a sore throat, a rash begins to spread from the head and neck down the body over the course of 3 or 4 days. Desquamation follows a few days later.

Patient problems

Patients are febrile and unwell. In some patients scarlet fever is followed by hypersensitivity reactions in the skin, joints, gut and kidneys.

Practical prescribing

Penicillin is essential. It is important to watch out for the complications listed above.

Erysipelas and cellulitis (Figs 15.6 and 15.7)

There is little point in trying to make a distinction between these two: they are both essentially infections of dermis and/or subcutaneous tissue by streptococci. The organisms require a portal of entry. These may be breaches in the skin (e.g. leg ulcers, eczema, tinea pedis) or deeper infections of sinuses or the middle ear.

Presentation

Erysipelas and cellulitis are most commonly seen on the head and neck and the legs. Besides having the local symptoms and signs of pain, redness and heat, patients are often pyrexial and unwell. Septicaemia may occur.

Practical prescribing

If the diagnosis needs confirmation, blood cultures are required. Surface swabs are of no value. However, treatment should not wait for test results and patients should be started on adequate doses of flucloxacillin and Penicillin V without delay. Patients who are systemically unwell should be admitted to hospital and started on high-dose parental therapy. In penicillin-allergic patients clarithromycin or sometimes cephalosporins are an alternative.

Necrotizing fasciitis

Necrotizing fasciitis is a highly dangerous state which occurs when streptococcal infection extends beyond the subcutis and into the fascia and underlying muscle. Nausea and malaise are common and the affected areas become very painful – often out of proportion to the

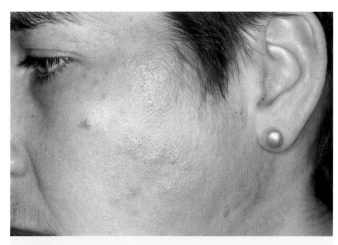

FIGURE 15.6 Erysipelas and cellulitis

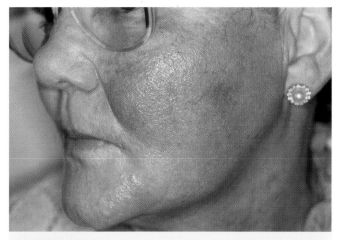

FIGURE 15.7 The hot, red cheek of facial streptococcal erysipelas/cellulitis

should be obtained for histology and culture although false negative results are not uncommon. A search should be undertaken to locate systemic infection.

Treatment consists in giving appropriate antituberculous chemotherapy, generally a combination of agents: rifampicin, isoniazid, ethambutol, pyrazinamide.

Cutaneous syphilis

Syphilis is making a return, having become quite rare for a while.

Primary syphilis results in chancres, which typically present as indurated painless ulcers usually on the male and female genitalia and the anus.

The secondary stage appears about 2–3 months later. Typically there is an asymptomatic eruption, often accompanying malaise, a low-grade fever and lymphadenopathy. The rash most commonly consists of a shower of reddish-brown, scaly papules. Lesions classically appear across the forehead (Fig. 15.8a). Lesions also occur on the palms and soles (Fig. 15.8b). Lesions are also frequently found in the anogenital area (condylomata lata) and in the mouth (snail-track ulcers). Sometimes, however, the eruption may closely resemble pityriasis rosea.

clinical signs. Superficial necrotic changes may appear but will normally indicate much more severe underlying damage, which results in rapid and widespread tissue destruction, septicaemia and, often, death. Urgent surgical debridement of all infected tissue, together with high doses of intravenous antibiotics and general support, is the only hope of cure.

Cutaneous tuberculosis

The cutaneous signs associated with active tuberculous infection are many and varied. The most common clinical pattern is *lupus vulgaris*. Lesions are almost always on the head and neck. Most are indolent, brownish-red patches, which may scar. If cutaneous TB is suspected, samples

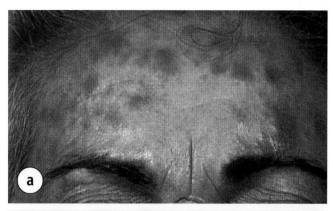

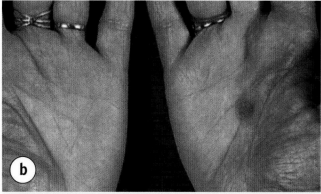

FIGURE 15.8 **(a)** Primary syphilis: lesions classically appear across the forehead. **(b)** Lesions also occur on the palms

209

Warts (human papillomavirus infections)

Viral warts are extremely common.

Common warts, plantar warts

Warts may occur at any age, although they are most prevalent in childhood and adolescence. The hands and feet are the most customary sites, with those on the plantar surface often being called verrucas. They can, however, occur virtually anywhere (Fig. 15.9). They may be a real nuisance around the nails and on the soles, where they may be painful or interfere with normal function.

Practical prescribing

Warts are not as easily treated as patients expect. Although a number of techniques appear to increase the clearance rate, results are often disappointing:

- Wart paints – containing salicylic acid, formalin, glutaraldehyde and other agents – require close attention to a daily regimen for several weeks; patience soon wanes, unless immediate visible gains are achieved.
- Cryotherapy works well for smaller, elevated warts, but is not as effective at dealing with deep plantar warts and can be excruciatingly painful; some authorities use longer freeze times, and regular treatments every 2–3 weeks.

Common warts resolve spontaneously over time and it may be reasonable to leave them completely alone unless they are causing significant symptoms or functional impairment: this is especially true in smaller children.

Some doctors use the age-old technique of 'wart charming'.

Plane warts (Figs 15.10 and 15.11)

Plane warts sometimes give rise to diagnostic difficulty. They are also a therapeutic problem, particularly when they occur on the face because they respond poorly to cryotherapy and most of the simple painting techniques. Although they do resolve eventually, they sometimes last for years.

Anogenital warts

Warts of the anogenital area are extremely common (Fig. 15.12). Most, but not all, are sexually transmitted. Occasionally, lesions become so large and numerous as to create cauliflower-like masses which interfere with normal functions. This may occur on the vulva during pregnancy.

In women, infection may be intravaginal or present only on the cervix. A proper examination should include

colposcopy wherever possible. Some patients with genital warts also have other sexually transmitted infections. Anogenital wart infection should generally be managed by experts in genitourinary medicine or by gynaecologists.

Treatment will normally involve some form of destructive technique such as cryotherapy, diathermy or snipping under local or general anaesthesia, but painting with podophyllin also works well for lesions of relatively

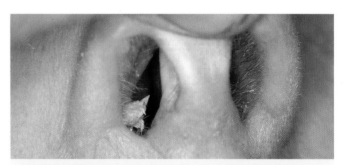

FIGURE 15.9 Wart in the nostril. Warts can appear anywhere: in this location they can be difficult to treat

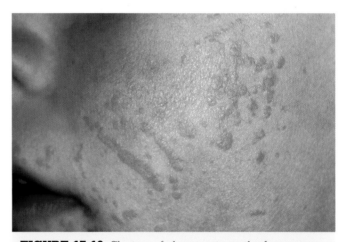

FIGURE 15.10 Clusters of plane warts on the face; many are clearly following the lines of previous scratches (Köbner phenomenon)

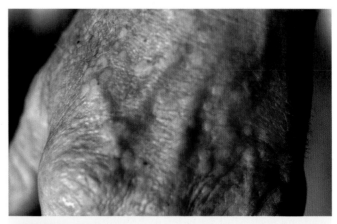

FIGURE 15.11 Plane warts on the back of the hand

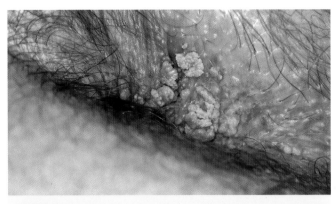

FIGURE 15.12 Perianal warts

limited extent. More recently imiquimod has been found highly effective.

Some genital warts induce dysplastic and neoplastic changes in cervical, vulval and penile epithelia.

Anogenital warts in children

Apart from the implications that this may have if the type of wart virus concerned is one of those associated with dysplastic or neoplastic changes, the possible source of such infections is a crucial issue.

In neonates, it seems likely that the main cause is direct transmission during birth. Infection may result from transfer from hand warts, but wart viruses can be transmitted sexually in children too. Childhood sexual abuse should always be considered as a possibility.

Molluscum contagiosum

Molluscum contagiosum is another extremely common superficial skin infection and, like warts, is most commonly seen in children. The infection is thought to be passed predominantly by direct contact, although the occurrence of outbreaks associated with swimming pools and other communal activities suggests that indirect transmission may also occur.

Infection may last from a few months to several years, but spontaneous resolution invariably occurs. However, lesions may become sore and infected, and parents often strongly desire some form of treatment.

Presentation

Lesions are papules with a typical appearance (Figs 15.13 and 15.14). They often appear in clusters.

Practical prescribing

Gentle cryotherapy is probably the most tolerable effective modality, although some authorities favour curettage and others opt for the time-honoured remedy of a phenol-impregnated pointed stick. Other options include topical salicylic acid, weak solutions of potassium hydroxide, cantharidin and imiquimod.

Herpes simplex

There are two strains of herpes simplex virus (HSV): HSV1 and HSV2. To some extent, these segregate by site of infection, with HSV2 being particularly common in genital infections, but both strains may occur anywhere. In common with the herpes varicella zoster virus (see below), HSV, once acquired, persists in nerve tissue throughout life. Attacks are therefore not new infection but recrudescences of existing disease. HSV2 is more prone to produce recurrent disease.

Active lesions are infectious both to others and to the patient, by direct inoculation of virus-containing material into the skin.

Presentation

Primary HSV

Most people have no memory of a 'first infection', although some develop acute symptomatic infections that can be

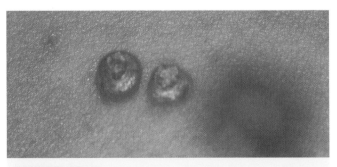

FIGURE 15.13 Good example of molluscum contagiosum

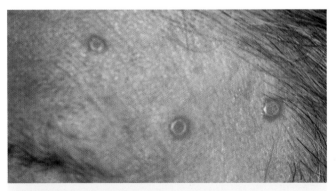

FIGURE 15.14 Molluscum contagiosum

quite dramatic. One of these is *herpetic gingivostomatitis*, which is most often encountered in children. The mouth becomes studded with small vesicles that rapidly break to leave ulcers. The child may be constitutionally unwell for a day or two beforehand, and lymphadenopathy is the rule. The lesions continue to crop for a few days before subsiding. A similar process may affect the genital area. Primary infection may also occur on other parts of the body, such as the finger or around the eye.

Recurrent disease (Figs 15.15–15.17)

The same area or areas are involved over and over again. The skin often tingles for a few hours before visible changes appear. Initially, the area becomes red and slightly swollen, before vesicles emerge on the surface. After a day or so, these become pustular and crust over. The lesion eventually settles after about 7–10 days, leaving mild erythema. Sites of predilection are well known – lips and face, male and female genitalia, and fingers and hands – but lesions may occur virtually anywhere. Recurrences may be triggered by minor infections (hence the name 'cold sore'), trauma, or sunlight.

Eczema herpeticum (*Kaposi's varicelliform eruption*) is covered in the Chapter 10.

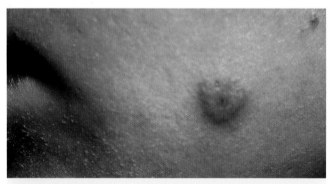

FIGURE 15.15 Example of herpes simplex infection in a less common site

Patient problems

Although people get used to having recurrent HSV, attacks are still very annoying and can be quite restricting. The virus can damage the cornea if it is inoculated into the eye.

Practical prescribing

If there is any doubt about the diagnosis, samples may be sent for electron microscopy and culture. It is important to try and obtain fluid from the lesions if possible and to place them in viral transport medium. Dry swabs or those handled as if for bacteria are useless.

Antiviral agents, such as acyclovir, reduce viral replication and may shorten attacks. If used topically they must be started early enough in the course of an attack.

Systemic treatment is seldom required for an acute episode unless there are complications, or in very extensive disease (e.g. eczema herpeticum). However, long-term prophylactic treatment may be indicated for recurrent disease which is occurring frequently, or in which the symptoms are very severe, and in immunosuppressed individuals.

Herpes varicella zoster virus

The herpes varicella zoster (HVZ) virus causes both chickenpox and herpes zoster, or shingles. After an attack of chickenpox, the virus rests in nerve ganglia and may re-emerge when conditions result in its reactivation.

Chickenpox (Figs 15.18 and 15.19)

Presentation

The incubation period is about 14 days. Chickenpox presents with mild prodromal symptoms (malaise, fever and headache). Occasionally, the systemic illness is more severe, with a high swinging fever and marked constitutional symptoms. A few days later the eruption appears: initial lesions are pink papules, but these rapidly

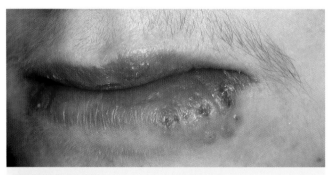

FIGURE 15.16 Herpes simplex infection

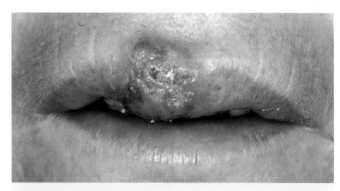

FIGURE 15.17 Herpes simplex infection

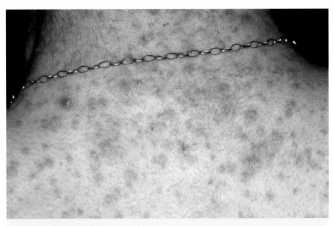

FIGURE 15.18 A mixture of papules, vesicles and pustules in chickenpox

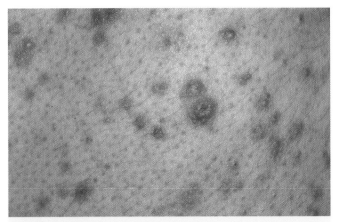

FIGURE 15.19 Chickenpox

become vesicular and then pustular, before a crust forms on the surface. Resolution and healing occur within 3–4 days, leaving a pink macule or depression. Further crops of new lesions continue to appear for several days.

Patient problems

Itching may be trivial or very unpleasant. Usually there is no significant scarring, but some lesions may become secondarily infected, which may result in small, permanent 'pock-marks'. The virus can also cause an encephalitis, pneumonia and thrombocytopenia, though this is very rare.

Practical prescribing

No treatment is generally needed. Antiviral agents may reduce the severity of a really nasty attack.

Herpes zoster (shingles) (Fig. 15.20)

Herpes zoster represents the re-emergence of varicella zoster virus from its resting place in a nerve ganglion.

Presentation

The clinical picture therefore depends on which nerve root is involved. Figure 15.20(c), for example, shows lesions in the perianal area, resulting from involvement of a lumbosacral nerve.

Initially, there may only be pain or discomfort in the 'to-be-affected' area. Crops of papules then develop in the area served by the affected nerve. These rapidly become vesiculopustular and crusted. Scattered lesions may occur elsewhere as well, but large numbers of disseminated lesions should suggest the possibility of underlying immunosuppression. Healing takes a further week or so if there are no complications, but can sometimes be significantly slowed by secondary infection and general ill-health.

Patient problems

The infection may be very painful, but this is not always the case, especially in younger patients. There are a number of

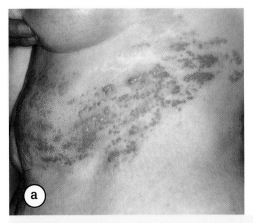

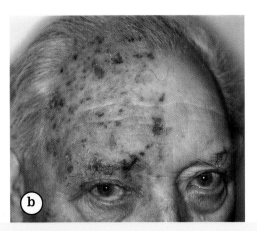

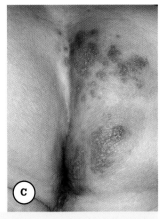

FIGURE 15.20 Herpes zoster in three different nerve distributions

complications that may accompany or follow an attack of shingles:

- Ocular damage.
- Motor involvement may lead to ocular palsies, facial nerve palsy (Ramsay Hunt syndrome) and difficulties with micturition/defecation.
- Scarring in the previously affected area.
- Nerve damage with dysaesthesia (neuralgia); this is especially common after trigeminal nerve involvement and may result in *trigeminal trophic syndrome*, where repetitive trauma to skin with impaired sensation leads to permanent loss of tissue.

Practical prescribing

There is some controversy over whether shingles should routinely be treated with antiviral medication. There is some evidence that a course of acyclovir, or one of the newer agents, may reduce the incidence and severity of post-herpetic neuralgia. However, doses need to be high (at least 800 mg five times daily for 7 days) to have any effect at all. If neuralgia occurs, this will need separate attention and often requires careful management by a specialist in pain control.

Measles, rubella, hand foot and mouth, fifth disease

Measles (Figs 15.21)

The rash follows a short prodromal illness in which upper respiratory symptoms, conjunctivitis and fever predominate. Classically, the rash starts behind the ears on day 4, and spreads to involve the whole body surface. Small punctate lesions appear in the mouth (Koplick's spots, Fig. 15.22). Most patients recover completely, but pneumonia, otitis and encephalitis may affect some.

Rubella (Fig. 15.23)

There is a very short illness, there often with no prodromal element. The rash often clears within 3 or 4 days. Tender lymphadenopathy is common. The major complication is that the virus wreaks havoc in pregnant women, causing severe handicaps in the unborn child.

Hand foot and mouth disease (Fig. 15.24)

This is a mild infection, characterized by vesiculopustular lesions in the mouth and along the sides of the fingers and toes. The lesions generally clear within a week of the onset.

Erythema infectiosum (fifth disease, slapped cheek disease) (Figs 15.25 and 15.26)

Caused by parvovirus B19, this disorder occurs in mini-epidemics, usually in the early spring. The typical patient is a child, who suddenly develops hot, swollen, red cheeks

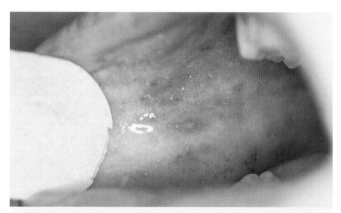

FIGURE 15.22 Koplick's spots, pathognomonic of measles

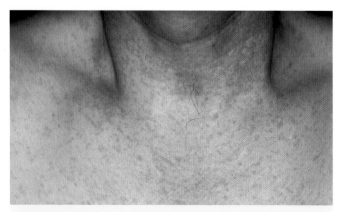

FIGURE 15.23 Rubella: the rash only lasts 3 days

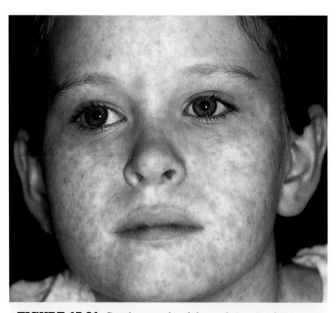

FIGURE 15.21 Good example of the rash in measles

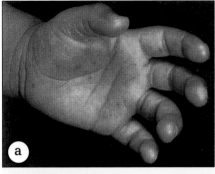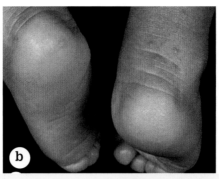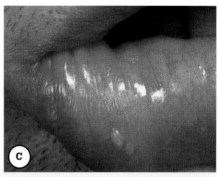

FIGURE 15.24 **(a)** Hand foot and mouth disease: hand. **(b)** Hand foot and mouth disease: feet. **(c)** Hand foot and mouth disease: mouth

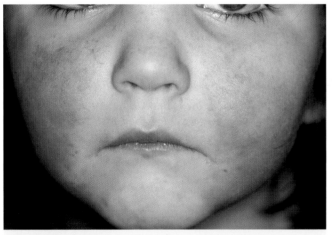

FIGURE 15.25 Bright red cheeks in fifth disease

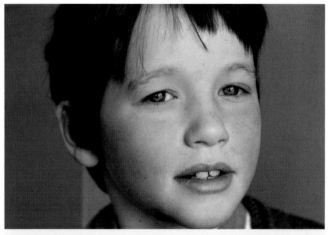

FIGURE 15.26 Bright red cheeks in fifth disease

(which look as though they have been slapped). A more widespread eruption follows over the succeeding 3–4 days, but this is quite variable in its extent. Older individuals may develop arthralgia. The main concern is if the infection is passed on to a pregnant woman, as the virus can be highly teratogenic.

Other viral rashes

A number of viruses cause rashes:
- Viral hepatitis: rashes are quite common during the early phases of infection with the hepatitis viruses A, B and C. They may be non-specific, maculopapular eruptions, but urticarial lesions due to a vasculitis also occur with hepatitis B virus.
- Coxsackie viruses can cause a wide range of cutaneous changes, including exanthematic eruptions, and are the cause of hand foot and mouth disease; rashes associated with Coxsackie viruses are generally mild and non-specific.
- HIV infection is associated with numerous skin problems, especially in advanced disease: xerosis, drug eruptions, infections and seborrhoeic dermatitis.

FUNGAL INFECTIONS

Two main groups of fungal organisms infect human skin: dermatophytes (which cause what the layman usually calls ringworm) and yeasts. The most widely used subclassification of the dermatophyte infections, however, is based on the region of the body that is affected.

DERMATOPHYTE INFECTIONS

Tinea capitis

Scalp ringworm is a disorder of children. There is hair loss with a variable degree of inflammation and scaling. In general, fungi caught from animals tend to cause more inflammation than those passed on from human to human. In some infections there may be virtually no inflammation at all.

In white UK residents the normal situation is either of a mildly inflamed area with broken hairs (Fig. 15.27) or a boggy, oozy mass called *kerion* (Fig. 15.28), in which the organism has usually been acquired from animals,

215

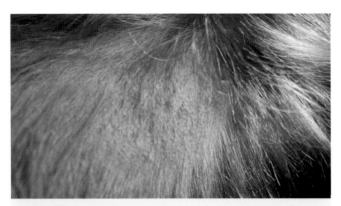

FIGURE 15.27 Tinea capitis: mildly inflamed area with broken hairs

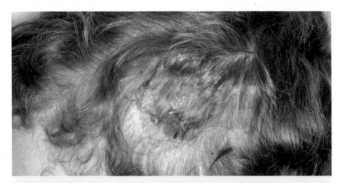

FIGURE 15.28 Tinea capitis: inflammation and induration known as 'kerion'

especially cattle. This form of the disease is often diagnosed as a bacterial infection and the failure of any such area to respond to simple antibiotics should suggest fungus.

In some populations with enduring contacts with Africa and Asia, a form of infection may occur in which the hair becomes very fragile and breaks very close to its emergence from the scalp. Sometimes there is marked swelling of the hair follicles, resulting in the appearance of 'black dots' across the surface.

Only one scalp ringworm fungus common in the UK fluoresces under Wood's light (*Microsporum canis*), so this test can be misleading.

Tinea barbae and tinea facei

Hair invasion is also seen in ringworm of the beard area (tinea barbae) (Fig. 15.29), where a patch or patches of inflammation, sometimes studded with follicular pustules, classically develop (Fig. 15.30). Outbreaks of tinea barbae have been associated with communal shaving arrangements in long-stay hospital patients.

Infection outside the beard area is known as *tinea facei*. This is frequently misdiagnosed – and therefore mistreated – as eczema.

Box 15.1 Dermatophyte infections	
Tinea capitis	Scalp ringworm
Tinea barbae	Ringworm of the beard area
Tinea facei	Facial infection outside the beard area
Tinea corporis	Ringworm of the body with annular (circinate) lesions
Tinea cruris	Ringworm of the leg but generally applied to infection in the groin and on the upper, inner thighs
Tinea manuum	Ringworm infection of the hand(s)
Tinea pedis	Fungal infection of the feet
Tinea unguium	Fungal invasion in nails
'Tinea incognito'	Ringworm infections with clinical features masked by treatment with topical or systematic steroids

Tinea corporis

Ringworm of the body may be due to animal or human ringworm fungi. Infections caught from animals are generally much more inflammatory. Lesions are often annular, or at least have a circinate border (Fig. 15.31). The use of topical steroids may confuse the picture considerably (*see tinea incognito*).

Tinea cruris

Literally, tinea cruris means ringworm of the leg, but the term is generally applied to infection in the groin and on

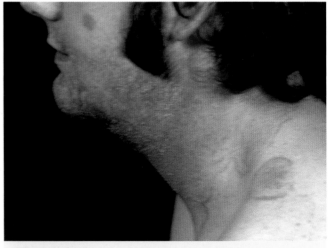

FIGURE 15.29 Tinea barbae

the dry, scaly, sweatless hand associated with the organism *Trichophyton rubrum* (Fig. 15.33). This can be mistaken for eczema but it is often unilateral. Inspection of the nails will often show changes of fungal invasion.

Tinea pedis

Fungal infections of the feet are extremely common. There are three quite distinct forms encountered in clinical practice:

- Toe–web space infection (athlete's foot), in which the interdigital toe clefts become fissured, macerated and itchy (Fig. 15.34); the fourth and/or fifth interspaces are the most commonly affected; the changes frequently recur endlessly. NB: Soft corns (Fig. 15.35) are commonly misdiagnosed as fungal infections.
- Vesicular patches, particularly on the soles and the sides of the feet (Fig. 15.36) may become

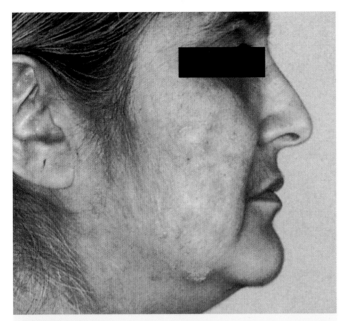

FIGURE 15.30 Tinea facei. Patch or patches of inflammation, sometimes studded with follicular pustules, classically develop

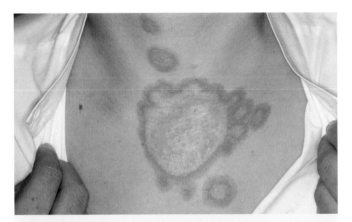

FIGURE 15.31 Tinea corporis: typical red rings with central clearing; the source of the infection was laboratory rodents

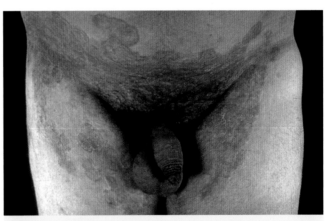

FIGURE 15.32 Extensive tinea cruris spreading onto the thighs and abdominal skin

the upper, inner thighs. Typically, the infection causes a scaly red, marginated eruption, which spreads outwards from the groin crease (Fig. 15.32) and may extend onto the buttocks and hips. Itching is a common feature. Tinea cruris is much more common in men than in women and tends to be recurrent, with autoinfection from accompanying disease elsewhere (especially the feet) being a factor.

Tinea manuum

There are several clinical patterns associated with ringworm infection of the hand(s), including blisters similar to those seen on the feet (see below). Perhaps the most striking is

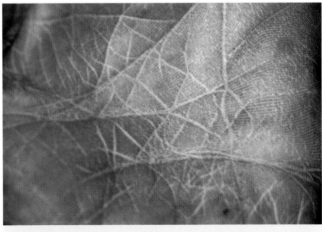

FIGURE 15.33 The typical dry, sweatless hand of chronic *Trichophyton rubrum* infection

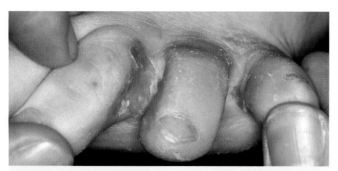

FIGURE 15.34 Tinea pedis: interdigital inflammation and peeling (often called 'athlete's foot')

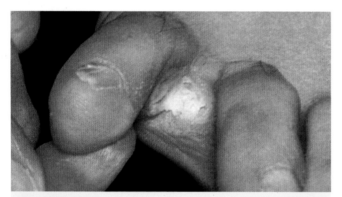

FIGURE 15.35 Soft corn: easily confused with tinea pedis

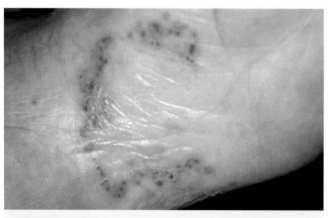

FIGURE 15.36 Tinea pedis: clusters of pustules are common

Tinea unguium

Nails, especially toenails, are frequently involved in fungal invasion, especially in association with chronic or recurrent *tinea pedis*. In fact, a reservoir of infection in the nails is an important cause of continued and recurrent fungal skin infections. One or just a few nail plates may be affected, but as time goes on there is a tendency for more to become involved. The nails become thickened and discoloured (Fig. 15.39), classically producing a yellowish-brown appearance. There may be a significant degree of subungual hyperkeratosis.

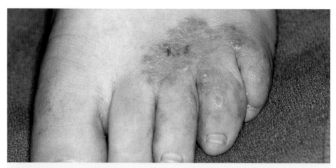

FIGURE 15.37 Tinea pedis: changes often extend on to the dorsum of the foot

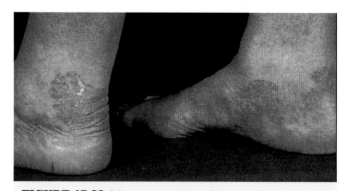

FIGURE 15.38 Moccasin pattern of tinea pedis

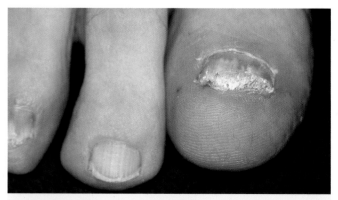

FIGURE 15.39 Typical nail changes due to fungal infection

widespread and confluent; big blisters occasionally develop; the areas are generally extremely itchy.
- Dry, scaly changes, which may extend from other areas to involve the sole, dorsum (Fig. 15.37) and around the sides of the feet – the so-called *moccasin pattern* (Fig. 15.38); the infection is frequently treated as eczema or psoriasis, leading to 'tinea incognito' (see below); accompanying nail disease is very common.

Tinea incognito

Tinea incognito is the name given to ringworm infections whose clinical features have been modified by treatment with topical or systemic steroids (Fig. 15.40). This may occur at any site, but is most commonly seen on the feet and lower legs, or in the groin. Occasionally the scalp is affected. There are some features that should alert one to this possibility:

- A history of initial improvement with topical steroids, but with subsequent relapse and extension.
- Persistent follicular nodules and pustules.
- The presence of signs of fungal infection in nearby areas (e.g. groin or nails).

Practical prescribing

The best way to be sure whether a rash is due to a fungal infection is to take specimens for microscopy and culture. Microscopic examination is simple enough to perform in a surgery or clinic with the right equipment and with some training and experience. In practice, however, scrapes and clips are most often sent to a laboratory.

Here are a few simple tips to ensure the best results:
- Scrape the *edge* of ringworm lesions on the skin.
- Cut the nail back and send along with scrapings from the undersurface of the nail.
- Cut out a piece of the blister roof of vesicular lesions.
- Send both scalp scale and hair in suspected scalp ringworm.

Mycological culture takes up to 6 weeks.

Once a diagnosis has been made, either clinically or with laboratory support, the only decision required is whether the patient needs systemic therapy, or whether topical agents alone will suffice.

As a rule of thumb, unless there is some compelling reason to avoid it, systemic therapy is indicated if:
- Disease involves hair or nails.
- More than one site is involved.
- Lesions are extensive.
- Topical treatment has already failed.
- The diagnosis is 'tinea incognito'.

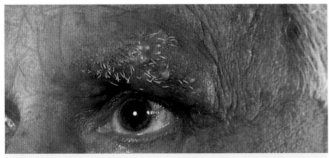

FIGURE 15.40 Tinea incognito. This lesion was due to a fungal infection but was treated with a topical steroid.

Topical treatment is satisfactory only for disease in one site and of limited extent. A number of topical agents are available:
- Undecanoate creams – generally weak.
- Tolnaftate creams – generally weak.
- Imidazole creams (e.g. clotrimazole, miconazole, econazole, ketoconazole) – these agents have for some years been the first choice for most infections; some are available in combination with hydrocortisone, which can help reduce inflammatory symptoms.
- Terbinafine cream – highly effective and possesses some anti-inflammatory properties.
- Amoralfine – available in paints for the treatment of nail disease, in combination with systemic therapy, or if it is not tolerated or is otherwise contraindicated.

The systemic therapies currently in use are:
- Griseofulvin – in use for over 40 years; it is safe and remains the only licensed drug for children with scalp ringworm, where the dose required is 20 mg/kg per day for 6–8 weeks; the cure rate for nail infections is poor, however, and treatment must be continued for over a year.
- Imidazoles (ketoconazole, itraconazole, fluconazole) are effective and generally safe; ketoconazole induces hepatitis in a small proportion of patients and liver function should be monitored in all patients on systemic imidazoles; the spectrum of activity includes yeasts (see below).
- Terbinafine – a very good drug, although it is ineffective against yeasts (see below).

Recommended regimens for nail infections vary around the world, but 3 months' treatment at adequate dosage (terbinafine, 250 mg daily; itraconazole, 200 mg daily) is usually satisfactory, as is 'pulsed' itraconazole. The use of terbinafine in children is unlicensed, but has become very common and is mentioned in the British National Formulary (BNF), with very helpful dose recommendations.

The addition of appropriate antibiotics may also speed up the response when treating a child with kerion.

YEAST INFECTIONS

Yeasts are capable of inducing human disease but many are also true commensals and only become invasive under certain conditions. For example, *Candida albicans* may only cause 'thrush' following a course of broad-spectrum antibiotics. The superficial infection known as *pityriasis versicolor* and the disease states caused by *Candida* are considered below.

Pityriasis (or tinea) versicolor

Pityriasis (sometimes 'tinea') versicolor is a very common, superficial fungal infection caused by a commensal yeast. Most commonly called *Malassezia furfur*.

Presentation

The most typical clinical picture is of slightly scaly patches on the upper trunk, upper arms and neck. In pale skin, the patches appear to be a slightly dirty-brown colour (Fig. 15.41), while in skin that is either genetically darker or has been exposed to ultraviolet radiation the areas are hypopigmented (Fig. 15.42).

Practical prescribing

Scrapes from affected skin can be directly examined under the microscope, but the organism will not grow in standard culture systems.

Treatment and clearance are relatively straightforward, but recurrence is common. The organism is sensitive to selenium sulphide and the imidazoles. One successful approach is to combine a topical imidazole cream twice daily, with a daily wash with half-strength selenium sulphide shampoo. Another widely used regime is ketoconazole shampoo, made into a lather and applied to the skin for 10 minutes before washing off. This should be done four times a week for 2 weeks.

If the infection is very widespread, a week's course of oral itraconazole, 200 mg daily, is highly effective. Recurrence may be prevented by using selenium sulphide or ketoconazole in the shower from time to time.

Patients should also be warned that the hypopigmentation will require longer to resolve.

Candidiasis (candidosis)

Defining the diseased state in candidiasis is sometimes difficult, since *Candida* spp. are found naturally in the mouth or lower intestinal tract in 50–60% of people, and are occasionally a commensal in the normal vagina as well. However, true invasion, with symptoms and signs, may occur in a number of sites:

- *Oral*. Candidal infection in the mouth may be seen at any age, but is most common in children, older adults with dentures, the immunocompromised and in patients receiving antibiotics or steroids, either orally, by inhalation or locally to the mouth itself. In the classic form, known as thrush, lesions consist of whitish, creamy patches, which peel off to leave a red, oozy and bleeding base; this may affect any part of the oropharynx. *Candida* is also involved in angular stomatitis (Fig. 15.43).
- *Vulvovaginal*. Vulvovaginal thrush is characterized by a creamy-yellow discharge, erythema, oedema and itching. Infection is often recurrent, with some women seeming to be much more prone to infection. The problem is also commoner in pregnancy and in those receiving courses of broad-spectrum antibiotics. Very occasionally, diabetes presents with vulvovaginal candidiasis.
- *Penile*. Candidal balanitis usually occurs in the partner of an infected individual, although oral and anal carriage may be the source in some patients. The glans becomes red and inflamed, with white, cheesy plaques developing on the surface.

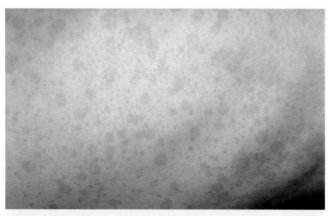

FIGURE 15.41 Brown, slightly scaly patches in widespread pityriasis versicolor

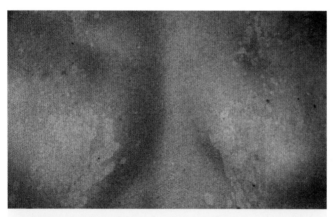

FIGURE 15.42 Pityriasis (or tinea) versicolor: in skin that is either genetically darker or has been exposed to ultraviolet radiation, the areas are hypopigmented

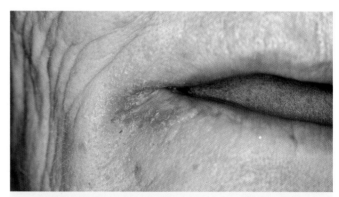

FIGURE 15.43 Angular chelitis

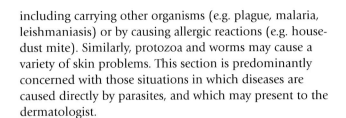
- *Perianal.* Infection of the perianal skin may occur alone or in association with genital infection, or infection of the groin and scrotum.
- *Paronychial. Candida* is probably involved, at least as a co-pathogen, in many instances of chronic paronychia.
- *Skin and flexures. Candida* is an important cause of skin inflammation in intertriginous areas (Fig. 15.44). *Candida* is also frequently isolated from intertrigo in the inframammary folds, axillae and groin, where the presence of small 'satellite' pustules around the edge of the characteristic glazed erythema of intertrigo should raise suspicion.
- *Nappy (diaper) infection.* Infants and young children are prone to rashes in the nappy area and *Candida* is a common secondary invader (Figs 15.45 and 15.46).

ECTOPARASITIC INFECTIONS

Humans, for the most part, live in peace with the arthropods, protozoa and worms in their environment. However, arthropods may cause disease in a variety of ways,

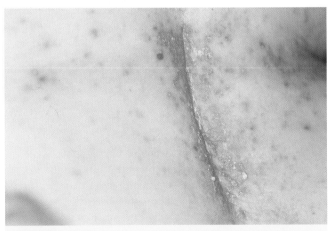

FIGURE 15.44 Candidal intertrigo: note the pustules around the areas of erythema

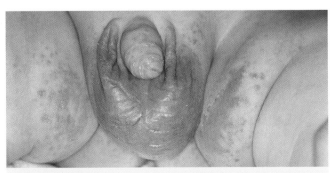

FIGURE 15.45 Nappy dermatitis with the characteristic peripheral pustules of superadded candidal infection

including carrying other organisms (e.g. plague, malaria, leishmaniasis) or by causing allergic reactions (e.g. house-dust mite). Similarly, protozoa and worms may cause a variety of skin problems. This section is predominantly concerned with those situations in which diseases are caused directly by parasites, and which may present to the dermatologist.

FLEAS, LICE AND OTHER BLOOD-FEEDERS

Many arthropods are adapted to feeding on the blood of homoiothermic creatures: for example, fleas, various mites, lice, bugs and flying insects such as mosquitoes. The puncture and penetration of the host by the creature often causes little or no significant injury and many people are completely unaware that they have been bitten. However, reactions may occur to chemicals or to insect parts (or to both), either as an irritant or an allergic response. The clinical picture varies with the arthropod concerned and with the site affected.

Fleas

Fleas are small insects that inhabit the dwelling-place of a particular species to which they are adapted. Infestation by the human flea (*Pulex irritans*) is rare in the Western world and is only seen in individuals living in highly congested conditions. Outbreaks do occur from time to time in refugee camps and other such situations. The human flea, together with the rat flea, are the vectors of plague. Most flea problems arise from the bite of animal fleas, most commonly those associated with domestic pets (Fig. 15.47a) or, occasionally, birds in adjacent nests.

The characteristic clinical picture is of recurrent crops of irritable papules (Fig. 15.47b). These are most common on the lower legs, but may occur elsewhere and may appear under clothing. This clinical picture is called papular urticaria. Occasionally, the reaction is so marked that blisters may form. The lesions are itchy and often continue

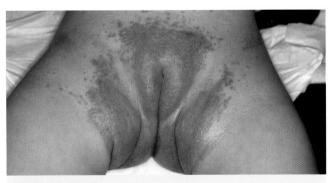

FIGURE 15.46 Nappy dermatitis with the characteristic peripheral pustules of superadded candidal infection

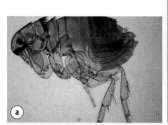

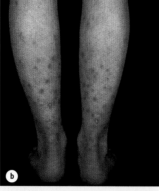

FIGURE 15.47 **(a)** Cat flea. **(b)** Papular urticaria of the legs

Courtesy of Dr D A Burns

to be symptomatic for some days, or even up to 4 weeks, with irritation coming in spasms. Secondary infection is quite common and lesions may heal to leave small depressions and pigmentary anomalies.

Examination of any domestic pet will usually reveal the presence of 'flea dirt' (small specks of brownish material) in the coat or fur. However, the fleas themselves are easier to find in the animal's bedding, as a flea colony contains many thousands of individuals at various stages of development, while the animal itself may carry only a few at any one time. Occasionally, the source of infestation is not immediately apparent, and a search of the local environment may be necessary. As an illustration, the authors offer this brief case history: a male patient presented one spring with typical flea bites on the upper trunk, neck and forearms; he kept no pets and had lived in the same house for 20 years; a search revealed a bird's nest, which had not been occupied as usual that year, in the roof of his garage; the fleas were activated by the starting of his car each morning and dropped down to bite him on the way to work!

Fleas need to be eradicated from the environment and not just from the animal source itself. There are a variety of agents and delivery systems available, but it is often useful to involve the local veterinary surgeon or the environmental health department.

Lice

Humans are unique in having more than one type of louse infestation. Lice are wingless insects and there are several different species. Some feed on the skin and hair of their hosts, but those that cause problems in humans are blood-feeders. There are three important clinical infections in humans:

- *Head louse infestation (pediculosis capitis)*. This remains an extremely common infection, occurring endemically in the developing world and epidemically in 'the

West', where outbreaks typically appear in schools and in other communities where children predominate. The infection is generally passed by direct head-to-head contact, although some authorities believe that hats and brushes may be vehicles of transmission. The most important symptom is pruritus, and any child with any itchy scalp should be examined very carefully for evidence of head lice. Sometimes there is a papular, excoriated eruption in the occipital area and on the nape of the neck. Secondary infection with *Staphylococcus aureus* is common and may be severe. The most important physical sign is the presence of 'nits', the egg cases of the insect which stick on to hair shafts (Fig. 15.48a) and are visible with a hand lens. They are often best seen at the back of the head. Occasionally, an adult louse may be seen scuttling away from the peering eyes of the examiner (Fig. 15.48b).

- *Body louse (clothing louse) infestation (pediculosis corporis)*. In developed countries, this infection is only seen in vagrants; however, like fleas, body lice will appear in overcrowded conditions such as refugee or prisoner-of-war camps, and infestation is still prevalent in poorer communities with bad housing conditions. The louse lives in the seams of clothing, but feeds on the blood of the wearer. Most patients complain of itching and are covered in scratch marks. Secondary bacterial infection is, again, very common. Once the clothes have been removed the problem subsides, unless the patient returns to the same living conditions. Body lice are important vectors of disease, especially typhus.

- *Pubic louse infestation ('crab lice', phthiriasis pubis)*. This infection is caused by an entirely separate louse (the head louse and body louse are essentially identical) known as *Pthiriasis pubis* (Fig. 15.49). It is seen almost exclusively among sexually active young adults. The lice are generally found in the pubic hair, on the lower abdomen or inner thighs, clinging to hair shafts along with their egg cases. Occasionally, lice are also found on the chest, in the axillae, on the scalp margins and in the eyelashes and beard hair. There may be little or no other sign of the infection, although most patients complain of some itching and there may be blood spots on underwear and other clothing.

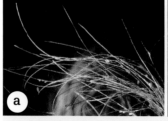
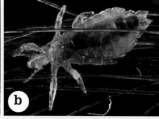

FIGURE 15.48 **(a)** 'Nits'. **(b)** Adult louse

Courtesy of Dr D A Burns

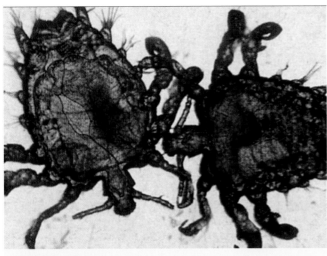

FIGURE 15.49 Crab lice

Lice are all susceptible to simple insecticides such as malathion, but do develop resistance. More recently, permethrin has been added to the range of available treatments. Scalp treatments should be carried out with lotions rather than shampoos. Body louse infection requires little more than a change of clothes.

Bed bugs

Bed bugs live in the furniture, floors and walls. At night they move out in search of food and may be attracted towards the warmth of the (usually) sleeping victim. They feed by sucking blood from exposed sites and may leave little or no trace. However, in a patient sensitized to the bite, large urticarial wheals develop. Occasionally, the reaction is severe enough to cause blisters. The bugs need to be eradicated from the dwelling, but can survive without food for over a year, as one of the authors can personally confirm!

Mosquitoes, gnats, and midges

Almost everyone will be familiar with the flying blood-suckers mosquitoes, gnats and midges. Apart from producing insect-bite reactions in sensitized individuals, many are vectors of diseases such as malaria, yellow fever, filarial infections and leishmaniasis. The insect-bite reactions are similar in nature to those seen with fleas and bed bugs: urticarial wheals, which may persist for some days or even 1–2 weeks. More extreme reactions may result in the swelling of parts of limbs or in blister formation. Lesions are most common on exposed sites, although the insects can penetrate hosiery and light clothing. The legs are frequently affected, especially in women. Sandflies may transmit leishmaniasis.

Ticks

Ticks are arachnids, belonging to the same group of arthropods as spiders and mites. They feed on their host by implanting their mouthparts into the skin and remaining attached for some considerable time. As they feed, they swell with blood, and they are often identified as small blobs on the skin surface, and urticarial reactions may occur around the site. They are generally acquired by humans passing through infested vegetation. Ticks should be removed with care, to avoid leaving mouth-parts behind.

The importance of these creatures for humans lies in their ability to transmit other diseases, particularly the rickettsial infections (e.g. Rocky Mountain spotted fever), some forms of viral encephalitis, relapsing fever, some forms of typhus and Lyme disease.

Fly larvae (maggots)

Some flies complete their life cycle in the skin of living animals. They have various ways of achieving this, and the infection is not always an essential part of their development. However, when the development of fly larvae (maggots) occurs in the skin, this leads to a condition called myiasis. Most parts of the world have flies that infect animals, particularly cattle, but human infections are generally acquired in the tropics. Typically, the patient develops a boil-like lesion, which breaks down and suppurates (Fig. 15.50a). Careful inspection may reveal the moving maggots within the lesion (Fig. 15.50b). The larvae can be removed surgically, but the condition will resolve itself naturally in due course as the maggots die or mature.

SCABIES AND OTHER MITE INFECTIONS

Humans can be affected by a large number of mites. One of the more common human–mite interactions is with *Dermatophagoides pteronyssinus*, the ubiquitous house-dust mite. Its role in some allergic processes (asthma, rhinitis) seems clear, and there is increasing evidence of a role for it in atopic dermatitis. Other problems are due to more direct involvement by the mite, but are also often associated with a significant hypersensitivity component.

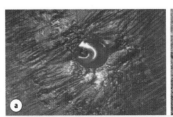 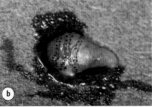

FIGURE 15.50 **(a)** Myiasis: an indolent, suppurating lesion on the upper arm. **(b)** Myiasis: moving maggot of the fly *Dermatobia hominis* within the lesion

Human scabies

Scabies is very common. The infection is due to the invasion of the host by the mite *Sarcoptes scabiei* var. *hominis* (Fig. 15.51), which passes from person to person almost exclusively by direct contact. The typical clinical picture begins with the onset of pruritus, usually about 6 weeks after exposure in a first attack. The itching is most severe at night. Characteristically, other members of the family are also affected by itch, but this is not always the case. There have been several reports of outbreaks in institutions, especially those caring for the elderly.

The onset of symptoms is accompanied by the appearance of a widespread, papular or eczematous rash which spares the head and neck in all except very small babies. The rash is often more pronounced around the anterior axillary folds. It may also become secondarily

infected. Careful inspection will also reveal the presence of the cardinal lesion: the burrow (Fig. 15.52a). These may be very numerous (especially if the patient has been treated with topical corticosteroids) or quite sparse (especially if the patient has received some, but not adequate, scabicidal therapy). The clinical features are sometimes obscured by inflammation (Fig. 15.52b). The sites of predilection are the sides and webs of the fingers, the palms, the soles and sides of the feet, and the male genitalia (Fig. 15.52c). Indeed, papules on the penis and scrotum in a male with itch will prove to be scabies in 99% of cases. In small children, the burrow may become vesicular and is more common on the palms and soles. Lesions may also appear on the cheeks and even the scalp in infants.

Very rarely, mites proliferate hugely without apparently giving rise to much itching or other symptomatology. This situation, known as crusted or Norwegian scabies, is usually seen in those with neurological, immunological or mental deficits. The clinical picture is variable, often simulating an eczema, psoriasis or another inflammatory skin disease.

Scabies is best diagnosed by the examination of scrapings of a burrow in 10% KOH under low-power microsocpy. Mites, nymphs, eggs and egg cases (Fig. 15.53; see also Fig. 15.52) are all confirmatory evidence of infection. Treatment should be undertaken with one of the proven acaricides:

- Benzyl benzoate, which has to be applied from chin to toes three times in 24 hours. It is an irritant and is unsuitable for small babies and patients with pre-existing eczema; treatment should not be repeated without further advice because irritation and sensitization become more troublesome with multiple applications.
- Gamma-benzene hexachloride, which should be applied to the same areas as for benzyl benzoate and left in place for 6–24 hours; there have been worries over its neurotoxicity in infants and in pregnant or lactating mothers.

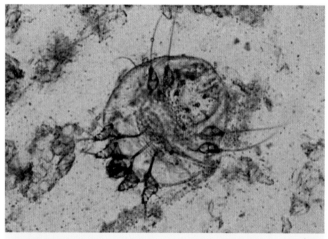

FIGURE 15.51 *Sarcoptes scabiei* var. *hominis*: microscopic view

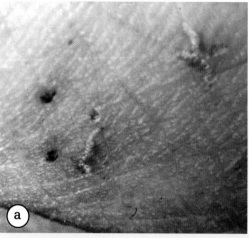
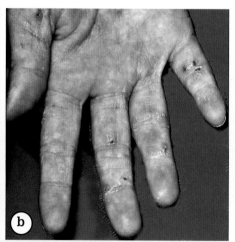
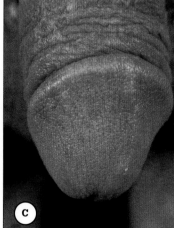

FIGURE 15.52 **(a)** Scabies burrow. **(b)** Scabies burrow: on the palm, hard to see here because of intense inflammation and secondary infection. **(c)** Scabies burrow: inflammation on the glans penis

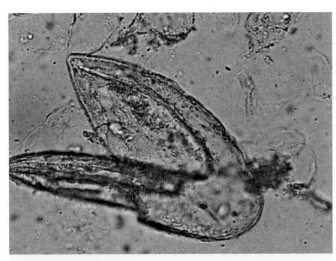

FIGURE 15.53 Egg cases

- Malathion, which should be used twice over the course of a week, being left on for 24 hours on each occasion.

- Permethrin, which has recently become the treatment of first choice in many centres; the cream is applied once to the trunk, limbs and genital areas; some authorities recommend a second application a few days later.
- Crotamiton (present in Eurax®), a weak acaricide but a useful general antipruritic which can be used to help relieve the symptoms both before and after treatment with a more active agent.

Resistant cases, particularly where there is an institutional outbreak, may be managed by the use of ivermectin orally in a single dose (200 µg/kg)

All those living and sleeping in the same house, all sexual contacts and, where appropriate, all close friends should be treated simultaneously. Patients should be warned that itching may persist for several days even after the live mites have been successfully eradicated. Occasionally, patients develop small irritable lumps which persist for weeks or months following scabies. These lumps, which are known as post-scabitic nodules, can be treated by intralesional steroid injection, but sometimes have to be excised.

Chapter 16

Leg Ulcers and Lymphoedema

Summary

- Leg ulcers
- Lymphoedema

LEG ULCERS

Diseases of arteries, veins, capillaries and lymphatics may all present with skin changes, of which leg ulceration is one of the most troublesome. Leg ulcers may also occur in rheumatoid arthritis and haemoglobinopathies (especially sickle cell disease, thalassaemia and spherocytosis).

Box 16.1 Skin signs commonly associated with vascular disease	
Arterial	
Chronic insufficiency	Loss of hair, cold extremities, ulceration, gangrene
Spasm	Raynaud's phenomenon
Venous	
Incompetence	Dermatoliposclerosis, pigmentation, dermatitis, atrophie blanche, varicose veins, ulceration
Lymphatic	
Obstruction	Lymphoedema, Stewart–Treves lymphangiosarcoma (see Ch. 4), elephantiasis
Hypoplasia	Lymphoedema, recurrent cellulites
Capillaries	
Inflammation	Pigmented purpuric eruptions

Presentation

Arterial insufficiency leads to trophic changes: tight, shiny skin with little or no hair. The skin is generally cold, and ulceration or gangrene may supervene (Fig. 16.1).

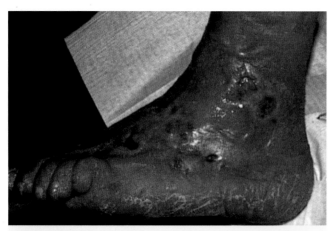

FIGURE 16.1 Multiple ulcers in a patient with arterial insufficiency due to atherosclerosis

Arterial insufficiency is common in atherosclerosis, where the arteries may be narrowed generally or may become embolized from plaques on the vessel wall. Diabetes is, of course, a major risk factor and the additional neuropathy so often seen in diabetics causes further difficulties.

Leg ulcers due to arterial disease are usually small, punched out and painful. They may occur anywhere on the lower leg or foot.

Venous disease has more protean manifestations (Figs 16.2 and 16.3) and may again affect both lower leg and foot, although the main focus of changes is the lower third of the leg and the ankle. External varicosities (either large bunches of tortuous veins or finer, 'star-burst' or 'thread' veins may be in evidence), but there may be none. The skin frequently may become gradually more sclerotic around the ankles and over the lower third of the leg – a change known as dermatoliposclerosis (Fig. 16.4a). Pigmentation and eczema are also common and the skin is liable to ulcerate after minor trauma (Fig. 16.4b). Another characteristic change seen in venous disease is atrophie blanche (Fig. 16.4c).

Once established, venous leg ulcers are very slow to heal. Treatment entails rest, elevation of the leg(s) and, if the arterial supply is good enough, compression bandaging.

Venous and arterial disease frequently coexist.

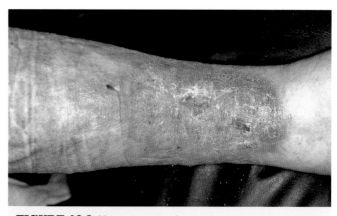

FIGURE 16.2 Venous stasis changes

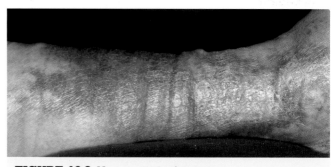

FIGURE 16.3 Venous stasis changes

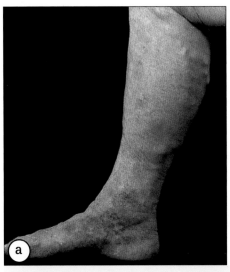
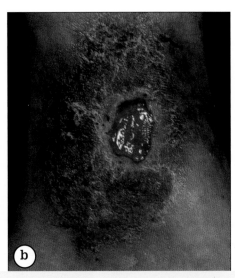
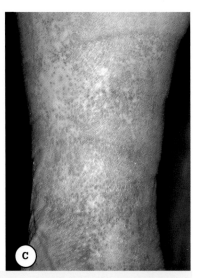

FIGURE 16.4 **(a)** Early dermatoliposclerosis, showing reddened, sclerotic plaques – note also the prominent, tortuous veins and the small patch of eczema over the medial malleolus on this woman's leg. **(b)** Pigmentation and eczematization around a typical venous leg ulcer. **(c)** Atrophie blanche is one of the changes seen in chronic venous disease

Patient problems

Whatever the cause, leg ulceration is greatly inconvenient and unpleasant and may lead to a significant reduction in mobility. The patient is generally in some pain, which is often worse when the ulcers are exposed. The presence of exudation, which may be considerable, is very distressing. Secondary infection often results in an offensive odour.

Practical prescribing

The focus in patients with leg ulcers is often on the dressings and in trying to establish which is best for the particular patient. In fact, it is more important to try and reverse, as far as possible, any underlying vascular problems – be they arterial, venous or both. Smokers should be urged to stop; diabetic control should be optimized. The opinion of a vascular surgeon is desirable if there is significant arterial disease.

Swabs should routinely be taken, although it is not always necessary to treat bacterial contaminants actively. Exceptions include beta-haemolytic *Streptococcus*, *Pseudomonas* and MRSA, where appropriate topical and systemic treatment may improve healing rates and reduce pain and morbidity.

In largely venous leg ulcers (which represent about 70–80% overall), assessment should start with an appraisal of the arterial supply, including Doppler studies (*Note*: these are unreliable in diabetics). If these are satisfactory the most successful treatment is the application of three- or four-layer compression bandages (Fig. 16.5).

LYMPHOEDEMA

Chronic lymphatic obstruction eventually leads to swelling of the limb distal to the blockage and lymphoedema, sometimes of astronomical proportions. This may follow any injury to the lymphatics, but is most common after surgery for breast cancer (when the swelling is in the arm) or pelvic disease (giving rise to problems in the leg or legs). Congenital hypoplasia of the lymphatics may also lead to the same problem.

Recurrent streptococcal cellulitis may complicate the situation, with each attack of infection further damaging an already parlous lymphatic network. Affected patients are best advised to stay on low-dose penicillin (or erythromycin in the allergic) for life.

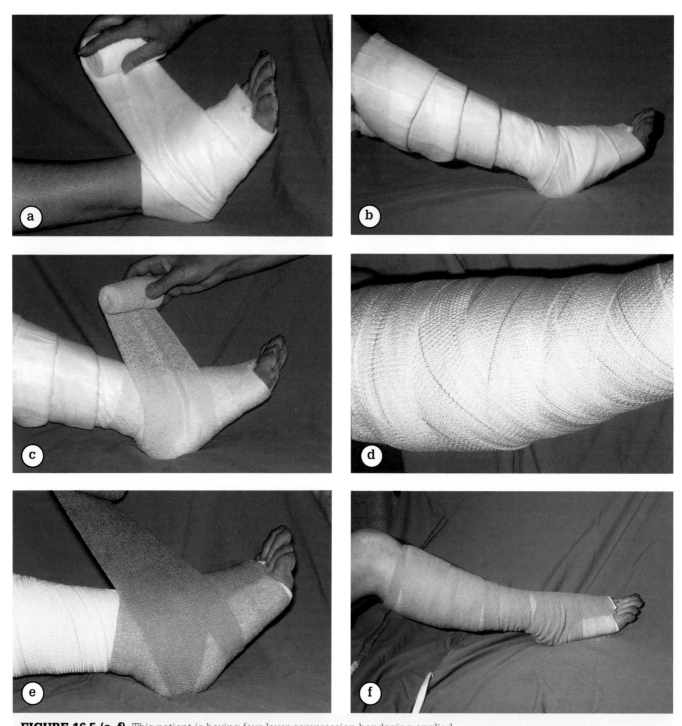

FIGURE 16.5 (a–f) This patient is having four-layer compression bandaging applied

Chapter 17

Skin Tumours

Summary

- Benign epidermal tumours
- Dysplastic and malignant epidermal tumours
- Naevi and tumours of melanocytes
- Naevi of dermal components
- Vascular naevi
- Disorders in which angiomas and vascular malformations are a feature
- Acquired benign dermal tumours
- Dysplastic and malignant dermal tumours
- Lymphomas
- Pseudotumours
- Subcutaneous tissue

There are hundreds of different types of skin tumour; some are very common (indeed there are some that probably affect the majority of us at some point in our lives); others are extremely rare.

This account covers those that are likely to be encountered in clinical practice and those which are important because they occur reasonably frequently and may cause significant problems.

They are listed as benign, dysplastic or malignant in groups based on the tissues that make up the majority of the lesion. Some tumours are naevi – essentially congenitally determined malformations of the skin.

For each tumour we aim to provide a core of essential information and, most importantly a guide as to what should and can be done.

Patient problems

For most patients skin lumps generally give rise to three main concerns that need to be addressed in deciding what, if any, action needs to be taken:

- The 'cosmetic' appearance.
- Some lesions are symptomatic or represent a significant nuisance (e.g. they catch or bleed).
- The threat of skin cancer.

This section will highlight only additional patient problems that arise with a particular lesion.

BENIGN EPIDERMAL TUMOURS

EPIDERMAL NAEVI

As with any other skin element, the epidermis may be subject to congenital anomalies. These take the form of various warty overgrowths, mostly present at birth.

They frequently follow a linear or pseudo-dermatomal distribution.

APPENDAGEAL NAEVI

Naevi may also arise from erroneous development of several epidermal appendages. Notable among these are:

- Naevus sebaceus (Fig. 17.1) – usually a yellowish/brown streak on the head and neck; hairless when in the scalp; may become warty over time; BCCs and other tumours may develop.
- Fordyce spots – small yellowish spots on the lips and inside the mouth; due to ectopic sebaceous glands; can give rise to undue anxiety when first spotted.

SEBORRHOEIC KERATOSIS (SEBORRHOEIC WART; BASAL CELL PAPILLOMA*)

Seborrhoeic keratosis is one of the most common benign skin tumours encountered in clinical practice. These tumours are much more common in the elderly, although in some families a genetic predisposition may result in lesions appearing at an earlier age.

Lesions may be solitary, but are frequently multiple, and numbers increase with age: there may be many hundreds (Fig. 17.2). They may occur anywhere, but are more common on the head, neck, and trunk. In black and Asian skin, multiple small lesions may appear on the face. This is often termed *dermatosis papulosa nigra*, but is essentially a variant of inherited seborrhoeic keratosis. On the limbs, lesions may be smaller and less pigmented.

---

*This term should probably be abandoned because of the unnecessary confusion it creates with basal cell carcinomas.

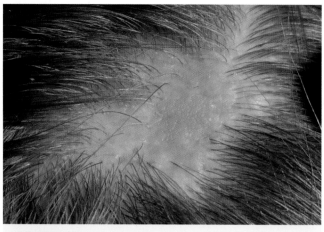

FIGURE 17.1 Naevus sebaceus

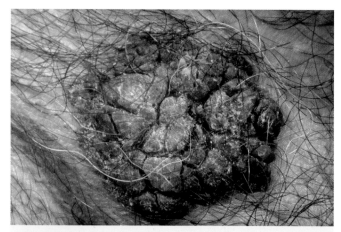

FIGURE 17.2 Seborrhoeic keratosis

Lesions are often pale, but become darker with time and may be very deeply pigmented. Lesions typically have a 'stuck-on' appearance. The surface is usually rather rough and warty and is often marked by plugged follicular orifices.

Patient problems

Very dark lesions can be very difficult to distinguish from malignant melanoma.

Investigation and treatment

Most lesions can be left alone. However, if there is diagnostic doubt, a biopsy (preferably excision) should be performed. If seborrhoeic keratoses are symptomatic, or if the cosmetic appearance is sufficiently annoying, they can be removed by curettage and cautery or treated with simple cryotherapy. They often recur.

CYSTS

There are three cysts of epidermal origin encountered commonly: milia, epidermoid cysts and trichilemmal cysts.

Milia

Milia (Fig. 17.3) are small keratin cysts which are seen in several different clinical situations:
* In newborn infants.
* As part of a familial trait.
* After physical trauma, blistering or inflammation in the skin.
* Arising spontaneously for no apparent reason.

Milia are small, rarely exceeding 2 mm in diameter. They are usually white or pale cream. In neonates, the lesions are scattered across the face. In adults, milia secondary to trauma or blistering may appear anywhere. Otherwise, by far the most common site for milia is the central face, especially around the eyes.

Investigation and treatment

The diagnosis is usually straightforward.

Neonatal milia disappear spontaneously. Those seen in adults may do so as well, although many persist. Although no treatment is necessary, the patient may wish the lesions to be removed, in which case they may be extruded following incision over the surface. A more practical solution for multiple milia may be the use of a fine needle and/or a hyfrecator.

Epidermoid cysts

Epidermoid cysts, are frequently called 'sebaceous cysts' (as are *pilar or trichilemmal* cysts, which are clinically identical), although neither has anything at all to do with sebum or sebaceous glands (Fig. 17.4). They often follow acne or some trauma to the skin, or may arise apparently spontaneously. They may be solitary or multiple. Each lesion is a dermal, cystic lump which can be felt to move over the subcutaneous fat but with the overlying epidermis. A punctum is frequently visible over the surface. The cysts may become red, inflamed and extremely painful. The most common sites for epidermoid cysts are the head and neck (especially around the ears) and the upper trunk, but they can occur anywhere.

Patient problems

Epidermoid cysts may rupture spontaneously, leading to considerable pain, swelling and discharging of purulent (though usually sterile) matter.

Investigation and treatment

Excision is usually curative as long as the sack is fully removed.

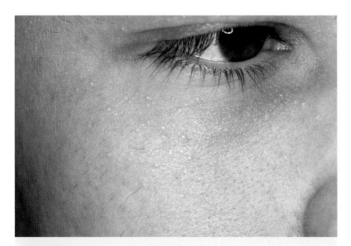

FIGURE 17.3 Multiple milia like these tend to run in families

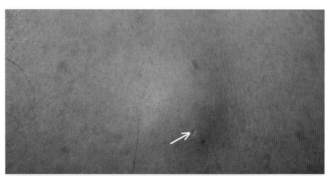

FIGURE 17.4 Fluctuant epidermoid 'sebaceous' cyst with punctum (arrow)

MALFORMATIONS/TUMOURS OF HAIR FOLLICLES

There are several malformations and true tumours of the pilosebaceous apparatus that result in skin lumps, mostly on the head and neck. Some are features of important genetic syndromes.

PILOMATRICOMA (CALCIFYING EPITHELIOMA OF MALHERBE)

It is worth mentioning this tumour, despite its rather exotic name, because it is commoner than is often appreciated. Classically a relatively deep-seated nodule in a child or young adult, the lesion feels very hard, almost stone-like, on palpation (Fig. 17.5). The surface will often reveal a faceted or tented appearance if the skin is stretched over the surface. They are usually found on the head and neck.

Patient problems

Apart from the obvious cosmetic concern, diagnostic uncertainty over a lump in a child, especially on the face, is sure to raise additional parental anxiety. It is quite common for such a lesion to be excised as 'lump ?cause' with the diagnosis emerging only from the pathology report. Patients and their parents can be reassured that the lesion is quite harmless.

Investigation and treatment

X-ray of the lesion may reveal calcification. Most patients/parents request excision of the nodule, but if the diagnosis is made on clinical inspection/palpation alone the decision will require a judgement about relative cosmetic outcomes of surgery or leaving well alone.

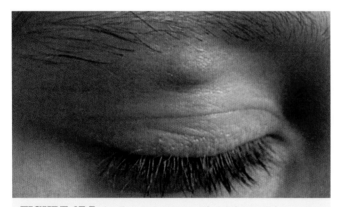

FIGURE 17.5 A pilomatricoma on the right eyelid

SEBACEOUS ADENOMA AND 'SENILE SEBACEOUS HYPERPLASIA'

These lesions are mostly seen in older patients (Fig. 17.6) and seem, for the most part, to represent one form of cutaneous ageing. There may be one or several lesions, usually on the forehead or cheeks, each of which is initially a soft, yellowish papule. As it enlarges, a rim may begin to form, which can make the lesion difficult to distinguish from a very small, early, basal cell carcinoma.

Investigation and treatment

Excision biopsy of a suspicious-looking lesion may be needed. Typical, multiple lesions may either be ignored or treated with simple destructive techniques, such as cautery, hyfrecation or cryotherapy. Cases confirmed as sebaceous adenoma should be discussed with a dermatologist as they ocasionally signify an underlying genetic disorder such as the Muir–Torre syndrome.

SYRINGOMA

Syringomas are said to be more common in women (Fig. 17.7). Most instances are sporadic, although familial cases have been described. Typically, the lesions appear as multiple, flesh-coloured, flat-topped papules around the eyes. They normally first arise in early adult life and gradually increase in size and number over the years. Very

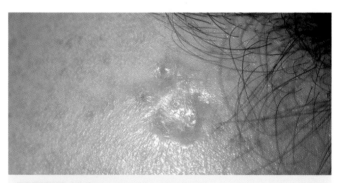

FIGURE 17.6 Sebaceous adenoma

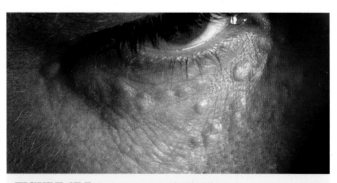

FIGURE 17.7 Syringomas in a typical site

occasionally lesions may develop on the neck and face and, even more rarely, over the lower abdomen or upper trunk.

Investigation and treatment

No treatment is very satisfactory, although gentle hyfrecation or cautery can produce reasonable results.

BENIGN TUMOURS OF SWEAT GLANDS

Sweat gland tissue may be the source of several different benign lumps. They may present as simple lumps, cystic swellings on the face, painful nodules or protuberant masses.

Investigation and treatment

They are often best excised and sent for histology.

DYSPLASTIC AND MALIGNANT EPIDERMAL TUMOURS

ACTINIC (SOLAR) KERATOSIS

Chronic exposure to solar and other ionizing radiation results in a number of changes in the skin, including a tendency for the epidermis to produce hyperkeratotic patches called *actinic keratoses*. They occur earlier in fair-skinned individuals and in those exposed to higher sunshine levels (Fig. 17.8). Actinic keratoses signal the fact that the skin has developed a significant degree of dysplastic change and that the patient is more likely to develop malignancy. Indeed, areas of actinic keratosis may progress to squamous cell carcinoma, although the potential for any individual patch to do this is low.

Actinic keratoses occur on any site that is chronically exposed to the sun: the face, ears (Fig. 17.9) and neck, the skin of the bald male scalp, the arms and hands, the lower regions of the legs. Similar changes occurring on the lip are known as actinic cheilitis. They present as scaly patches,

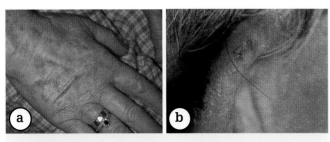

FIGURE 17.8 **(a)** Typical crusted solar keratoses on the back of the hand, ear, nose and forehead. **(b)** Crusted solar keratoses on a typical site: the back of the earaA

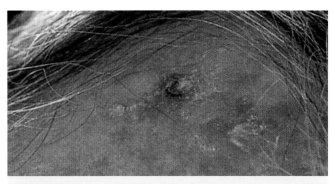

FIGURE 17.9 Actinic keratosis: multiple lesions on the forehead

often on an erythematous background. Most remain fairly flat and static in size, but some slowly spread laterally. Some become large, significantly elevated, and hypertrophic. They tend to wax and wane, and may disappear spontaneously. There may only be one lesion or there may be several, especially on severely sun-damaged skin and on the bald scalp.

Patient problems

The key issues for patients are:
- Ensuring that there is no skin malignancy present – and not just in the area of the index lesion(s).
- Dealing with patients affected by multiple lesions over large areas of skin.

Investigation and treatment

Remember that actinic keratoses = epidermal dysplasia. A more generalized inspection of sun-exposed sites is wise in any patient with actinic keratoses, especially when there are several present.

The next steps depend on the level of confidence in the diagnosis. If there is any doubt, it is best to send samples for histology. If the diagnosis is certain, individual lesions respond well to cryotherapy, although large lesions may be best curetted or excised. Minor lesions may be left alone as they often regress. It is when there are many lesions, over wide areas of skin, that difficulties occur. One alternative to multiple freezes or surgery is the use of the topical agents such as 3% diclofenac gel and 5-fluorouracil (5-FU) cream. These are both quite irritant, but, if used correctly, may be highly effective – especially 5-FU. A standard approach for 5-FU is to ask the patient to apply the cream to the affected area(s) of skin once daily for 3 weeks. A brisk irritant reaction usually develops during the treatment period, but this settles rapidly once treatment ceases. Repeat treatment cycles may be required to eradicate multiple keratoses. Recently, imiquimod has been granted a licence for the treatment of actnic keratoses. This causes very brisk reactions, but may find a role.

BOWEN'S DISEASE

Patches of Bowen's disease – which may be solitary or multiple – are red, scaly and well demarcated, and appear on any sun-exposed area (Fig. 17.10). They represent squamous cell carcinoma in situ and the risk of transformation into invasive carcinoma is low (approx. 5%).

Investigation and treatment

It is appropriate, in most instances, to take a biopsy to confirm the diagnosis, following which there is a choice of therapeutic interventions: excision of small areas; cryotherapy; curettage; radiotherapy. The decision as to which is best relates to the size and site of the lesion, and the age of the patient. Lesions on the leg, in particular, need to be treated gently, especially in older patients, because of problems with healing. On the lower legs an effective treatment is 5-FU cream applied every night for 4 weeks. Topical mupiricon ointment can be applied between weeks 4 and 8 to aid healing.

Some variants/parallels to Bowen's disease

There are three conditions which are essentially the same process as Bowen's disease:

* *Bowenoid papulosis*. This term has been used to describe the features seen in a group of patients who develop multiple lesions resembling flat seborrhoeic keratoses or plane warts, usually, but not exclusively, on the genitalia (Fig. 17.11). Histology shows the changes of Bowen's disease, but the lesions may resolve in time without treatment. The cause is almost certainly infection with human papilloma virus (HPV).
* *Vulval intraepithelial neoplasia* (VIN). A full discussion of the occurrence of vulval in situ squamous cell carcinoma will be found in good gynaecology textbooks. The clinical appearances may vary considerably, from a few flat lesions to gross epithelial irregularity and warty hyperkeratosis. The conventional classification, VIN I, II, and III, is based on the degree of histological 'atypia' present. Again, wart virus is probably involved in many cases. Any patient with such changes requires full investigation, including colposcopy and cervical smears.
* *Erythroplasia of Queyrat* (Fig. 17.12). This is the equivalent of Bowen's disease on the glans penis. There is no doubt that much dysplastic change on both male and female genitalia is associated with infection with HPV. Red, well-demarcated patches develop on the glans. There is a variable amount of scale, but often very little in the uncircumcised. Instead, the surface is often said to be 'velvety', but may be quite shiny and moist-looking.

KERATOACANTHOMA

Keratoacanthomas (often abbreviated to KA) are relatively common (Fig. 17.13). They are mostly seen in the middle

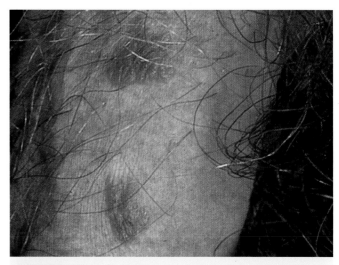

FIGURE 17.11 Bowenoid papulosis: two areas of lesions

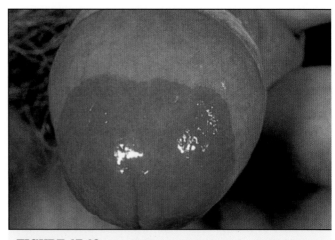

FIGURE 17.12 A well-circumscribed patch of squamous cell carcinoma in situ (erythroplasia of Queyrat)

FIGURE 17.10 A typical patch of intra-epithelial squamous cell carcinoma (Bowen's disease)

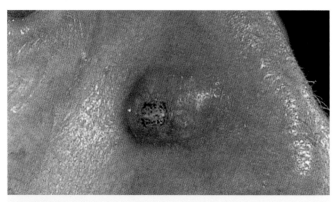

FIGURE 17.13 A typical keratoacanthoma

and later years of life, and chronic exposure to sunlight is likely to play a role in their pathogenesis. Other carcinogens, including tars and hydrocarbons, may be important causative agents in some patients.

Lesions present with several highly characteristic features:

- A short history of rapid growth, usually over 4–6 weeks.
- Initially, a small papule appears and is often dismissed by the patient as 'just a spot'.
- As the lesion grows, it becomes rounder, the edges become more rolled, and a keratotic plug develops in the centre.
- If left alone, the lesion shrinks and disappears – *this is an essential component of the diagnosis* – healing often leaving a small, puckered area in its wake.

Other key features:

- Size – most keratoacanthomas reach a maximum diameter of 1–2 cm, but very occasionally may be much larger (and in consequence are called 'giant').
- Number – they are usually solitary, but there are rare situations in which multiple tumours arise.
- Site(s) – keratoacanthomas typically occur on sun-exposed sites; most frequently on the face, neck, and ears, but they can occur on the limbs; giant keratoacanthomas are usually found on the arms.
- Pathology – this is not the place for a dissertation on histopathology, but the pathologist should be confident *if* the whole lesion is submitted for histology; with incisional biopsies – even quite generous ones – however, there can be real difficulty being confident that the lesion is not a squamous cell carcinoma (see below).

Investigation and treatment

An early keratoacanthoma can be difficult to distinguish from several other lesions, such as a viral wart, hypertrophic actinic keratosis, and giant molluscum contagiosum. The main issue, however, is to avoid missing a squamous cell carcinoma, some of which may closely resemble

a keratoacanthoma. Note, though, that squamous cell carcinomas usually have a longer history.

There are only two ways to be certain: one is to wait expectantly for spontaneous resolution; the other is to remove the lesion and submit it for histology. In the very elderly and frail, the former course may be reasonable. However, in most instances we would recommend formal excision. This probably produces the best cosmetic result, reduces anxiety and removes doubt from the minds of the patient and relatives, and provides useful histopathological information.

INVASIVE SQUAMOUS CELL CARCINOMA

Like its in situ counterpart, most areas of invasive squamous cell carcinoma (SCC) on the skin develop in older patients, particularly on skin exposed to high cumulative doses of ionizing radiation or other carcinogens. Particularly important are chronic exposure to radiation (e.g. ultraviolet radiation, X-rays) and to tar-derived compounds. SCC may also arise in areas of chronic injury, such as ulcers and scarred areas following burns or chronic infections. Another, increasingly important factor is chronic immunosuppression (e.g. transplant recipients).

SCCs may present a number of clinical appearances: small, scaly patches, very similar to actinic keratoses; larger masses; ulcers (Fig. 17.14). In chronically damaged skin,

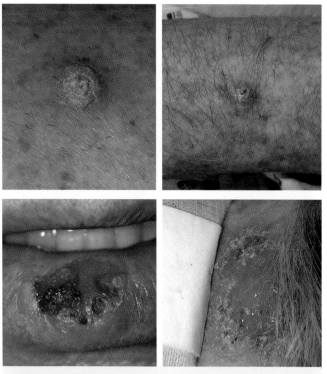

FIGURE 17.14 The spectrum of SCC is considerable, varying from nondescript warty papules to fungating ulcerative masses

the presence of SCC must be suspected if any new change develops: for example, an ulcer or nodule arising in old scar tissue or the elevation of the edge of an established leg ulcer. Sun-exposed sites are the most common areas involved in clinical practice: the head and neck (especially the front and rim of the pinna and the lips, the arms and hands, the lower parts of the legs. But beware! Occupational or other exposure to ionizing radiation may result in lesions in unusual sites. Genital SCC may be HPV-related.

Investigation and treatment

A biopsy is essential if there is any doubt, but, if the lesion is reasonably small the most appropriate action is excision with primary closure. Larger lesions may require plastic surgery. An alternative approach is to obtain a tissue diagnosis and then treat with radiotherapy. All patients with SCC or suspected SSC should be referred to secondary care.

SCCs are capable of metastasis and, while cutaneous SCC is, fortunately, not associated with a high rate of spread, lesions of the lip and ear, and those induced by radiation and other carcinogens, are more aggressive. It is important, therefore, to check for draining lymph nodes and to refer patients with any suspicious lumps for further attention.

BASAL CELL CARCINOMA ('RODENT ULCER')

Basal cell carcinoma (BCC), like other skin cancers, has become increasingly common over recent decades, especially in fair-skinned races. In some countries (including the UK), it is now the most common single malignancy in both sexes. The single most important factors are age and sun exposure, but there are also some who are more prone to develop BCC and may develop multiple tumours. Rarely, BCCs may be seen as part of genetically determined syndromes.

A number of clinical patterns of BCC can be distinguished:

- Solid/nodular – these lesions begin as small papules with a translucent quality, but, as they expand, a central depression frequently develops, often resulting in an annular appearance. A highly characteristic feature of these lesions (and of cystic BCCs) is the presence of telangiectatic vessels coursing over the surface of the lesion (Fig. 17.15).
- Cystic – in some BCCs, cystic change may result in a lesion of particular translucence.
- Morphoeic – some BCCs have a much greater stromal, connective tissue element which results in a flat or depressed area, closely resembling a scar or a small area of localized scleroderma. It can be extremely difficult to identify the edges of these tumours clearly.
- Superficial – BCCs, especially those occurring on the trunk, may exhibit a very superficial growth pattern.

Lesions present as indolent, reddish areas with a fine, serpiginous edge, often flecked with pigment (Fig. 17.16). The area continues to expand for years, leaving irregular, roughened skin centrally, but larger nodular elements may occasionally arise in these tumours.

- Pigmentation in BCCs: lesions are often partly pigmented and are sometimes markedly so, giving rise to diagnostic difficulties, particularly in distinguishing them from nodular melanomas (Fig. 17.17).

Solid, cystic and morphoeic BCCs typically affect the head and neck, specifically the face, the neck, and the ears and retroauricular area. However, lesions may occur in the scalp and on the limbs, and superficial BCCs are

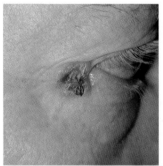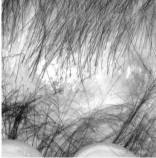

FIGURE 17.15 Typical basal cell carcinoma with telangiectasia

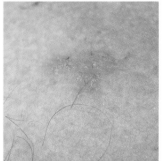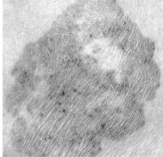

FIGURE 17.16 Superficial BCC

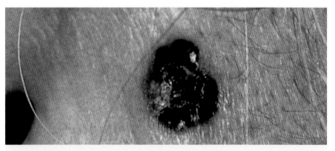

FIGURE 17.17 Pigmented BCC

most prevalent on the trunk. They may even occur in the perineum, although this is very rare.

Most BCCs are rather indolent, slow-growing tumours. Some (especially the superficial variety) rarely, if ever, create more than a minor inconvenience. However, occasional tumours exhibit a much more aggressive growth pattern, with rapid extension and invasion. This is particularly troublesome in tumours arising around the eyes, nose and ears.

Investigation and treatment

If there is any diagnostic uncertainty, an incisional biopsy should be performed. Small tumours are easily excised with the added benefit of cure. In experienced hands, curettage and cautery or cryotherapy are options for dealing with large superficial BCCs on the trunk, but there is a relatively high rate of recurrence. More recently, 5% imiquimod cream and photodynamic therapy have been found to be effective in the treatment of superficial BCCs.

Larger lesions may require the attentions of a dermatologic or plastic surgeon, although radiotherapy is an alternative, especially in the very elderly. For very large lesions, for those adjacent to the nose, eyes and ears, or for some morphoeic lesions, microscopically controlled surgery (Mohs' surgery) may be appropriate. This is a technique widely used in the USA and gaining ground in Britain, in which horizontal slices are removed and processed immediately. Areas with residual tumour islands are excised and re-excised until demonstrably clear. The resulting defects may be left to heal by secondary intention or repaired by flaps or grafts.

PAGET'S DISEASE OF THE SKIN

Paget's disease of the skin is rare but important. It occurs on the breast (when it is always associated with an underlying intraductal carcinoma) or at extramammary sites (notably in the anogenital region, where underlying cancers may also be found).

On the breast, the disease is unilateral. There is a fixed plaque of (usually) non-itchy skin over the nipple, or the areola, or both. The surface may be scaly or glazed, or may resemble eczema (Fig. 17.18). The area gradually extends and may occasionally ulcerate. There is no response to topical steroids. It is sometimes, but by no means always, possible to feel an underlying lump in the breast.

Extramammary sites are less easily diagnosed clinically, largely because there are many more differential diagnoses. On the skin, the changes may be very similar to those described for breast disease, but the lesion may also resemble a superficial epidermal lesion such as a seborrhoeic keratosis. In vulval and perianal skin, however, the areas become moist and reddened and more often multifocal. Lesions may extend into the vagina and anus.

Investigation and treatment

A biopsy is essential. A diagnosis of Paget's disease of the breast necessarily involves a mastectomy and it is crucial that the diagnosis is made as early as possible. In extramammary Paget's disease, a search for underlying tumours should also be undertaken: carcinoma of the rectum, cervix, vagina and ovary; rare skin tumours such as sebaceous and sweat gland carcinomas.

NAEVI AND TUMOURS OF MELANOCYTES

NAEVI OF MELANOCYTES

Melanocytes are derived from the neural crest. During embryonic life, they migrate and spread along the dermo-epidermal junction. In most of us, some aggregate to produce discrete lesions that may become visible to the naked eye and palpable to the probing finger: we call these melanocytic naevi. For the vast majority of people, this poses no problem apart from minor cosmetic inconvenience or discomfort. However, in a few people, the lesions have a greater significance, especially when they are precursors to, or markers of a genetic tendency to malignant melanoma. Conventionally, these lesions are classified as congenital and acquired. There is some overlap here because birth is an event with no specific relationship to melanocyte development. Some melanocytic naevi that appear in the early years of life are very similar to those that are present at birth – and may have the same significance. Conversely, some of those present at birth are small and behave in very much the same way as do those that arise later.

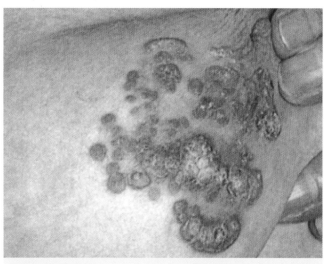

FIGURE 17.18 Paget's disease of the nipple

Congenital melanocytic naevi

Melanocytic naevi are present in approximately 1% of all live births. They are of significance because the giant type (>20 cm diameter in an adult or >5% body surface area in a child) carries a substantial increase in the risk of malignant melanoma. It is impossible to estimate the risk associated with smaller naevi but it is generally accepted that the larger they are, the greater the probability of malignant transformation – though it is nowhere near the risk with the giant type.

Smaller lesions are well-circumscribed papules or plaques whose surface may be smooth or rougher and quite verrucous. Hair follicles are frequently found within the naevi. Occasionally, several lesions may be present.

Larger naevi can vary in size, from a few centimetres across to the enormous giant melanocytic or bathing-trunk naevus (Fig. 17.19). In the latter, a huge area of the body surface is involved, and there may be multiple (sometimes thousands) smaller lesions present.

Patient problems

All forms can cause major cosmetic disturbance.

Giant naevi need specialist management and careful follow-up. Some authorities believe that very early interventions may be helpful.

The key issue in smaller lesions is whether to intervene and excise the lesion or not. In the absence of clear data on the risk of melanoma it is hard to justify excision if the cosmetic result will be poor, but parents and patients may want to discuss this in detail.

Investigation and treatment

Children with the rare giant naevus should probably undergo MR scanning because of associated defects (especially neurological), although it is debatable as to what action would follow. A photograph and recorded measurement of smaller lesions is useful.

A decision to excise requires careful consideration.

Junctional, compound and intradermal naevi

'Acquired' melanocytic naevi (AMN) arise, by definition, after birth. They represent abnormal collections of melanocytes. As they mature they pass through three sequential phases: junctional, compound, intradermal. Mostly, the junctional phase is predominant in children, adolescents and young adults, whereas compound and intradermal naevi are more evident in later life. Ultimately most, if not all, simple acquired melanocytic naevi disappear. The absolute number of naevi is important in that a very large number is, of itself, a statistical risk factor for melanoma. The presence of large numbers of odd-looking naevi raises the risk still further (see below – atypical naevi).

The clinical features depend on the phase in their development at which they are examined:

- *Junctional naevi* (Fig. 17.20). These may be slightly raised, but are largely flat, brown or black marks, varying in diameter from about 1 to 10 mm. The edge of a naevus is generally smooth and even, but may be quite irregular. There is a point at which the clinical appearance becomes sufficiently marked for the label 'atypical' or 'dysplastic' to be applied (see below); no matter how unusual the shape of the naevus, the normal skin markings on the surface are generally preserved.

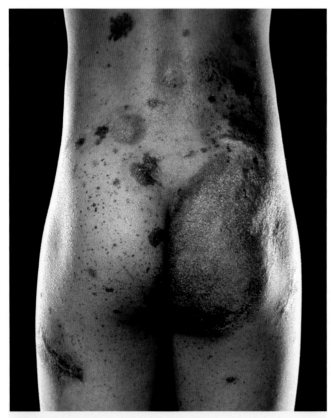

FIGURE 17.19 Giant congenital naevus

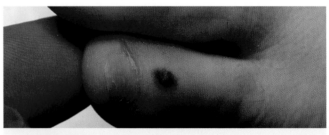

FIGURE 17.20 Junctional naevus

- *Compound naevi* (Fig. 17.21). These are fleshier and have an obvious dermal component on palpation. They may retain their pigment, but it is common for the lesions to become progressively paler and more flesh-coloured.
- *Intradermal naevi* (Fig. 17.22). The most common clinical appearance is of a flesh-coloured or pale-brown lesion that protrudes from the skin surface, sometimes to a significant extent.

AMN may occur anywhere, although some sites are only involved relatively rarely: palms and soles, genitalia, ears. The presence of several naevi in unusual sites is another feature that marks the patient out as having 'atypical' features.

Patient problems

The cosmetic appearance of AMN may cause concern but by far the biggest issue is the anxiety that they may be transforming into malignant melanoma.

Investigation and treatment

Excision of an acquired AMN is only justified on pathological grounds if there is a suggestion of malignancy, although there may be a case for taking some samples from a patient with the (rare) atypical mole syndrome phenotype (AMS) or (even rarer) familial atypical mole melanoma syndrome (FAMM) (see below).

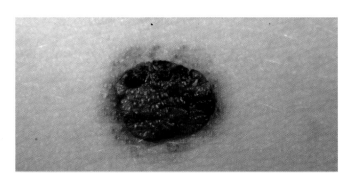

FIGURE 17.21 Compound naevus

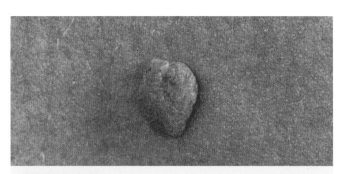

FIGURE 17.22 A pedunculated intradermal naevus

IMPORTANT VARIANTS OF AMN

'Atypical' or 'dysplastic' naevi

There is, as yet, no true consensus as to the status of AMN that fulfils the criteria laid down by various authorities under these headings.

Lesions described as either clinically 'atypical' or histologically 'dysplastic' are seen:

- Sporadically, as single lesions, in otherwise entirely normal people.
- In large numbers in people with, at the time of presentation, no other significant problems (and in particular with no personal or family history of melanoma). This is known as the '*atypical mole syndrome phenotype*'.
- In large numbers in people with a strong family history of melanoma (Fig. 17.23) and in whom melanomas occur with enormously increased frequency – the '*familial atypical mole melanoma syndrome*'.

Naevi are generally considered to be 'atypical' if they are over 5 mm in diameter and have an irregular outline. There are also some histological changes that cause a pathologist

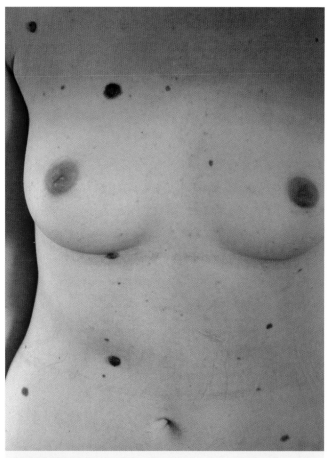

FIGURE 17.23 Familial atypical mole and melanoma syndrome

to describe a naevus as dysplastic. *The clinical and histological appearances do not necessarily coincide.*

Some people have several naevi that would fit this description and often large numbers of relatively banal melanocytic naevi as well. Such patients may also have naevi in relatively unusual places, such as the scalp, buttocks, and hands and feet, and melanocytic lesions in the iris. This phenomenon was first noticed when it was realized that these changes represented a cutaneous marker for a genetically determined tendency to melanoma, in the familial atypical mole melanoma syndrome.

However, the same clinical features occur with no family or personal history of melanoma, and the concept of the 'atypical mole syndrome phenotype' has been promulgated.

Investigation and treatment

There are disagreements about how to manage the individual with atypical naevi, but as a rule:

- For one or two: removal under local anaesthesia is probably the simplest way of providing reassurance and eliminates the problem.
- In FAMM the most practical solution is to arrange excision of some representative naevi; the patient should be counselled and followed up, and asked to look out for new lesions between visits; it is best practice to take an initial set of good clinical photographs and examine these at each successive visit, alongside the patient.
- In AMS patients should be referred for assessment and photography.

Education is important but long-term hospital follow-up is often not needed.

Sutton's halo naevus (leucoderma centrifugum acquisitum)

Quite commonly, a ring of white skin appears around a melanocytic naevus. The depigmented area is indistinguishable from a patch of vitiligo, with which this phenomenon may also be associated. Several moles may behave in this way. Different courses are possible:

- The pale patch may persist for a few months and then disappear.
- The central naevus may diminish in size and thickness, and even disappear completely, following which the area usually repigments.
- The changes may persist indefinitely.

Investigation and treatment

No specific treatment is required. Some parents and patients request removal of the mole.

These naevi may occur anywhere.

Spitz naevus

Spitz naevus is seen relatively often in children. In older texts and papers, these lesions were sometimes labelled benign juvenile melanomas.

The classical Spitz naevus is brick-red, elevated and firm (Fig. 17.24). Pressure results in a degree of blanching, but not to the same degree as is seen in a vascular lesion. Although usually solitary, multiple lesions may occur, and rarely a group of these naevi may be found (a situation known as 'agminate'). Spitz naevi are commoner on the head, neck and upper trunk, but may occur virtually anywhere.

Investigation and treatment

If the diagnosis is certain clinically, no further action is needed. However, in practice, biopsy and/or excision is often necessary to confirm the diagnosis and some experts recommend excision because of the very rare occurrence of malignancy in these lesions.

Blue naevus

Blue naevi are relatively common and consist of circumscribed collections of functioning melanocytes within the dermis (Fig. 17.25).

The lesion has a highly characteristic dusky-blue/black colour, with a smooth surface; it is rarely more than a centimetre in diameter. Although they may occur anywhere, blue naevi are most common on the extremities (feet, hands), the buttocks and the scalp.

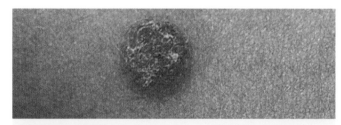

FIGURE 17.24 Spitz naevus: the typical 'brick-red' colour is well illustrated

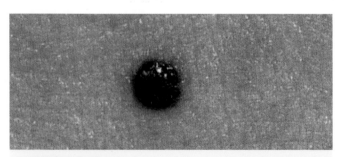

FIGURE 17.25 Blue naevus

Investigation and treatment

Clinical diagnosis is usually straightforward, but excision and pathological examination may be a sensible approach if there is any doubt.

DERMAL MELANOCYTOSIS

Mongolian blue spot

Mongolian blue spot occurs in over 90% of children of Mongolian extraction, but is also seen quite commonly in Indo-Asian and Afro-Caribbean infants. It is rare, however, in white European babies.

A bluish-grey patch of skin with otherwise entirely normal surface markings is present. The area may be quite small or may be very extensive; it normally fades during the early years of life, but may persist. The most common sites by far are the lower back and buttocks. However, very extensive lesions may cover large parts of the torso.

Patient problems

Patches are reported to have created suspicion about bruising and, therefore, child abuse in the unwary.

Investigation and treatment

Nothing needs to be done apart from reassurance that all is well. As it is, most affected families are familiar with the appearance and do not present for medical attention.

BENIGN ACQUIRED MELANOCYTIC LESIONS

Freckles (ephelides; singular = ephelis) and lentigines (singular = lentigo)

There is some overlap between what is congenital, naevoid, inherited and acquired in the classification of melanocytic lesions. Freckles and lentigines are descriptive terms for flat (macular) brown or black patches due to melanocytes in normal numbers but with increased reactivity (freckle) or increased absolute numbers (lentigo).

Everyone must be familiar with freckles that occur on the face, across the cheeks and nose, and on the upper trunk and arms.

Lentigines collectively occur most frequently as an isolated phenomenon, but are occasionally a feature of some rare genetic disorders, such as the LEOPARD and the Peutz–Jeghers syndromes. Some lentigines are seen in patients with sun-damaged skin and are termed solar lentigines.

Investigation and treatment

There is nothing to be done with or for freckles.

Investigation for lentigines is only required in the following circumstances:
- If there is any diagnostic doubt, particularly if lentigo maligna is a possibility, in which case a biopsy should be taken. Biopsy may occasionally miss an early lentigo maligna and, if the lesion is suspicious or continues to change, specialist referral is recommended.
- If there are a large number present, when the possibility of associated abnormalities must be considered and investigated accordingly.

Labial melanotic macule

The cause of these lesions is unknown.

Labial melanotic macules are what their name suggests: flat, pigmented areas on the lips. They can be quite large. Similar lesions have been reported on the genitalia.

Investigation and treatment

The major differential diagnosis is malignant melanoma. Therefore removal – or at least biopsy – is often appropriate.

DYSPLASTIC AND MALIGNANT MELANOCYTIC LESIONS

Malignant melanoma

There has been a dramatic increase in the incidence of malignant melanoma (MM) in white populations over the last 40 years. In many countries (e.g. Australia) MM is now one of the major cancers, accounting for a very significant morbidity and mortality. It is now the most common cancer of younger adults in the UK, although it is numerically more common in older age groups.

It is generally agreed that much of this increase is due to exposure to sunlight, and there is a large body of epidemiological evidence supporting this hypothesis. In particular, it seems that childhood sun exposure and a pattern of intermittent bursts of sun, accompanied by sunburn, may be important. There are also a number of individual risk factors that may determine any one person's chance of developing an MM in their lifetime:
- Heredity – there are some rare families with a vastly increased risk (see section on atypical/dysplastic naevi, above). A family history of MM also increases an individual's risk independently.
- The presence of large numbers of melanocytic naevi (whether 'atypical' or not) – this may also be linked to heredity and to childhood sun exposure.
- Skin colour/type – those with very fair skin, especially with red hair and freckles, are at an increased risk,

whereas those with genetically brown or black skin have a very low risk.

The prognosis of an individual tumour is closely related to its initial cross-sectional area and its level of invasion at first excision. Most pathology laboratories will provide a report indicating both the 'Clark's level' and a measurement (in millimetres) of the depth of tumour from the granular cell layer to the deepest visible point in the dermis (known as the 'Breslow' depth or thickness).

Broadly speaking the statistics are:

Breslow in millimetres	Percentage 5-year survival
<0.75	>95%
0.76–1.49	>80%
1.5 –3.49	60–70%
>3.5	<40%

There are two pre-invasive forms and four recognizable 'histogenic' types of MM that are seen in clinical practice:

Lentigo maligna (pre-invasive)

Lentigo maligna is seen in sun-damaged skin (Fig. 17.26). It is therefore predominantly found in older patients, although the lower end of the age range is reducing. The lesion begins as a small, brown smudge and gradually extends to produce an irregular-edged area of unevenly distributed pigmentation, often reaching a considerable size. Most lesions occur on the face. Exceptionally sun-damaged skin on the upper arm or trunk may also be affected.

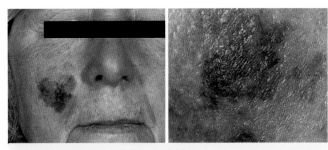

FIGURE 17.26 Lentigo maligna

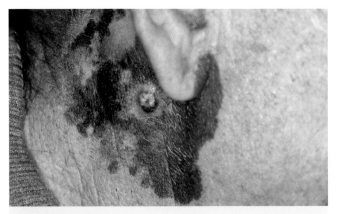

FIGURE 17.27 A nodule has developed in an area of lentigo maligna

Investigation and treatment

An incisional or punch biopsy will confirm the diagnosis. Although lentigo maligna can be eradicated clinically by the use of cryotherapy, excision should be advised for all but the largest lesions because of the risk of recurrence and the development of invasive change. It may be reasonable to be less draconian in a very frail patient.

Lentigo maligna melanoma

This term is used for invasive melanoma developing within a lentigo maligna (Fig. 17.27).

A nodular or thickened area develops within a pre-existing lentigo maligna.

Investigation and treatment

The whole lesion should be excised and sent for histology and assessment of the level of invasion.

In situ superficial spreading melanoma (pre-invasive) (Figs 17.28 and 17.29)

Superficial spreading malignant melanoma (SSMM) represents the most common 'type' seen in white-skinned individuals in most countries. SSMM begins with a phase of gradual extension along the dermo-epidermal junction, in a manner similar to lentigo maligna, before invasion into the underlying dermis occurs. This so-called radial growth phase may last for some years.

It is not possible to determine whether invasion is present on clinical grounds alone and both should be treated in the same way (see below).

Invasive superficial spreading melanoma.

This term refers to the point at which there is a distinct vertical element, with malignant melanocytes invading the dermis. It is at this point that there is a real danger of metastasis.

Superficial spreading malignant melanoma (SSMM) varies in size from a few millimetres to, rarely, several centimetres across. More typically, a lesion will be a centimetre or so in diameter by the time the patient presents. Most lesions have a degree of irregularity in their edge, and this feature is often marked. Irregularity of pigmentation is also a cardinal feature, often accentuated by areas of spontaneous regression, which are common. When the lesion is *in situ* it is macular. In invasive SSMM, or when a nodular component has developed within SSMM, the lesion may become more raised, and the surface characteristics may alter: there may be some scaling, bleeding, or ulceration.

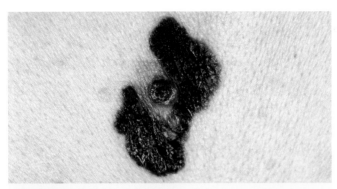

FIGURE 17.28 Typical examples of superficial spreading melanoma

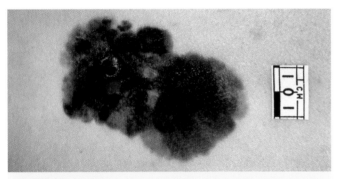

FIGURE 17.29 Typical example of superficial spreading melanoma

SSMM is most commonly seen on the legs in women. When it occurs in men, it is most common on the trunk, particularly the back. Lesions, however, may arise anywhere.

Investigation and treatment

Any lesion suspected of being SSMM should either be excised immediately with a clear margin with subsequent specialist referral for further investigation, or referred urgently to Dermatology. There is a considerable debate about the necessity for wide excision, which some protocols still advocate, especially for thicker lesions with deeper invasion. However, the most important treatment is an adequate primary removal. A debate on further surgery can be held once this has been achieved. All pathology reports should therefore contain an indication of the depth of invasion, usually using both 'Clark's levels' and 'Breslow thickness'. The role of other investigations, including scans, sentinel node biopsy and others, and the advisability or effectiveness of adjunctive therapies, remain a controversial and specialist area. Some dermatologists advocate special techniques for aiding the diagnosis SSMM. These include use of the dermascope, which is becoming a very popular addition to most specialist clinical assessment, and epiluminescence microscopy, which is only available in a few centres at present.

Nodular melanoma

Lesions present as nodules, sometimes smooth and dome-shaped, sometimes more irregular, and sometimes quite crusty and verrucous (Fig. 17.30). Nodular melanoma is not always pigmented, and a small halo of pigment can often be seen around the base of the tumour. Lesions usually arise and grow rapidly, and may be quite large at presentation.

Although nodular MM is said to be more common on the upper back, the lesion may arise anywhere.

Investigation and treatment

Treatment consists of immediate excision and histopathology, including depth of invasion. See the section on SSMM for further comments on what is necessary.

Acral, lentiginous melanoma

This is the rarest form of MM in white-skinned populations. However, it is relatively more common in Asians and in Afro-Caribbeans. Although originally subclassified to account for lesions on the palms and soles and under the nails, it has been pointed out that MM of oral, anal and genital epithelia present similar histological features.

The most typical presentation is of a flat, pigmented area on the palm or sole or a pigmented area under a fingernail or toenail (Figs 17.31 and 17.32). Pigmentation of the nailfold is suspicious of melanoma – Hutchinson's sign.

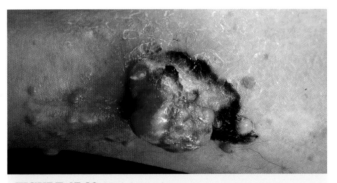

FIGURE 17.30 Nodular melanoma

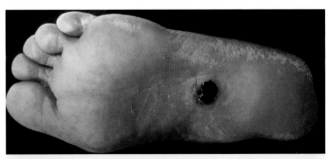

FIGURE 17.31 Acral melanoma

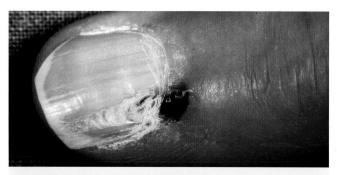

FIGURE 17.32 Acral melanoma

If it is not possible to distinguish between a subungual haematoma and an early acral MM clinically, the only way to tell is to take a biopsy, either by lifting the nail plate and sampling the underlying nailbed, or by performing a full-thickness nail biopsy.

Investigation and treatment

A biopsy is essential. If the diagnosis is confirmed, adequate excision is required. This may involve the amputation or partial amputation of a digit.

Prevention of death from MM

Efforts have been made in many countries to educate the populace about the links between sun exposure and skin cancer, especially MM. The pioneers in this area have been the Australians, who have been very successful in altering sun-exposure behaviour. Similar efforts will no doubt continue over the coming decades in all countries with fair-skinned people which have the resources to do so.

Primary prevention, however, will take time. Meanwhile, patients with MM must receive treatment as promptly as possible because, as indicated previously, the prognosis is related to the depth of invasion and, therefore, the sooner the tumour is excised the better. Education campaigns on early diagnosis have been run in several countries, with some apparent success in bringing patients forward earlier than would otherwise have been the case.

Treatment of late-stage, recurrent MM

MM is capable of metastasis to local lymph nodes and to distant sites, such as bone, brain, lungs and liver. Most dermatologists and surgeons keep patients with primary melanoma under surveillance for a period of time (usually a minimum of 5 years) and monitor their progress. Enlargement of nodes or the appearance of other symptoms should initiate appropriate surgery or investigations. Distant metastases are more difficult to treat because MM is not particularly radiosensitive and is notoriously resistant to most chemotherapeutic regimens. However, there have been

some remarkable apparent successes and most specialists can recall the occasional case where a patient has lived for long periods after therapeutic intervention. Immunotherapy has had its advocates and has recently been revisited, again with claims of success.

NAEVI OF DERMAL COMPONENTS

CONNECTIVE TISSUE NAEVI

As with other components of the skin, malformations and hamartomas may occur in the dermal connective tissue. Some of these are seen as one feature of multisystem syndromes (e.g. tuberous sclerosis, where the shagreen patch is a collagen naevus).

VASCULAR NAEVI

Vascular blemishes are very common indeed. Most cause no trouble or present relatively minor cosmetic problems, but some are very disfiguring and a few cause major difficulties. The classification of vascular birthmarks is by no means uniform and we are adopting a relatively simple approach.

TELANGIECTATIC NAEVI

There are two main forms of these lesions, which are both composed of dilated and tortuous, but otherwise essentially normal, vessels:
- The superficial capillary type.
- The deep capillary type (port-wine stain).

The superficial capillary type

Approximately 50% of all neonates have a salmon patch (at the nape of the neck), a stork mark (at the nape of neck or on the forehead) or angel's kisses (on the eyelids). It is often stated that lesions on the neck disappear, but in fact many persist, hidden by hair. Lesions on the face usually fade quite quickly and cause no further problems.

No investigation or treatment is needed.

The deep capillary type (port-wine stain)

Here there are vessels much deeper in the dermis and the vascular abnormalities may extend further, and deeper, during life. These lesions are permanent and are often very unsightly. They may also be associated with intracranial vascular malformations (the Sturge–Weber syndrome). Lesions may vary in size from a few millimetres to many centimetres in diameter and, very occasionally, may cover whole limbs or more. The colour also varies: some are a relatively pale pinkish-red, whereas others are very dark purple. All port-wine stains tend to darken as the years pass, and lesions may also become thicker with time. Lesions on or near the eyelid may be associated with glaucoma.

Many port-wine stains affect the head and neck (Fig. 17.33), but other parts of the body may be involved as well or alone. When a port-wine stain involves the area supplied by the trigeminal nerve there may be an ipsilateral intracranial vascular malformation, and this can result in mental retardation and long-tract neurological signs.

Any child with a facial port-wine stain should be assessed neurologically. Any child with a persisting vascular blemish on or near the eyelid should be referred for an ophthalmic opinion because of the risk of glaucoma. The treatment of choice is obliteration of the aberrant vessels using one of the modern lasers.

Deep arteriovenous malformations

Aberrant vascular development may also occur within subcutaneous tissues, with or without cutaneous involvement. The area is usually soft and warm. Many of these lesions are small and of no real consequence, but others lead to significant distortion of normal architecture and may need surgical correction.

Haemangiectatic hypertrophy

Occasionally, a patient presents with a vascular port-wine type birthmark or deep arteriovenous malformation associated with hypertrophy of the affected area, usually a whole limb, but occasionally a digit.

Angiomas (haemangiomas)

These vascular tumours are seen in infancy (Figs 17.34 and 17.35). They are slightly more common in premature babies. Some lesions are relatively superficial, while others are deeper, involving the subcutis. Very rarely, a child develops multiple lesions, sometimes in association with angiomas in internal organs (diffuse neonatal angiomatosis).

The most common presentation is of a rapidly growing, obviously vascular swelling in a baby a few days or a few weeks old, although some are present at birth. Most superficial angiomas are relatively soft, and somewhat irregular in outline. The deeper type presents as rather more diffuse swellings, and can be seen to have relatively normal skin overlying part of the area, at least at the outset. However, in many children, a deep component is accompanied by a superficial element on the surface. The size and extent are extremely variable, with some lesions reaching their maximum size quite quickly, but with others (especially those with a significant deep component)

continuing to grow and becoming very large. In the case of the deep type, large lesions may grossly distort normal anatomy.

Both types continue to grow for a few months (generally no more than six) and then stabilize. The majority also undergo spontaneous regression and may resolve completely. In superficial angiomas, this process often results in areas of necrosis within the lesion, which can look quite alarming. Just as lesions grow at different rates, the time taken for resolution to occur is also very variable. Superficial lesions usually start to resolve more rapidly than deeper lesions, but either type may last for some

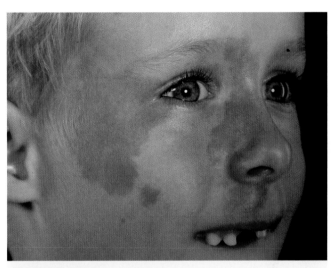

FIGURE 17.33 Port-wine stain

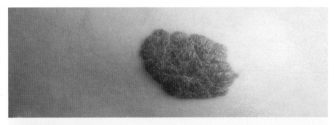

FIGURE 17.34 Haemangioma

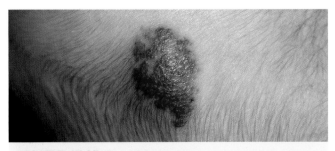

FIGURE 17.35 Small infantile haemangioma

247

years. An oft-quoted rule of thumb is probably not far out: 40% gone by the age of 4 years; 50% by 5 years; 70% by 7 years; and 90% by 9 years. Resolution may be complete, but larger lesions, in particular, often leave a significant cosmetic abnormality, either as a result of residual atrophic areas, or loose, redundant skin over the affected area, or a combination of both.

Angiomas may occur anywhere on the body surface, but superficial lesions seem to occur more frequently on the head and neck, and on the buttocks and perineal area, than elsewhere.

Patient problems

Apart from the obvious issue of parental anxiety over the prognosis and the best treatment, it is important to recognize that several complications may arise. Superficial lesions often ooze, especially after trauma. Ulceration is also common and may be part of the process of regression. Occasionally, this is complicated by infection, and cases of severe, life-threatening infections have arisen. If bleeding occurs within some rare forms of angioma, coagulation factors and platelets may be sequestered, leading to full-blown consumption coagulopathy.

More importantly, lesions on the face may obstruct breathing or feeding by distortion of the nose and mouth, and may interfere with vision. If this happens, and the eye is deprived of visual signals for more than a few weeks, complete amblyopia will result. Angiomas overlying the lower back, sacrum and buttocks may be associated with tethering of the spinal cord.

Investigation and treatment

In most instances nothing needs to be done apart from reassuring the parent and keeping a watchful brief. It is helpful to have available a picture or two of a child whose lesion has disappeared. However, many authorities now recommend that a scan be performed in a child with an angioma overlying the lower back or sacrum.

The main indications for immediate intervention and urgent specialist referral are: uncontrolled bleeding; excessive size; interference with feeding, breathing or vision. The treatment of first choice is a short course of systemic steroids (at no less than 2 mg/kg per day, and possibly up to 4 mg/kg per day), following which many lesions will shrink dramatically. The treatment must not be tailed off too quickly and care must be exercised in watching for systemic side effects. Injected steroids may be an alternative for smaller but troublesome lesions. Other options include sclerosant injections, embolization and laser therapy. Vincristine has been used.

Some patients will require surgical attention to correct deformities.

DISORDERS IN WHICH ANGIOMAS AND VASCULAR MALFORMATIONS ARE A FEATURE

Vascular malformations and angiomas are also a feature of a number of disorders and syndromes.

ACQUIRED BENIGN DERMAL TUMOURS

Dermatofibroma (histiocytoma, sclerosing haemangioma)

It is not clear how or why these extremely common tumours arise, although many authorities still cling to the notion that they may occur following minor scratches or insect bites.

On inspection, there may not be much to see apart from a degree of surface elevation and some discoloration (varying from a light-brown colour to quite deep pigmentation – Fig. 17.36). On palpation, however, a small dermal mass shaped like a lentil is found, which moves with the overlying epidermis. Gentle squeezing often evokes an apparent 'dimple' on the surface. It is not uncommon to see patients with several of these lesions. Less commonly, the tumour protrudes from the surface and, very occasionally, may be polypoid.

Dermatofibromas are much more common on the limbs, especially the lower legs. Women are particularly affected.

Investigation and treatment

Very dark lesions may need to be excised because of concern that they may be malignant melanomas. However, most lesions are innocuous and can safely be left alone.

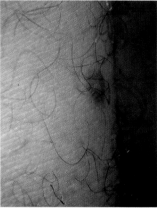

FIGURE 17.36 Dermatofibromas: firm, pea-sized, varying in colour from pink to brown

Fibrous papule of the nose

These small, firm, dome-shaped papules are nearly always found, as their name suggests, on the nose. They consist of a mixture of abnormal connective tissue and cells, some of which resemble naevus cells. They may bleed on contact and are often confused with cellular naevi and basal cell carcinomas.

Acrochordons (skin tags)

Skin tags are very common, increasingly so from middle-age onwards, and affect both sexes (Fig. 17.37). They are more prevalent in the obese and may arise during pregnancy. Skin tags are also seen in association with acanthosis nigricans.

Small, pedunculated, fleshy outgrowths are seen around the axillae, groin and the side of the neck.

Investigation and treatment

Tags can be removed easily by diathermy or hyfrecation or even snip excision with a pair of sterile scissors.

Acquired benign angiomas and angiokeratomas

Acquired simple angiomas and angiokeratomas are relatively common. Some rare angiomatous tumours should also briefly be mentioned here:

- *Simple angioma*. A reddish or purple papule that may appear anywhere on the body surface. It may be dark enough to be confused with malignant melanoma.
- *'Cherry' angioma*. Red or purple in colour, it is, strictly speaking, an angiokeratoma. It appears with advancing years and is often known as Campbell de Morgan spot. It has no sinister significance (Fig. 17.38).
- *Angiokeratoma of Fordyce*. These lesions are extremely common in older men and women and often pass unnoticed until one bleeds. Small, verrucous, purple papules appear on the penis, scrotum, or vulva (Fig.

17.39). They gradually increase in number and persist indefinitely.

Investigation and treatment

Lesions can be treated by cryotherapy, diathermy, hyfrecation, laser or excision.

Pyogenic granuloma

The term *pyogenic granuloma* is a misnomer. The lesion is essentially a rapidly growing mass of capillaries enmeshed in connective tissue. They are most common in childhood, adolescence and early adulthood, but may occur at any age. Trauma may be an important initiating factor.

The lesion arises suddenly, often beginning as a small red spot but quickly enlarging into a lump some millimetres across. The surface is initially smooth, but often becomes eroded and bleeds easily on contact. Many pyogenic granulomas appear to arise on a short stalk, with a collarette of hyperplastic epidermis around the base (Fig. 17.40).

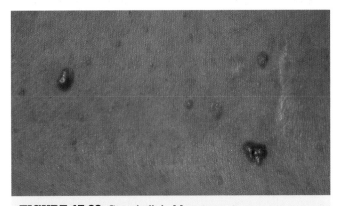

FIGURE 17.38 Campbell de Morgan spots

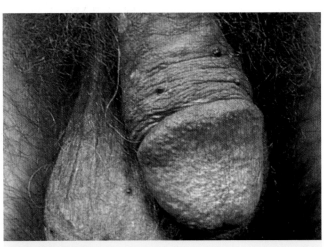

FIGURE 17.39 Angiokeratoma of Fordyce

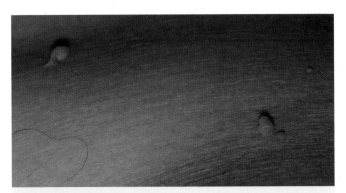

FIGURE 17.37 Skin tags

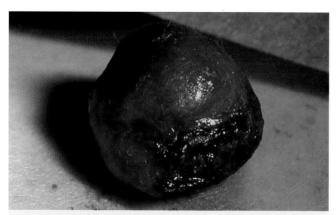

FIGURE 17.40 Pyogenic granuloma: bleeding painful lump

If left alone, many begin to organize, with an epithelium spreading over the surface. Some fibrose and disappear, but most persist as small angiomatous nodules.

Pyogenic granulomas are most common on the digits, but may appear anywhere. Multiple pyogenic granulomas around the nailfolds and on the upper trunk occasionally occur in patients with acne who are treated with retinoids. One of the important, if uncommon, differential diagnoses is an amelanotic melanoma which can look similar although tend not to bleed as easily.

Patient problems

These lesions bleed profusely, often with minimal trauma, and can be a real nuisance.

Investigation and treatment

Although pyogenic granulomas can be destroyed in a variety of ways, the simplest approach is to remove the lesion by curettage and cautery. By doing this, some tissue can be preserved for histology, which may be important if there is any diagnostic doubt. Lesions sometimes recur.

Neurofibroma

Neurofibromas are the main cutaneous feature of neurofibromatosis. However, patients without this multisystem genetic disorder occasionally present with solitary lumps that prove, on histology, to be neurofibromas.

Solitary neurofibromas usually present as flesh-coloured, dermal or subcutaneous nodules (Fig. 17.41). They may appear anywhere.

Investigation and treatment

250 Simple excision and pathology are all that is required.

DYSPLASTIC AND MALIGNANT DERMAL TUMOURS

MALIGNANT BLOOD VESSEL TUMOURS

Kaposi's sarcoma

Kaposi's (haemorrhagic) sarcoma was first described in elderly Jewish patients. However, this tumour has now been described in several different settings:

- The 'classical' form, largely restricted to elderly Ashkenazy Jews and northern Italians.
- In relation to HIV infection and AIDS.
- As a complication of immunosuppressive therapy, especially in patients with organ transplants.

In the classical form, purplish-brown patches appear on the extremities, particularly the feet, and very slowly grow into small, vascular tumours. Lesions can become quite widespread but this normally takes years.

In patients who are immunosuppressed, due to either chemotherapy or AIDS, the lesions crop up almost anywhere (Fig. 17.42), but often occur on the head and neck and in the mouth. They may resemble the lesions seen in the classical form, but can begin as very subtle, dusky, purplish patches similar to bruises, only later becoming thicker and more indurated.

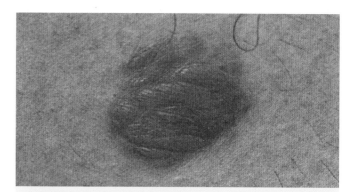

FIGURE 17.41 Solitary neurofibroma

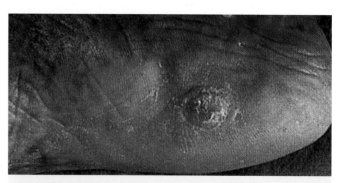

FIGURE 17.42 Kaposi's sarcoma: on the foot

Investigation and treatment

This is a specialized area.

The skin may be the primary site of a lymphoma, which, in almost all cases, is of T-cell origin, or be infiltrated by various haematological malignancies, including B-cell lymphomas (see also Ch. 6).

CUTANEOUS T-CELL LYMPHOMA (MYCOSIS FUNGOIDES)

A huge array of terms has been applied over many years to early phases in the evolution of this disorder (e.g. parapsoriasis-en-plaque, parakeratosis lichenoides, poikiloderma atrophicans vasculare), with the later stages often being called mycosis fungoides (MF). Many authorities now prefer the term cutaneous T-cell lymphoma (CTCL) to cover all the different manifestations of the disease.

In the early years, the lesions can be really quite non-descript, but are notoriously indolent and tend to be asymmetrical. Diagnosis in the early stages is often difficult because of the non-specific appearance of the rash and also the histology is frequently equivocal. Several biopsies may be necessary for different areas to confirm the diagnosis. In later phases of the disorder, tumours and ulceration may develop (Fig. 17.43). This may be accompanied by, or precede, systemic involvement, with lymphadenopathy and hepatosplenomegaly being prominent features.

Investigation and treatment

Any patient with lesions suggestive of CTCL should be managed by a member of a multi-disciplinary lymphoma team and a member of a secondary care dermatology department.

B-cell lymphomas

The skin may be infiltrated by B-cell lymphomas and other haematological malignancies.

A number of swellings may occur within the skin or the subcutis that are not true tumours: the so-called pseudotumours.

Chondrodermatitis nodularis helicis (or antihelicis) chronicus (painful nodule of the ear)

This very common lesion affects mostly older patients. It is thought to result from a degenerative and inflammatory process of the ear, probably with pressure acting as an initiating factor or as a cofactor. The individual lesion is a papule, often with a central plug which is tender on pressure (Fig. 17.44). Men are affected much more often than women. It is most common for the lesion(s) to appear

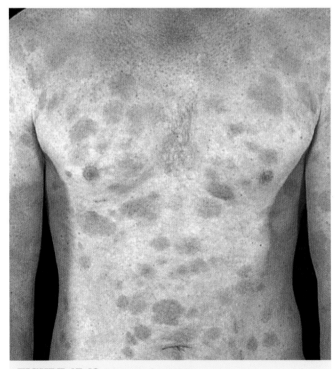

FIGURE 17.43 Mycosis fungoides

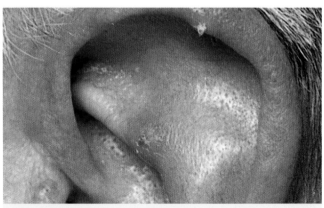

FIGURE 17.44 Chondrodermatitis nodularis helicis (or antihelicis) chronicus

251

on the rim of the helix, but they can also occur on the antihelix if this is particularly prominent.

Patient problems

The main problems with these lesions is the pain they cause, and the fact that they can be confused with dysplastic lesions such as basal or squamous cell carcinomas.

Investigation and treatment

Reasonable results can be obtained with injected steroids and cryotherapy. Taking pressure off the lesion at night by means of a ring pillow or similar appliance may also help. If there is any diagnostic doubt, however, the simplest approach is to excise the area under local anaesthesia.

Keloids and hypertrophic scars

Both of these conditions represent abnormally proliferative scar tissue. There is a degree of confusion about what differentiates a hypertrophic scar from a keloid scar. One authoritative textbook considers that the defining point is that a *hypertrophic scar* remains confined to the original dimensions of the injury, whereas a *keloid* extends beyond it. Another considers that the term *hypertrophic scar* is appropriate if the lesion ultimately undergoes a degree of spontaneous resolution. Use of either definition therefore means that the diagnostic distinction can only be made with a degree of retrospection and most lesions have to be treated *ab initio* as one and the same.

Hypertrophic and keloid scars usually follow some form of trauma (which may be remarkably trivial) or be a sequel to inflammation, such as that accompanying acne (see Ch. 14). Some keloids appear to arise without any preceding trigger.

Young people are much more prone than the middle-aged or elderly, although site may override this. Certain anatomical sites are particularly susceptible: the chest (and cardiac surgery scars are notorious for this), the upper back, the shoulders and upper arms down to the insertion of the deltoid, the suprapubic region and the ears. Afro-Caribbeans are particularly predisposed to keloid formation, although any ethnic group may be affected.

Hypertrophic and keloid scars present as smooth swellings in the line of a previous scar, injury or inflammatory episode (Figs 17.45 and 17.46). They are often itchy and may become quite red and livid. The area may continue to expand over many weeks or months until, in most instances, the process becomes quiescent. Large keloids, such as those following burns, may also produce significant contractures and deformity.

Investigation and treatment

The most satisfactory solution is to do as little as possible. Certainly, excision is highly likely to result in a recurrence, often larger than before. Some surgeons, however, maintain that postoperative radiotherapy or intralesional steroid/ haelan tape injections produce better results. A more conservative approach involves the use of intralesional steroid injections with or without cryotherapy. Furthermore, formulations of silicon can now be prescribed and can be used to treat early scarring or as a prophylaxis following surgery in high risk cases.

SUBCUTANEOUS TISSUE

Lipomas

Solitary lipomas are extremely common. Occasionally, multiple lesions are inherited as an autosomal dominant trait.

The individual lesion is a soft, lobulated, subcutaneous mass (Fig. 17.47). Some lesions appear to have a slight

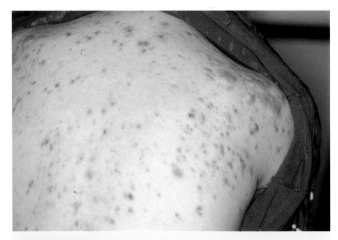

FIGURE 17.45 Extensive acne of the back, leading to scars, some of which are hypertrophic

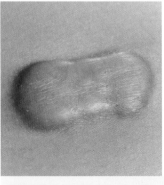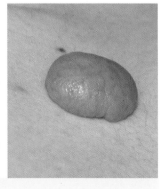

FIGURE 17.46 Keloid scar

increase in surface vascularity. Such lesions are sometimes painful when knocked. Lipomas can occur anywhere.

Investigation and treatment

Solitary tumours are easily excised. Multiple lesions are best left untouched.

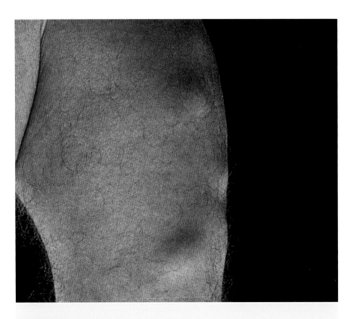

FIGURE 17.47 Multiple lipomas

Chapter 18

Disorders of Hair and Nails

Summary

- Disorders of hair
- Disorders of the nails

Hair and nails are formed from invaginations of the epidermis. Both may be affected by congenital abnormalities or by acquired diseases.

In some instances, both hair and nails are affected by the same process, but either may be affected independently.

DISORDERS OF HAIR

Three basic problems with hair result in patients seeking attention:

* Disorders of texture and colour.
* Too much hair.
* Too little hair.

DISORDERS OF TEXTURE AND COLOUR

A number of congenital syndromes exist in which hair texture and colour are abnormal.

Textural and colour changes may also be acquired:

* *Greying of hair*. A natural process; in some, greying occurs at a much earlier age than usual; this may be an inherited tendency; it may be associated with pernicious anaemia.
* *Kinking*. Acquired kinking of the hair occurs in some males as an early feature of male pattern balding.
* *'Dryness'*. Weathering and damage by chemicals, heat and harsh hairdressing techniques (including bleaching and back-combing) may lead to permanent changes in the texture of the hair.

TOO MUCH HAIR

Society dictates certain 'standards' regarding the normal amount of hair that is acceptable. It is conventional to consider 'excessive' hair growth under two broad headings (hirsutism and hypertrichosis), although 'excessive' may in reality be physiologically normal.

Hirsutism: excess hair in a sexual distribution

Essentially a problem in women, the presence of too much hair on the upper lip, face, chest and abdominal wall is usually 'normal' for that individual and the women in her family. Sometimes, however, there are underlying factors, the most common of which is the polycystic ovary syndrome. In addition to excess hair in a 'male' secondary sexual distribution, there may be acne and a tendency to a male body shape.

Much less commonly, there may be a significant endocrinological problem, such as congenital adrenal hyperplasia, androgen-secreting tumours or Cushing's syndrome. Hair in unusual sites, or recent, rapid hair growth should act as an alert.

Appropriate investigations should be considered if there is any doubt. Most clinicians request a full sex hormone screen, involving at least FSH, LH, SHBG, prolactin, testosterone and DHEA. The interpretation of results should be undertaken with care.

Practical prescribing

The hair can be destroyed physically in a variety of ways: shaving, plucking, depilatories, electrolysis and laser treatment. Cyproterone acetate may also reduce the excessive hairiness gradually.

A cream containing a hormone-blocker, eflornithine (Vaniqa), has recently appeared on the market, claiming to reduce hair density, thickness and growth.

Hypertrichosis: excess hair in a non-sexual distribution

This is also frequently genetically determined (Fig 18.1). However, hypertrichosis is a feature of some congenital disorders.

Some drugs – notably ciclosporin, hydantoins and steroids – induce hypertrichosis, sometimes quite marked.

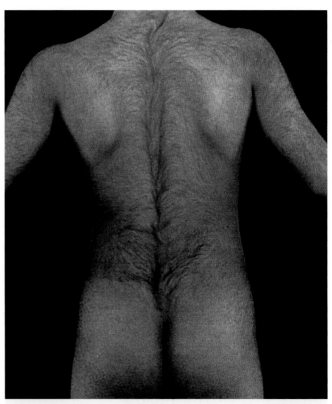

FIGURE 18.1 Generalized hypertrichosis in a teenage girl – this was normal for this family

It is also a feature of cachexia and of advanced anorexia nervosa. Localized areas of hypertrichosis are seen in pretibial myxoedema and overlying spina bifida occulta.

TOO LITTLE HAIR

Scalp hair density may be abnormal from birth, due to localized failure of development of the hair-bearing skin, naevi on the scalp or scarring from injury.

The normal density of hair for any individual is maintained by the fact that normal hair loss is matched by an equivalent rate of hair replacement.

Alopecia (a generic word for hair loss or thinning) may affect any part of the body, but is most noticeable and most frequently symptomatic when it affects the scalp.

Androgenetic alopecia

This is the most common form of alopecia. It affects both men and women, although it is worse and more likely to begin at an early age in men.

Presentation

In men, the appearances are well known and there is often a strong family history. Typically, the hair loss begins with temporal recession and is followed by a thinning and loss of hair over the crown. A rim of hair is retained around the parietal and occipital regions.

In women, the condition seldom progresses to such an extreme degree, at least before the menopause. However, thinning of the crown may commence early in life (Fig. 18.2a) and may become quite marked (Fig. 18.2b), particularly if there is a strong family tendency.

Patient problems

Despite the general familiarity with the condition, it is still a cause of great distress, particularly if the onset is at a very young age.

Practical prescribing

Treatment is difficult.

Minoxidil, if used daily over long periods, has been shown to improve matters, but it needs to be started early and used pretty much for good. It is not available on the NHS, but a topical lotion is commercially available. The 5α-reductase inhibitor, finasteride, is available for men on a private basis only in the UK at present. There is evidence that it works, but has the side effects that one would associate with anti-androgens.

Various replacement techniques using artificial hair are available, including hair transplantation (which relies on the permanence of the occipitoparietal follicles), hair weaving, and toupées and wigs.

Telogen effluvium

Human hair grows completely asynchronously – i.e. hairs are all growing independently. However, some 'life events' are capable of accelerating a rapid transition of many hairs into 'telogen' (the resting phase) together. This is followed some weeks later by a moult, as the old hairs are released from the follicles to allow their replacements to succeed them.

Presentation

The patient experiences a sudden and alarming shedding of hair known as a *telogen effluvium*.

Patient problems

There are few more upsetting experiences than a sudden loss of large amounts of hair, especially as the likely outcome is generally assumed to be that all hair will be lost.

Practical action

It is important to know that there are a number of common triggers: childbirth, coming off oral contraceptives, severe feverish illnesses, operations, extreme stress.

An explanation may be all that is required because the condition will settle over time, but it can unmask an underlying androgenetic alopecia, and scalp hair density may never return completely to pre-effluvium levels.

Drug-induced alopecia

A number of drugs can induce hair loss.

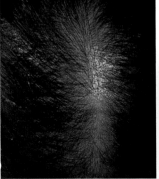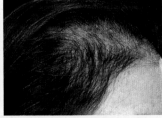

FIGURE 18.2 **(a)** Androgenetic alopecia – hair thinning over the crown in a 30-year-old woman. **(b)** More marked thinning in a young woman whose father was bald

257

Other causes of generalized hair loss with a normal scalp

A patient presenting with a generalized loss of hair should be screened for evidence of thyroid dysfunction and for iron deficiency. Both secondary syphilis and systemic lupus erythematosus are associated with a rather patchy, but diffuse, alopecia.

Trichotillomania

The term *trichotillomania* describes the deliberate pulling or twisting of hair, leading to fracture of the hair shafts and consequent alopecia (Fig. 18.3). It is most commonly seen in children. Scalp skin is usually normal, but may be mildly inflamed and scaly. There may be serious psychopathology present.

Traction alopecia and other physical causes of hair loss

Constant tension on hair follicles also results in damage, breakage and potentially permanent loss of follicles. This may result from particular hairdressing styles (Fig. 18.4).

Some people with very curly hair may damage the hair follicles with hot waxes and combs designed to straighten the hair shaft.

Some chemicals (such as perming solutions) can damage hair shafts, resulting in breakage, but permanent loss is very unusual.

Repetitive trauma to the scalp may occur if sensation is abnormal. One cause of this is postherpetic neuralgia, and the resulting damage is known as the *trigeminal trophic syndrome*.

Inflammatory causes of alopecia without scarring

Severe scalp psoriasis and dermatitis may result in temporary hair loss. Occasionally, psoriasis or seborrhoeic dermatitis may present with an extreme accumulation of scale, known as *pityriasis amiantacea* (Fig. 18.5). If the scale is removed, hair comes away too. This hair loss is generally temporary.

Cicatricial alopecia

Scalp hair loss with loss of follicles or with scalp atrophy is known as cicatricial alopecia (Fig. 18.6). The cause of such changes is not always apparent. However, the two most important primary skin disorders that give rise to this appearance are lichen planus and chronic discoid lupus erythematosus.

A careful clinical examination for evidence of skin disease elsewhere or nail changes should be undertaken. A

FIGURE 18.3 Trichotillomania – this girl had developed a habit of pulling and twisting the hair over her right temple

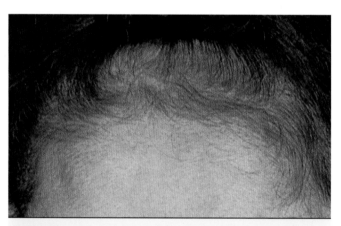

FIGURE 18.4 Traction alopecia – this Sikh boy has lost follicles around the front of his scalp. Similar changes occur with ponytails

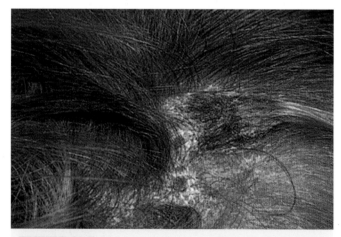

FIGURE 18.5 Pityriasis amiantacea – there is thick, adherent scale appearing to cling to a bunch of hair follicles. When this scale is lifted away, the hairs usually come away too

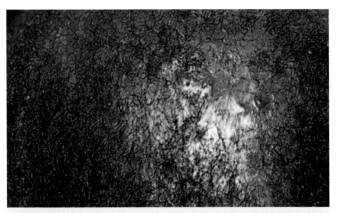

FIGURE 18.6 Cicatricial alopecia, showing widespread hair loss and loss of follicles

biopsy for histology, immunofluorescence and a screen for lupus erythematosus should be performed.

Treatment is mostly symptomatic, but some patients respond well to topical, intralesional or systemic steroids.

Alopecia areata, totalis and universalis

Alopecia areata is a very variable disorder and is thought to be an autoimmune process; organ-specific autoantibodies are found in some patients and there is an association with vitiligo. Alopecia areata is more common in patients with Down's syndrome.

Presentation

The typical appearances are of circumscribed patches of hair loss with no cutaneous alteration at all (Fig. 18.7), but there may occasionally be mild redness. The cardinal sign of this condition is the presence, usually at the edge of the area, of short, stubby hairs that taper towards the base – so-called exclamation-mark hairs (Fig. 18.8). Areas other than the

scalp are often involved, especially the eyebrows (Fig. 18.9), eyelashes and beard.

If the condition affects the whole scalp, it is known as *alopecia totalis*.

If the whole body is affected, it is called *alopecia universalis* (Fig. 18.10).

This nomenclature may seem somewhat artificial, since these clinical manifestations are really due to one and the same process. However, prognostically, the more extensive the process becomes, the less likely it is that it will resolve.

Patients often have fine pits in the nails (Fig. 18.11), especially in more extensive disease.

Patient problems

As with other causes of hair loss, patients are usually emotionally disturbed. The natural history of limited

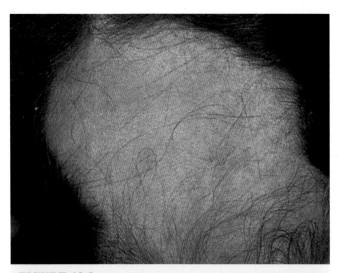

FIGURE 18.8 Alopecia areata – exclamation-mark hairs can be seen at the right edge of this area

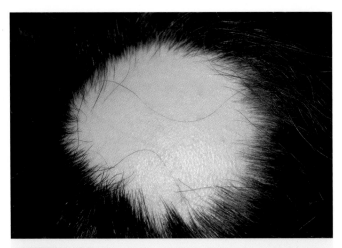

FIGURE 18.7 The characteristic complete loss of hair with normal scalp skin seen in alopecia areata

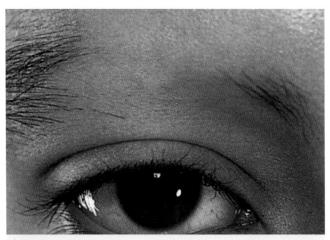

FIGURE 18.9 Alopecia areata – eyebrow involvement is common

outweigh the benefit since the hair nearly always falls out as soon as the treatment ceases. Topical sensitization therapy with diphencyprone (DCP) may be of value, but is restricted to widespread, resistant alopecia. A contact dermatitis is deliberately induced with the DCP, and the skin is repeatedly challenged with the antigen.

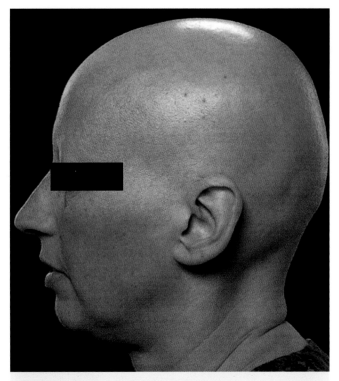

FIGURE 18.10 Alopecia universalis – this woman has no hair anywhere

DISORDERS OF THE NAILS

CHANGES OF TEXTURE AND SHAPE

Nails are subject to repeated trauma in normal daily life. It is hardly surprising, therefore, that they may be texturally abnormal or become physically damaged.

However, there are some changes that are worthy of specific mention because they are encountered frequently or because they represent significant pathology:

- *Onychogryphosis.* The nails become grossly thickened and distorted, usually in older patients (Fig. 18.12).
- *Koilonychia.* This classical sign of iron deficiency (Fig. 18.13) is more commonly seen as an inherited tendency.

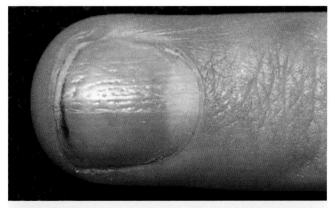

FIGURE 18.11 Fine pits in the nails are characteristic of alopecia areata

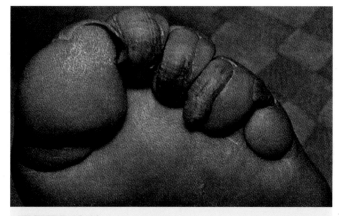

FIGURE 18.12 Onychogryphosis

disease is actually pretty good: smaller areas will regrow in most instances. Exceptions, where the prognosis is generally poor, include very extensive alopecia and areas around the nape of the neck.

Practical prescribing

Treatment with intralesional steroids may help and, while there is no concrete proof that topical steroids are of value, they are frequently offered. Systemic steroids may bring about temporary hair growth, but the risks probably

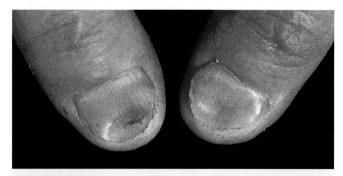

FIGURE 18.13 Koilonychia – this woman's mother and daughter had similar nails

- *Median nail dystrophy*. A habit-tic of 'fiddling' with the central paronychial area can lead to permanent nailplate changes (Fig. 18.14).
- *Pits*. Seen in psoriasis and alopecia areata.
- *Coarse dents and ridges*. May occur in the ezcemas.
- *Beau's lines*. Arrested nail growth, due to systemic illness or upset, may lead to a horizontal depression (Fig. 18.15). Occasionally, the nails may be lost temporarily.
- *Clubbing*. This is really an expansion of the finger end, but is an important sign of malignancy and of liver and cardiopulmonary disease.
- *Onycholysis*. Lifting of the nailplate is common in psoriasis and fungal infections; it may occur as an isolated phenomenon or, very rarely indeed, may be seen in thyrotoxicosis.
- *Leuconychia*. White marks in the nails are almost universal.
- *Black areas*. Especially if there is involvement of the nailfold (Hutchinson's sign), is an important sign of subungual melanoma.

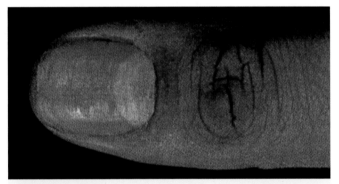

FIGURE 18.14 Median nail dystrophy – there are horizontal ridges down the centre of the nail – sometimes known as washboard nail. The appearance is due to habitual minor trauma to the paronychium

CONGENITAL ABNORMALITIES OF THE NAILS

Almost any change may occur as a developmental defect, from relatively trivial abnormalities to complete absence of all nails.

NAIL CHANGES ASSOCIATED WITH ACQUIRED DISEASE

The nail changes of psoriasis and lichen planus are discussed elsewhere. Those seen in alopecia areata are illustrated in Figure 18.11. There are a number of other conditions with relatively characteristic nail changes which deserve specific mention.

The yellow-nail syndrome

The yellow-nail syndrome is seen almost exclusively in adults. The nails in this disorder are overcurved, yellow and hardly grow (Fig. 18.16). Patients notice a gradual change in their nails. However, once the changes are established, the nails remain unchanged for the rest of the patient's life. There are a number of important associations: lymphoedema, pleural effusions and bronchiectasis. This syndrome has also been described in AIDS.

Trachyonychia and twenty-nail dystrophy

Children occasionally present with an onset of roughness (trachyonychia) that affects all twenty nails – although not always all at once (Fig. 18.17). The appearances are very similar to those seen when there is very extensive pitting, and some children have had, have, or will develop, alopecia areata. The histology in some instances is lichenoid.

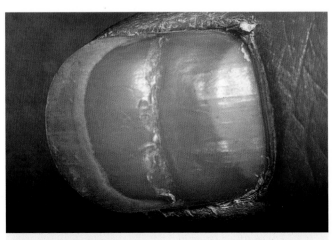

FIGURE 18.15 Beau's lines

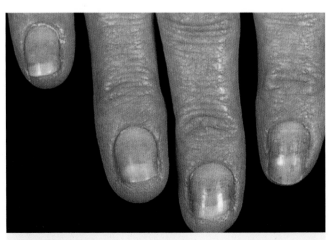

FIGURE 18.16 Yellow-nail syndrome

Exostoses and other space-occupying lesions of the nail bed

Any tumour or mass beneath the nail may cause it to lift from its base. One very common lesion is an exostosis of the terminal phalanx (Fig. 18.18), which can easily be seen on X-ray. Surgical excision cures the problem. Other tumours may also develop under the nail. Melanoma has been discussed in Chapter 4. Naevi can arise in the nailbed and give rise to longitudinal brown streaks. Glomus tumours, although rare, are also classically found in the nails. They are usually exquisitely painful.

Paronychial disorders

Acute paronychia (or 'whitlow') is usually due to a staphylococcal infection. Herpetic infections may occur in the periungual area, as may warts. Large masses of viral wart in the paronychium can be a real nuisance and are very difficult to treat.

Ingrowing toenails are painful and unpleasant. They are due to lateral overcurvature of the nails, with the edges digging into the paronychial tissue, and cause chronic or acute-on-chronic sepsis. Most cases can be managed conservatively and the patient encouraged to let their nails grow out and be cut straight. However, if the problem is recurrent , surgery is required: a wedge excision may help, but complete nailplate ablation may be required.

Chronic swelling and inflammation of the paronychium (Fig. 18.19) is often due to a combination of factors. Repeated damage and friction from occupational activities (packing, washing up, catering), especially if associated with damp conditions, predispose to the development of chronic paronychia. Candidal superinfection may also be important. Treatment is very difficult. Gloves often make matters worse by causing the hands to sweat. Anti-candidal agents may help, but the condition frequently persists, despite the best endeavours of patient and physician alike.

Myxoid cysts

Another common presentation is of a small lump (or lumps) near the nail (or nails) of either hands or feet. If punctured, these exude a clear, gelatinous fluid. There is often a longitudinal depression in the nail (Fig. 18.20).

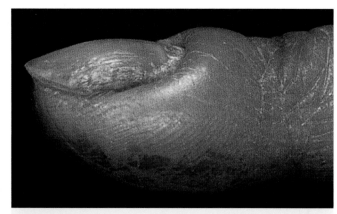

FIGURE 18.19 Chronic swelling and inflammation of the paronychium

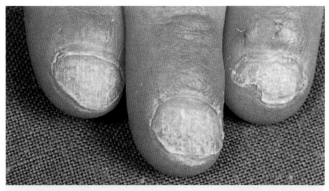

FIGURE 18.17 Trachyonychia – this girl's nails cleared spontaneously after about 3 years

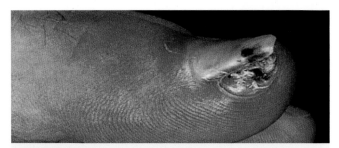

FIGURE 18.18 An exostosis of the terminal phalanx

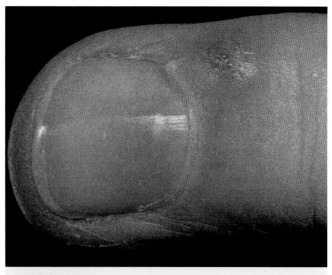

FIGURE 18.20 A slightly inflamed myxoid cyst with a depressed proximal nail and a longitudinal groove in the nailplate

Chapter 19

Drug Eruptions

For a comprehensive and very useful manual of cutaneous drug eruptions, the reader is referred to *Litt's Drug Eruption Reference Manual*, published by Taylor & Francis.

Presentation

There are numerous different cutaneous drug eruptions, and there is a vast array of potential triggers. Most occur within 3 weeks of the start of the offending agent, but that is not an invariable feature.

They are more common in patients with altered immunity, especially AIDS.

Patient problems

The key problem is usually deciding which, if any, of a cocktail of drugs might have been the trigger for a skin eruption. In practice this remains an inexact art, because allergy testing is largely unreliable, with the notable exception of patch testing for suspected contact sensitivity to topical therapies (see Ch. 10).

Decisions are therefore largely based on an intelligent assessment of which drug is the most likely to be responsible. The key factors to consider are:

- The nature of the eruption – as a general rule, any drug may cause any type of reaction; however, particular drugs are more commonly associated with specific reactions (see Box 19.1).

- The relationship between the eruption and the introduction of the possible drug or drugs – it is most likely (though not certain) that any given reaction is due to the most recent addition.
- The track record of a particular drug – some (e.g. sulfonamides) are much more common causes of reactions than others.

Practical prescribing

In most instances it is simply sufficient to identify the offending agent and stop it. In the case of a severe reaction, it may be necessary to offer some treatment. Antihistamines

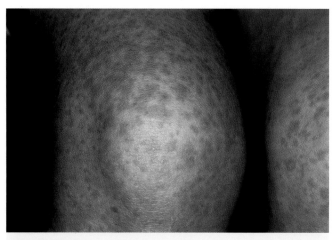

FIGURE 19.1 Morbilliform

BOX 19.1 Important patterns of drug eruption and causes

Morbilliform (Figs 19.1 and 19.2)	Antibiotics; antihypertensives; NSAIDs; barbiturates; hydantoins
Urticaria/anaphylaxis	Penicillin; vaccines; toxoids; aspirin; codeine
Fixed drug eruption	Phenolphthalein; tetracyclines; sulfas; quinine; paracetamol
Lichenoid	Beta-blockers; antimalarials; thiazides; gold; penicillamine; phenothiazines
Vasculitis	Thiazides; allopurinol; penicillin; sulfas; quinolones
Erythema multiforme (including Stevens–Johnson syndrome) (see Figs 13.8 and 13.9)	Barbiturates; sulfas; hydantoins; thiazides, NSAIDs; phenothiazines; rifampicin
Toxic epidermal necrolysis	Sulfas; NSAIDs
Bullous eruptions	Penicillamine; rifampicin; barbiturates; nalidixic acid; induction of porphyria cutanea tarda by oestrogens, etc.
LE-like syndrome	Hydantoins; hydralazine; grisefulvin; isoniazid; minocycline
Photosensitivity	Amiodarone; phenothiazines; nalidixic acid; tetracyclines, thiazides, quinolones; sulfas
Acneiform	Steroids; androgens; lithium; iodides
Pigmentary anomalies (Fig. 19.3)	Minocycline; mepacrine; chloroquine; silver; gold;
Eczema/contact dermatitis	Aminoglycosides; anaesthetics; antihistamines; ingredients in topical preparations (see Ch. 10)

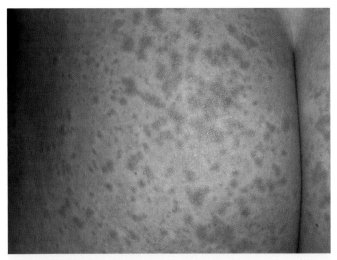

FIGURE 19.2 Morbilliform

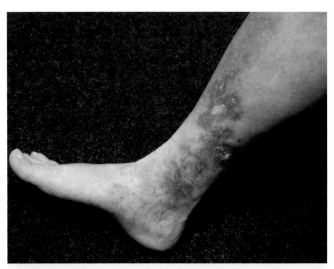

FIGURE 19.3 Minocycline hyperpigmentation in a patient with vasculitis

are useful in urticaria and sedative agents may reduce the itch of other eruptions. Similarly, topical steroids may be symptomatically helpful. It is only rarely necessary to prescribe systemic steroids, while anaphylaxis, of course, requires urgent interventions with adrenaline (epinephrine) and other life support.

Patients should be informed that they are intolerant of, or allergic to, a drug or group of drugs. They should be advised to pass this information on to their next of kin, and to carry something that will assist others in the event that they are too ill to talk – e.g. an alert bracelet.

Chapter 20

Less Common Disorders

Summary

- Pityriasis rosea
- Bullous disorders
- Lichen planus
- Cutaneous lupus erythematosus
- Lichen sclerosus
- Granuloma annulare and necrobiosis lipoidica
- Photosensitivity – light-induced disorders
- Skin signs of systemic disease

PITYRIASIS ROSEA

Pityriasis rosea is one of the most striking eruptions seen in clinical practice.

Presentation

The history and clinical features are almost always the same. An otherwise healthy child or young adult may feel slightly 'under the weather' and develops a scaly red patch somewhere on the trunk, upper thigh or shoulder (Fig. 20.1). This may be mistaken for a fungal infection or a patch of eczema, but is, in fact a *herald patch – larger than the other lesions*, which is followed some days later by a florid eruption of pink (hence, rosea), oval patches (Figs 20.2 and 20.3). These are nearly always on the trunk, upper arms and legs only. It is rare for lesions to involve the forearms, lower legs and face. On the trunk, the lesions are arranged with their longer axis seeming to follow the spinal nerves around the trunk. This sign (the 'inverted Christmas tree') is pathognomonic of the disorder.

On the surface of each oval patch there is a light, scurfy scale which appears centrally and rapidly spreads across the patch to produce the classical *peripheral collarette* (see Fig. 20.2).

Patient problems

The eruption lasts for approximately 6–8 weeks before disappearing, usually for ever. Some patients experience significant itching but many have no symptoms.

Practical prescribing

It may be worth considering syphilis serology if the appearance of the eruption is somewhat atypical – certainly if there are lesions on the palms and soles, and the patient is in a risk group. Treatment only needs to be symptomatic as the eruption inevitably settles spontaneously. Mild topical corticosteroids offer relief to some patients.

BULLOUS DISORDERS

The most common causes of blisters are trauma (burns – chemical/mechanical/thermal) and infections (impetigo, zoster, tinea, insect bites etc.). Inflammatory disorders such as severe dermatitis and drug reactions are also relatively common causes. These conditions are dealt with in the relevant section of this book.

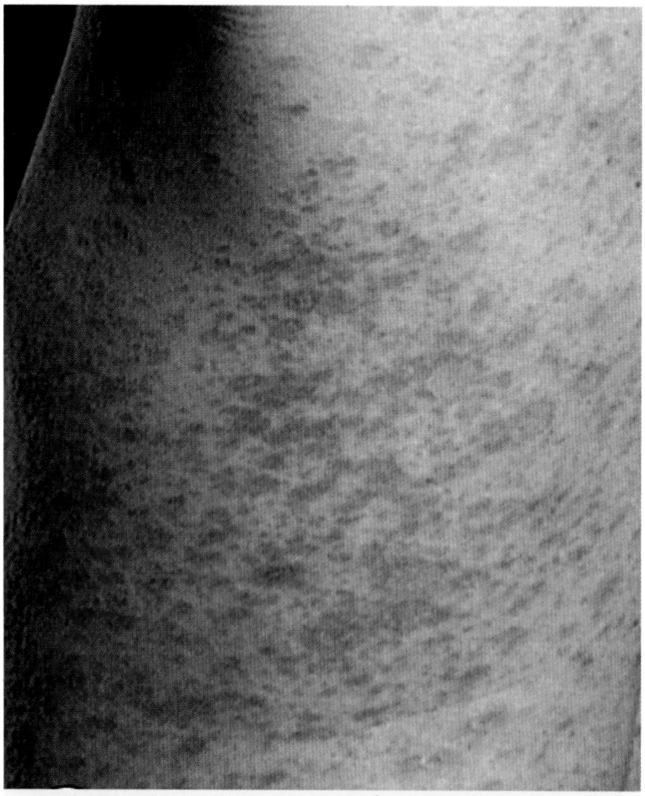

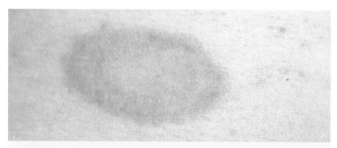

FIGURE 20.2 Pityriasis rosea – herald patch showing characteristic peripheral collarette of scale

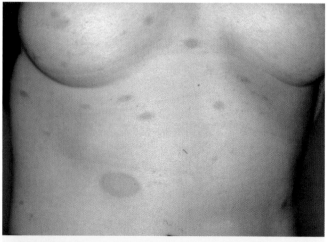

FIGURE 20.3 The eruption of pityriasis rosea; this example is not particularly florid

FIGURE 20.1 Pityriasis rosea – typical distribution following the lines of the ribs, on the sides of the trunk

Autoimmune blistering diseases are important causes of widespread blistering and we deal with the three key conditions here.

Pemphigus

Presentation

Pemphigus is a very rare disease. It presents with erosions and, sometimes, a few flaccid blisters (Figs 20.4 and 20.5). The process often begins in the mouth and may affect the genitalia and the conjunctivae. The erosions are very slow to heal, with new areas 'stripping off' around existing patches.

Patient problems

Patients often feel poorly – they certainly do if skin loss has become extensive. Eating can be troublesome if oral involvement is significant, and there may be dysuria.

Untreated there is a high mortality.

Practical prescribing

The disease needs aggressive treatment after diagnostic confirmation. High-dose steroids (40–60 mg prednisolone daily) and immunosuppressive medication is almost always required: azathioprine is probably the most commonly used drug (100–200 mg daily). This may need to be maintained for many months and years. Patients also need good acute and long-term nursing support to provide good skin care.

Pemphigoid

Presentation

Pemphigoid (or bullous pemphigoid, BP) is much more common. A disease of the elderly, BP is also less threatening than pemphigus, although it can be a real nuisance.

Typically tense blisters (which may be blood-filled) appear on an itchy, eczematous background (Fig. 20.6). Sometimes the pre-pemphigoid rash is present for weeks before blisters appear. The blisters emerge in crops and burst or resorb, with reasonably good healing.

Patient problems

Despite its fairly benign nature, BP can be one problem too many in an older, frail person. Secondary infection is common and general health may suffer as a result of the

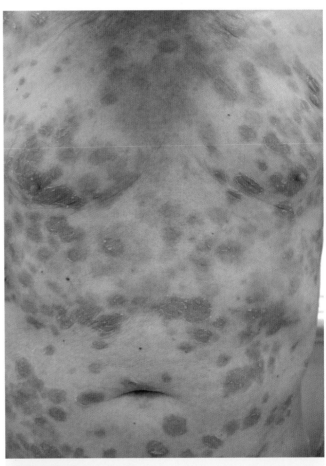

FIGURE 20.5 Pemphigus

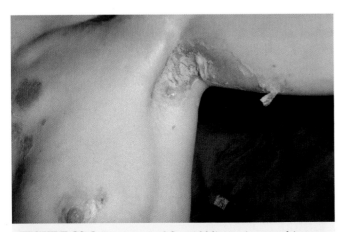

FIGURE 20.4 Erosions and flaccid blisters in pemphigus

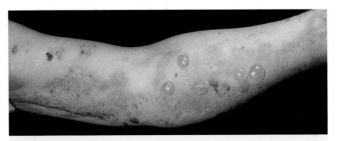

FIGURE 20.6 Tense blisters of an erythematous background – bullous pemphigoid

decreased mobility and the protein loss from the blister fluid.

The itchy background rash can be most annoying.

Practical prescribing

It is best to refer the patient to a dermatologist, because optimal treatment includes confirmatory biopsies for histology and immunofluorescence, but the diagnosis is often plain enough clinically. Oral steroids are usually very effective and in lower doses than pemphigus. In diabetics it is sometimes possible to gain control with antibiotics (especially erythromycin), careful nursing and the addition of a sulfone or azathioprine alone. Localized or relatively small areas may be controlled with topical clobetasol. The disease may burn itself out.

Dermatitis herpetiformis

Presentation

Most patients present with itching, associated with pink papules over the classical sites: forearms and elbows, knees and shins, base of spine/buttocks, scalp and shoulders (Fig. 20.7). Blisters are often not a prominent feature, although very small tense blisters are usually visible if sought really carefully.

It is rare for there to be any overt gastrointestinal symptoms at presentation.

Patient problems

The itch is always the main complaint. It usually fails to respond to even quite powerful steroids.

Practical prescribing

Diagnostic tests are a must: biopsy of a very early, pre-blister lesion; biopsy of normal skin for immunofluorescence; jejunal biopsy (if the skin diagnosis is confirmed) due to the association with coeliac disease.

Treatment consists of dapsone (starting at 50 mg twice daily). If there is any abnormality in the gut the patient should commence a lifetime gluten-free diet. On occasions diet alone may control the skin.

LICHEN PLANUS

Presentation

Lichen planus (LP) may present in a number of ways. Three are relatively common:

- A papular eruption varying in extent from a few lesions on the wrists and ankles (Fig. 20.8), to a very widespread and intensely irritable rash.
  - The lesions are flat-topped, polygonal, shiny, mauve/red in colour and are surmounted by lacy lines (Figs 20.9 and 20.10).
  - There is often significant staining left as lesions involute.
- Oral lesions that may be rough or ulcerating and sore.
- Indolent, highly itchy plaques, often on the lower legs (hypertrophic LP) (Fig. 20.11).

Rarely LP may affect the hair and nails. LP may also involve the genitalia.

Patient problems

When it is itchy LP is very, very itchy. Strangely, it is sometimes almost completely asymptomatic, although this is never the case with the hypertrophic variant.

Oral LP can be very difficult. It may alter taste as well as making it uncomfortable to eat and drink anything hot or remotely spicy.

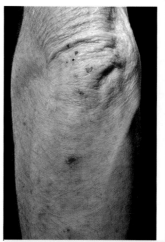
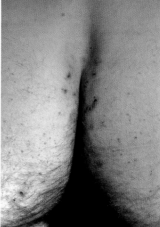

FIGURE 20.7 Dermatitis herpetiformis

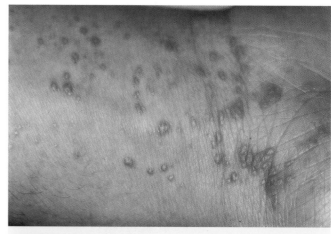

FIGURE 20.8 The papules of lichen planus on a classical site (the wrist)

FIGURE 20.9 White lines (Wickham's striae) visible on the surface of lesions

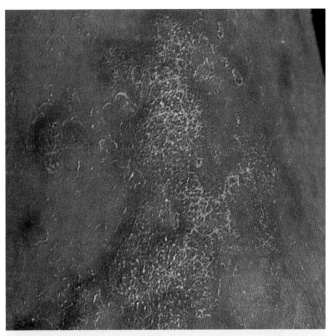

FIGURE 20.11 Hypertrophic lichen planus on the shin

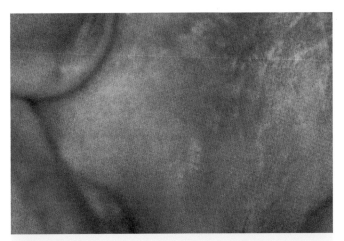

FIGURE 20.10 Lacy white lines in the mouth in lichen planus

Practical prescribing

Corticosteroids are the mainstay of treatment.

Potent or very potent agents are required for cutaneous lesions, and even they may fail to control the disease. It is also difficult to apply creams or ointments to a very widespread eruption. Occasionally, therefore, oral steroids are indicated and they work well. A dose of 20–30 mg daily is appropriate for an average adult.

Scalp involvement needs aggressive treatment, starting with a very potent scalp application, such as clobetasol, but systemic therapy with steroids or ciclosporin may be required to prevent scarring.

The mouth can be much more difficult. None of the topical steroid presentations for intra-oral use are all that successful, largely because they are hard to use. The use of squirts of asthma inhalers (deliberately *not* inhaled) may be the best of them, but secondary oral candidiasis is a nuisance. Oral therapy may be required, but chronic oral LP tends to recur and recur. Some authorities use preparations of topical tacrolimus, while systemic ciclosporin and mycophenylate mofetil are also options, but would require a specialist dermatological or oral surgical opinion.

Chronic oral LP is a precursor to squamous cell carcinoma and surveillance should include an oral check.

CUTANEOUS LUPUS ERYTHEMATOSUS

Skin changes occur commonly in the multisystem disorder systemic lupus erythematosus (LE). However, in some patients, skin lesions, classified as being in the LE family, are the predominant feature, with no systemic manifestations associated with LE.

Chronic discoid lupus erythematosus

Presentation

Chronic discoid lupus erythematosus (CDLE) causes erythematous plaques predominantly on the face (Fig. 18.12), neck, ears and scalp. Lesions may be photo-provoked or exacerbated. Two important features are the presence of follicular plugging and scarring. In the scalp, this leads to permanent hair loss.

Practical prescribing

A skin biopsy is generally considered an essential part of the routine work-up, but it may not be necessary in very typical lesions, especially on the face. If a biopsy is

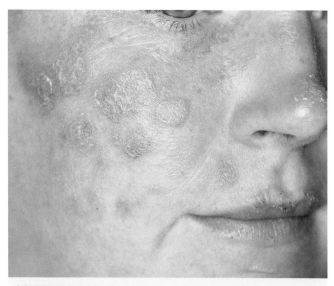

FIGURE 20.12 Chronic discoid lupus erythematosus

taken it should preferably be sent for both histology and immunofluorescence. Blood should be sent for routine haematology and biochemistry, as well as autoimmune serology.

Treatment should start with potent topical corticosteroids. Intralesional injections of steroids may also be useful in smallish areas.

In many patients lesions continue to spread despite intensive topical therapy. The drugs most commonly used in this situation are:

- Antimalarials, of which hydroxychloroquine, at a dose of 200–400 mg daily, is the best; mepacrine colours the skin an unpleasant orange stain and is less effective.
- Some authorities find the retinoid acitretin helpful.
- Dapsone has its advocates.
- Occasionally, a short course of systemic steroids may be required.

All patients with cutaneous lupus should be advised to use sunscreens and avoid excessive sun exposure.

LICHEN SCLEROSUS

Presentation

Lichen sclerosus (LS) may appear in several different guises:
- On the genital and perianal skin of adult females.

Here, the condition produces white, plaque-like changes (Fig. 20.13) in which erosions are common. Lichen sclerosus sometimes results in loss of tissue and fusion of vulval folds, particularly if lesions are long-standing.
- On the genital and perianal skin of prepubertal females.

LS in prepubertal girls is characteristically well circumscribed, often assuming a figure-of-eight distribution around the vulva and anus (Fig. 20.14). Surface areas of

purpura are commonly seen, which may break down to leave erosions.
- On the male genitalia.

In adult males, the equivalent changes caused by this condition are also called *balanitis xerotica obliterans* (Fig. 20.15). The glans, prepuce, or both, become white and

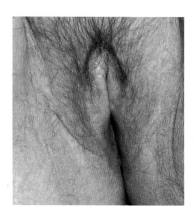

FIGURE 20.13
Ulcerated white plaques in lichen sclerosus of the vulva

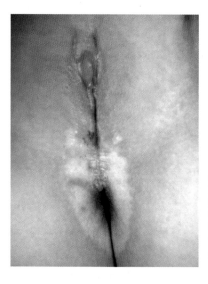

FIGURE 20.14
Prepubertal lichen sclerosis around the vulva and anus

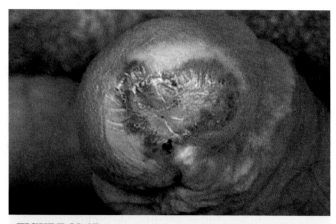

FIGURE 20.15 Balanitis xerotica obliterans

there may be significant fibrosis in longer-standing disease. This can lead to occlusion of the meatus, or to phimosis. In young boys, lichen sclerosus probably presents as phimosis but is not even diagnosed in most cases, since the troublesome prepuce is simply removed surgically and discarded.

• On non-genital skin.

Lichen sclerosus may occur on sites other than the genitalia, either alone or in combination with genital disease. It has a predilection for the wrists and the flexures, but may arise anywhere. The lesions are white and feel rather like cigarette paper, but there may be difficulty differentiating LS from areas of morphoea (localized scleroderma).

Patient problems

The changes of LS can give rise to significant discomfort. Children are often especially uncomfortable and may complain of soreness, dysuria and pain on defecation. LS has been mistaken for evidence of vulval damage from sexual abuse.

Practical prescribing

Clobetasol propionate is generally the agent of choice. While this is a very strong steroid, the results can be remarkable. There is obviously a need for careful surveillance of anyone using such powerful steroids.

All adult female patients should be advised to attend for a regular check-up and to report anything unusual, as LS may predispose to vulval carcinoma.

GRANULOMA ANNULARE AND NECROBIOSIS LIPOIDICA

These conditions have some important common features – notably that the histology of both is characterized by a very specific change in collagen known as *necrobiosis*. Furthermore, both disorders have been linked with diabetes, although it is really only of significance in necrobiosis lipoidica.

Granuloma annulare

Presentation

Typically granuloma annulare (GA) appears as small, ring-like areas over the knuckles, elbows, knees and feet (Fig. 20.16). Occasionally the lesions are much more widespread and do not form much in the way of rings.

Patient problems

The main issue is the look of the lesions – they seldom itch or hurt.

Practical prescribing

Topical or injected steroids may help, but lesions often recur and treatment may be very unrewarding for both doctor and patient.

Necrobiosis lipoidica

Presentation

Waxy yellow/brown plaques with a purple rim appear, usually on the shins (Fig. 20.17). The lesions may ulcerate.

Patient problems

The main issue that concerns patients is the unsightliness of the plaques.

Practical prescribing

It is essential that the patient is screened for diabetes if this is not already established. Although it is actually quite

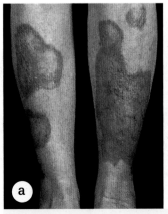
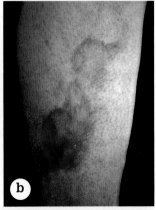

FIGURE 20.16 **(a)** Typical granuloma annulare in a typical site. **(b)** More extensive granuloma annulare

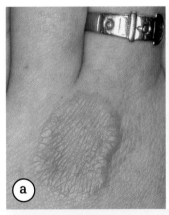
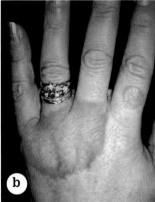

FIGURE 20.17 **(a)** Necrobiosis lipoidica – extensive lesions on the shins. **(b)** Necrobiosis lipoidica

rare in diabetics, two-thirds of patients with necrobiosis lipoidica are diabetic.

Treatment is generally very unrewarding. Injections of steroid around the active edge early in the development of lesions may be helpful.

PHOTOSENSITIVITY – LIGHT-INDUCED DISORDERS

Many conditions exist in which light plays a role in the induction or exacerbation of skin changes. Examples include photosensitive eczema and chronic actinic dermatitis, lupus erythematosus, rosacea, solar urticaria, a number of rare genetic disorders including the porphyrias, and polymorphic light eruption.

Some of these are dealt with in other sections of this book.

Sunburn

Most of us are familiar with the acute effects of sun exposure. Severe sunburn can be very unpleasant, with blistering and skin loss. It is rare for the changes to require anything more than simple, soothing lotions but occasionally a period of intensive nursing is needed.

Polymorphic light eruption

Presentation

Many people develop a rash that they may call 'prickly heat' following sun exposure. This may occur early in the summer in temperate climates, or only with light of greater intensity than normally encountered at home. The diagnosis can be made on history alone (and may have to be, because the eruption only appears on holiday and has long since vanished when seen by the doctor). The most common story is of the onset of a papular eruption on light-exposed surfaces within some hours of exposure to sunlight (Fig. 20.18).

Patient problems

The rash is usually intensely itchy. Blisters can form in very severe reactions. In most patients the reaction subsides and, if sun exposure continues, the rest of the summer is trouble-free, suggesting some degree of 'conditioning'.

Practical prescribing

All patients should be screened for lupus erythematosus (with which polymorphic light eruption shares many histological features). If there is any doubt about the diagnosis, a referral for porphyrin screens should be considered.

The most successful form of active therapy is probably prophylactic PUVA in a pre-season course, but oral hydroxychloroquine 200 mg twice daily is an alternative, and helps many patients to enjoy their holidays without their rash. Some authorities recommend narrow-band UVB (TL-01).

SKIN SIGNS OF SYSTEMIC DISEASE

There are some specific skin changes that may indicate an underlying disease process. Pruritus and vasculitis are considered elsewhere, but three others require further elaboration.

Erythema nodosum

Although not common, the classical features are unmistakable: tender, red nodules appearing in crops on the lower legs, especially the shins (Fig. 20.19), which fade through the colours of a bruise.

Conditions to consider:
- Streptococcal infection.

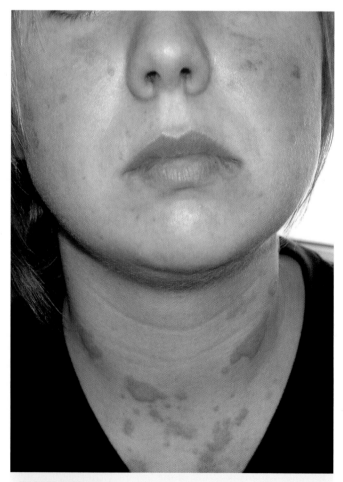

FIGURE 20.18 Polymorphic light eruption

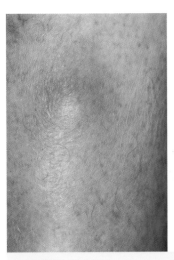
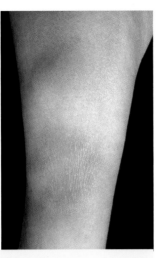

FIGURE 20.19 Erythema nodosum

- Sarcoidosis.
- Inflammatory bowel disease.
- Drugs.
- TB.

Treatment depends on the cause. Often, though, there is none identified, in which case bed rest, non-steroidal anti-inflammatory therapy and systemic steroids need to be considered.

Acanthosis nigricans

Although famously associated with cancer, this combination is actually exceptionally rare. The changes of acanthosis nigricans (AN) (Fig. 20.20) are, however, quite commonly seen in the overweight and in association with conditions characterized by insulin resistance. A young woman with AN may also have signs of polycystic ovary syndrome.

No treatment really helps, although weight loss should be encouraged.

Pyoderma gangrenosum

Pyoderma gangrenosum (PG) (Fig. 20.21) is seen predominantly in patients with inflammatory bowel disease, rheumatoid arthritis and in association with

paraproteinaemia. However, there is occasionally no apparent trigger and PG may complicate scars following surgical procedures.

A biopsy is essential, and swabs for culture are sensible. Oral minocycline may bring control, but most patients require oral prednisolone beginning at around 30 mg daily.

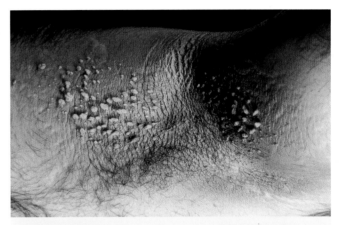

FIGURE 20.20 Typical acanthosis nigricans with skin tags; this is relatively common and usually associated with obesity

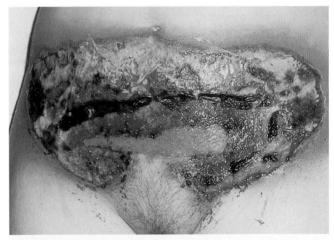

FIGURE 20.21 Pyoderma gangrenosum – the typically undermined, purplish edge

Chapter 21

Disorders of Pigmentation

Summary

- Normal pigmentation
- Hyperpigmentation
- Reduced or absent pigmentation
  - Congenital causes
  - Acquired causes

NORMAL PIGMENTATION

Humans produce two main types of pigment. The main agent responsible for the colour of skin, hair, and eyes is *eumelanin* (brown). The other is *phaeomelanin* (red). The amount of both pigments is genetically determined, but exposure to ultraviolet radiation increases the amount of pigment concentrated in the skin and causes a darkening of the skin – the much-glorified tan.

Normal skin colour is conventionally classified into six 'skin types':

- I – genetically 'white' but burns easily, never tans.
- II – genetically 'white' but burns easily, tans with difficulty.
- III – genetically 'white' but burns occasionally, tans well.
- IV – genetically 'white' but tans well, never burns.
- V – genetically brown (Asian, Indo-Asian, Chinese, Japanese).
- VI – black (Afro-Caribbean).

The presence of phaeomelanin modifies the phenotype by adding a reddish hue, most commonly seen in fair-skinned individuals – who often also have greenish eyes and many freckles.

Genetic defects or acquired disease processes may produce two types of pigmentary disturbance: increased (hyper-)pigmentation and reduced (hypo-) or no pigmentation.

Alteration to the 'normal' range of pigmentation has major social and psychological effects.

HYPERPIGMENTATION

By no means all hyperpigmentation is due to excess melanin.

Exogenous pigments

Skin colour may be altered by pigments other than melanin:

- Exogenously applied materials – both on the surface (make-up, decorative paints, hair dye) and within (tattoos).
- Ingested pigments (e.g. carotenes).
- Endogenously produced pigments such as bilirubin and haemosiderin.

Postinflammatory hyperpigmentation is extremely common following trauma to the skin and in inflammatory skin disorders, especially those, such as lichen planus, that affect the dermo-epidermal junction. Dusky, rather ill-defined pigmentation appears in the distribution of previous cutaneous damage or inflammation. Patients with darker skins are more severely affected and may need much reassurance that lesions will fade in time.

Chloasma (melasma) (Figs 21.1–21.3)

Presentation

Increased pigmentation is typically seen across the forehead, and on the cheeks, upper lip and chin. It is more frequently seen in women than in men, and may occur spontaneously or be associated with pregnancy or oestrogen consumption.

Patient problems

The main problem is psychological, and the pigmentation deteriorates in summer months with UV exposure.

Practical prescribing

It is reasonable to refer a patient who is very upset for a specialist opinion. It is also sensible to recommend cessation of oral contraception or HRT, although this does not often improve matters of itself. Some patients benefit from the use of agents that hypopigment the skin, notably hydroquinone (usually in a mixture: hydroquinone 2% + retinoic acid and dexamethasone). The effects are, however, unpredictable, and may make matters worse. There is no way of knowing in advance and it is very much trial and error – something that patients should be warned about. Sun protection may help to reduce the cosmetic impact.

Pregnancy

Pregnant women usually notice some increase in pigmentation, especially of the nipples and the linear alba/ nigra, and chloasma is common.

Haemosiderin

Haemosiderin is deposited in the skin in any situation in which red cells are extravasated and break down: bruises, petechiae, including senile purpura (Fig. 21.4), and in venous stasis and accompanying vasculitis (Figs 21.5 and 21.6).

Carotenes

Carotenes are naturally occurring pigments. Beta-carotene is found in carrots, peppers and many orange or yellow fruits and vegetables. Some people have a relative deficiency of the hepatic enzyme responsible for metabolizing beta-carotene and find that their skin becomes tinged with yellow or orange pigment. This is harmless. Beta-carotene is responsible for the yellowish tinge in the skin in myxoedema and pernicious anaemia.

The distribution of the pigmentation is characteristic: palms and soles are typically noticeably high-coloured, as is

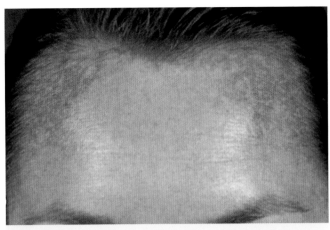

FIGURE 21.1 Chloasma: hyperpigmentation around the hairline

the area around the nose and mouth. The sclerae, however, are spared.

Drugs and chemicals

Several drugs and chemicals can pigment the skin, including chloroquine, mepacrine, minocycline (see Fig. 19.3) and amiodarone.

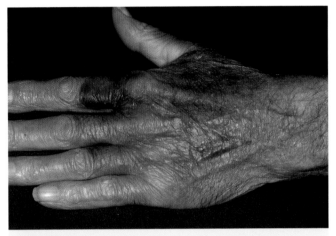

FIGURE 21.4 Skin thinning and purpura in a patient on long-term systemic steroids

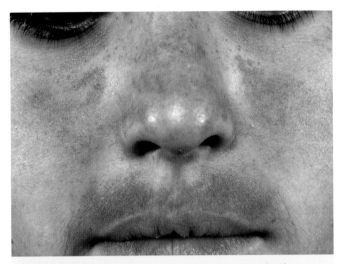

FIGURE 21.2 Chloasma: most marked on the cheeks, across the nose and on the upper lip

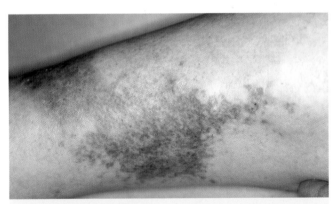

FIGURE 21.5 vasculitis

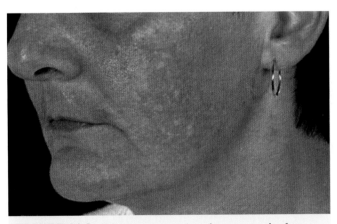

FIGURE 21.3 Chloasma: extensive changes on the face

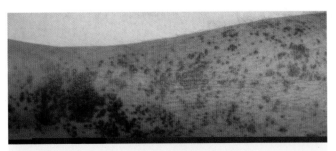

FIGURE 21.6 Pigmentation with vasculitis

279

REDUCED OR ABSENT PIGMENTATION

CONGENITAL CAUSES

Albinism

The term *albinism* is applied to genetic disorders in which the normal enzyme pathways involved in the production of melanin are defective. Patients may be grouped into those in whom the enzyme tyrosine is absent and those in whom it is present but defective. Most forms are inherited as autosomal recessive traits. In tyrosinase-negative albinism the skin is pink and remains pale throughout life. The eyes are severely affected, with complete absence of pigment and marked nystagmus. Skin cancers are very common in patients living in sunny countries.

Patients with tyrosinase-positive albinism are less pale. The hair is yellow and the eyes may show some pigmentation, and skin, hair and eyes darken gradually as the patient ages. However, nystagmus and ocular problems are still common and skin cancers occur more frequently than among other individuals of the same ethnic background.

Tuberous sclerosis

Pale macules are one of the key markers of tuberous sclerosis (Fig 21.7).

Similar lesions may occur in isolation, when they are known as *achromic naevi*.

Practical prescribing

With the exception of phenylketonuria, there is no satisfactory treatment for any of these genetic disorders other than symptomatic control of associated problems and sun protection as appropriate.

ACQUIRED CAUSES

Acquired hypopigmentation is a common problem. In some ethnic groups, *leucoderma* (usually due to vitiligo) is associated with severe stigmatization and has major cultural connotations.

Postinflammatory hypopigmentation is due to alteration of the normal pigment balance in the immediate aftermath of an inflammation or damage to the skin. Normal colour will usually return unless the damage is very severe. Psoriasis is particularly prone to do this, especially if the patient is treated with ultraviolet radiation, as is eczema. Indeed the condition known as *pityriasis alba* is essentially a hypopigmenting form of eczema. In more significant injuries, including burns or freezing, the melanocytes may be permanently destroyed and the depigmentation may persist indefinitely.

Pityriasis versicolor

The lesions in this disorder are often paler than the surrounding skin in sunny months and on pigmented skins, but are a faint brown on pale, untanned skin.

The key features to look out for are:

- Rarely appears before puberty.
- More common on upper trunk.
- May have fine scale.
- Treatment depends on extent:
  - Limited disease can be managed with ketoconazole shampoo alone; make into a lather, apply and wash off after 10 minutes; this should be used four times a week for at least 2 weeks.
  - More extensive disease may require a short burst of oral itraconazole.
  - The condition is notoriously recurrent; wash periodically with ketoconazole or selenium sulfide as prophylaxis.
- The pale areas take many months to repigment.

Pityriasis alba

Presentation

Pityriasis alba is a common cause of hypopigmentation, most typically seen on the cheeks (Fig. 21.8) and the upper outer arms in children. The lesions become more noticeable in the summer months. Other changes can be very subtle, with only very fine scale.

Patient problems

The key issue for the patient and parents is whether the pale patches are actually due to vitiligo. Unfortunately, it

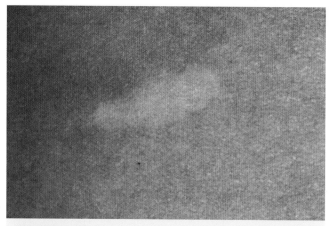

FIGURE 21.7 Tuberous sclerosis: a typical pale macule on the trunk of an infant

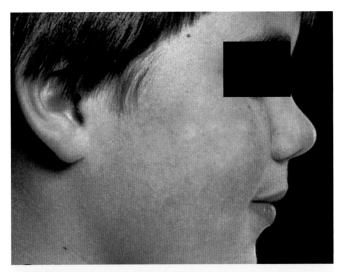

FIGURE 21.8 Pityriasis alba: typical pale patches on the cheeks

is not always possible to be absolutely certain and vitiligo occasionally develops from a previous inflammatory process. It may be sensible to take a cautious line.

Practical prescribing

The condition usually responds to mild topical steroids or moisturizers, or both. It also seems to improve at or around puberty and is really not seen in adults.

Vitiligo

This is the most important of the disorders that cause loss of cutaneous pigmentation.

Presentation

The appearance of a white patch immediately requires a decision as to whether the problem is vitiligo or one of the mimics we have already discussed (postinflammatory hypopigmentation, pityriasis versicolor, pityriasis alba).

Key signs that point towards vitiligo are:
- There is total loss of pigment in affected areas – and occasionally a peripheral rim of increased pigmentation.
- Although it is not always the case in vitiligo, symmetrical involvement, often around both eyes, on both hands is highly characteristic.
- A family history of vitiligo, alopecia areata, thyroid disease and some other autoimmune disorders.

Once made, the diagnosis brings with it the prospect of continued distress, as only a proportion of patients will see significant repigmentation – whether spontaneous or as a result of active treatment.

Patient problems

Vitiligo can be a most distressing condition. It is much more noticeable in pigmented skin, but even in white skin can be very unsightly, especially in the summer if there is any degree of tan in the 'normal' skin (Fig. 21.9).

Patients are also upset by the sunburn that occurs in the white patches.

Practical prescribing

There is no guarantee that any treatment will work but it is certainly important to give every patient a chance. There is good evidence that treatment works, although not in

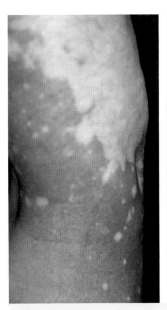
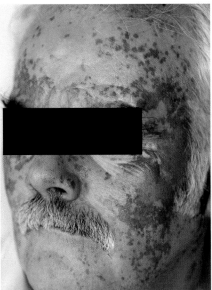
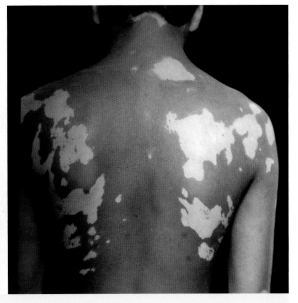

FIGURE 21.9 Vitiligo

everyone, and less often in adults than children and in extensive, symmetrical disease.

Sun care advice is important. Patches of vitiligo will burn badly and need extra protection.

First-line therapy is usually a potent topical corticosteroid, but the calcineurin inhibitor tacrolimus is catching up fast. There is a case for using both in rotation, because the tacrolimus will not thin the skin, and neither will steroids as long as they are used strictly intermittently. Caution and common sense regarding steroids need to be exercised too on facial skin (especially around the eyes). Care still needs to be taken, though, to assess the quantity of steroid being used and over what period.

If this approach is unsuccessful (and it is important to allow a good length of time to elapse – say, 3–6 months), then a referral for PUVA may be considered if such facilities are available, but treatment is very prolonged and many centres cannot accept patients because there just is not enough capacity without restricting opportunities for other disorders, such as psoriasis.

Some patients benefit hugely from advice on cosmetic camouflage, which is prescribable on the NHS for vitiligo. If patients have access to a branch of the Red Cross Society, they are able to give invaluable advice on the use of the range of agents.

Chapter 22

Genetics

Many skin disorders have a genetic basis and skin changes are present in many genetic diseases, with important manifestations in other organs. In some of these the genetic abnormalities have been fully characterized; in others there is yet much to discover.

Atopic eczema

The strong family history and the high concordance between identical twins clearly indicate a genetic basis for atopic eczema. The nature of this is still unknown in is entirety, although it seems likely that several genes may be involved. Most of the attention has, until recently, been focused on looking at the genetics of the abnormal immunology (e.g. IgE production), but the recent discovery of abnormalities in the production of the epidermal component *filaggrin* has widened the search considerably.

It does seem from epidemiological studies that something is needed to unmask or release the underlying genetic tendency and it remains a mystery that atopic eczema apparently clears in 60–70% of children. There are also some genetically inherited diseases in which atopic eczema is a key component (e.g. Netherton's syndrome).

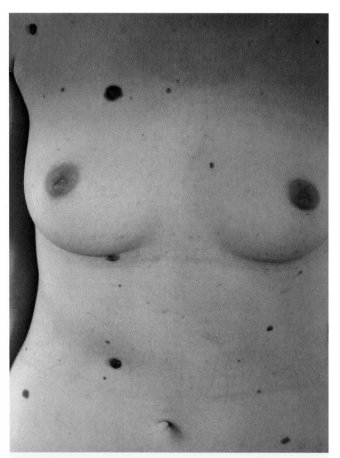

FIGURE 22.1 Familial atypical mole and melanoma syndrome

BOX 22.1 Genetics and the skin

Common skin diseases where genetics are important

Atopic eczema

Psoriasis

Vitiligo

Alopecia areata

Melanoma (Fig. 22.1)

Common genodermatoses

Ichthyosis (Fig. 22.2)

Palmoplantar keratodermas (Fig. 22.3)

Albinism

Hereditary angioedema

Darier's disease (Fig. 22.4)

Common genetic diseases with skin manifestations

Down's syndrome

Neurofibromatosis

Tuberous sclerosis

Ehlers–Danlos syndrome (Fig. 22.5)

Psoriasis

Strong family histories and the close association of younger-onset disease with HLA-Cw indicate a genetic background in psoriasis. Like atopic eczema it seems likely that the disease is multifactorial.

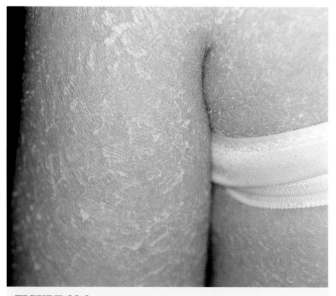

FIGURE 22.2 Ichthyosis vulgaris

Vitiligo and alopecia areata

These disorders cluster in families and are associated in some with organ-specific autoantibodies.

Melanoma

There are well-described family pedigrees with an autosomal dominant pattern of inheritance of multiple atypical moles and (sometimes) multiple melanomas. Some family pedigrees have been reported with no abnormal moles.

Ichthyosis

Common ichthyosis (ichthyosis vulgaris) is inherited as an autosomal dominant disease. There is a rarer form, seen

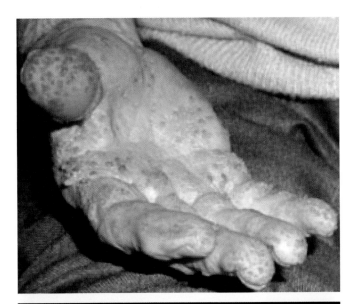

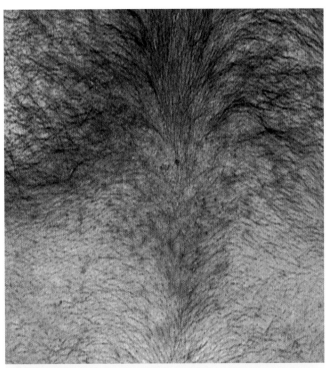

FIGURE 22.4 Darier's disease – typical greasy papules on the chest

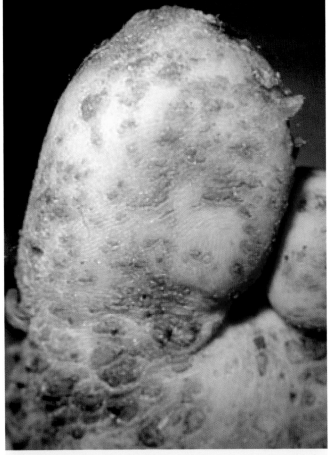

FIGURE 22.3 Palmoplantar keratoderma

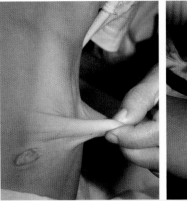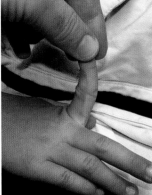

FIGURE 22.5 **(a)** Ehlers–Danlos syndrome: skin laxity. **(b)** Ehlers–Danlos syndrome: joint laxity

only in boys, that is X-linked. They often have a delayed onset of labour owing to the absence of a critical enzyme.

Palmoplantar keratoderma

There are a number of patterns of hyperkeratosis on the palms and soles, most of which are genetically inherited. Much is made of an association with oesophageal cancer, but this is extraordinarily rare and relates only to some families with their roots in the Liverpool area.

Albinism

The skin is clearly abnormal in oculocutaneous albinism, a group of inherited conditions in which tyrosinase is absent or ineffective.

Hereditary angioedema (see Ch. 13)

This rare disorder is inherited in an autosomal dominant manner.

Darier's disease

Another autosomal dominant condition, this is characterized by multiple scaly lesions.

Down's syndrome

Individuals with Down's syndrome are prone to several skin abnormalities – most importantly a tendency to chronic infections.

Neurofibromatosis

Skin manifestations of neurofibromatosis are often the presenting feature. Café-au-lait patches and axillary freckling are the most common, but small nodules (the neurofibromas themselves) may cause trouble.

Tuberous sclerosis

The earliest marker of tuberous sclerosis is usually the white macular patches (often 'ash-leaf' shaped). Other skin markers are: periungual fibromas, angiofibromas on the face (Fig. 22.6) – the *shagreen* patch.

Ehlers–Danlos syndrome(s)

There are now a number of defined genetic syndromes with different collagen defects. A number result in marked cutaneous abnormalities, notably hyperlaxity and poor healing.

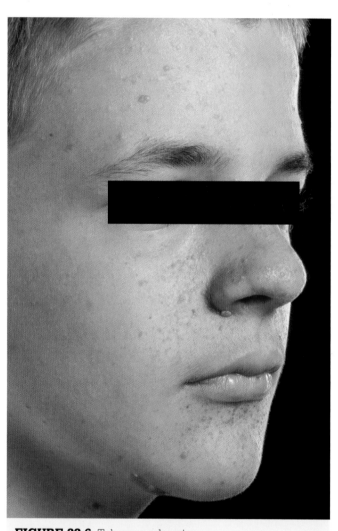

FIGURE 22.6 Tuberous sclerosis

3
Section

Management

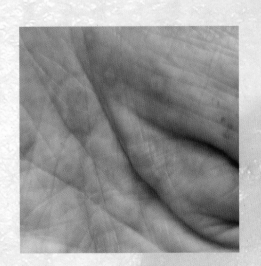
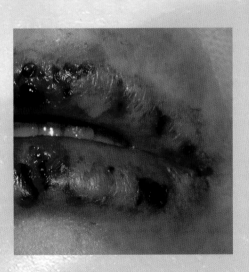
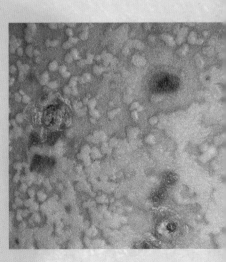

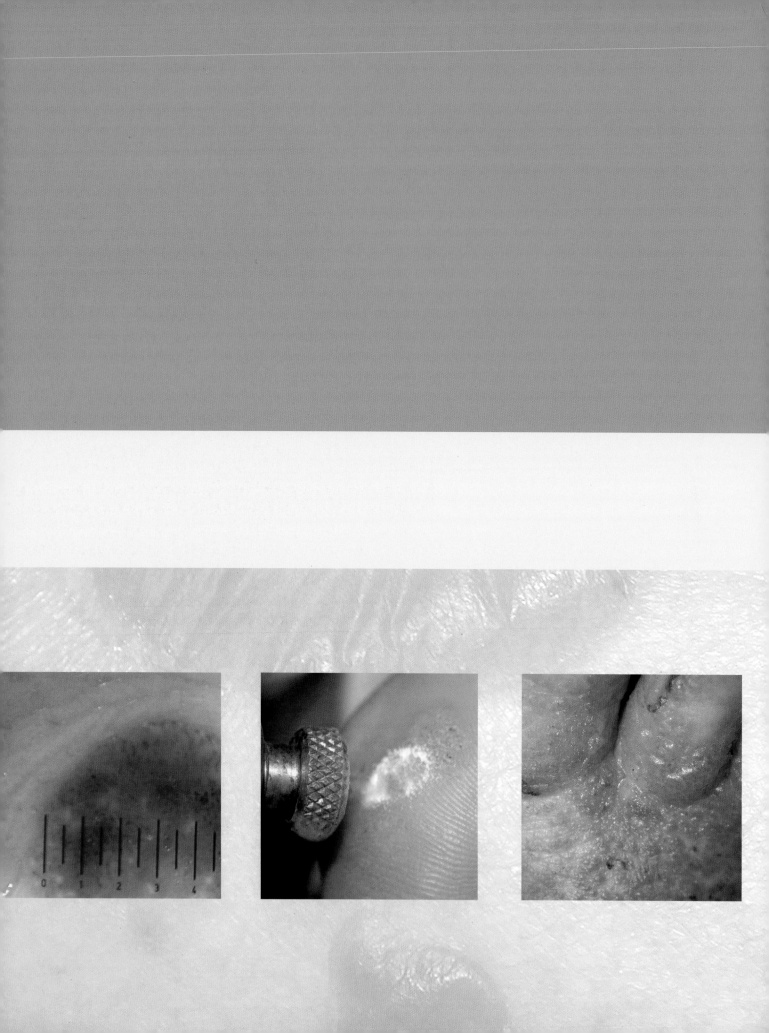

Chapter 23

Investigations

Summary

- Psychological aspects
- Dermatological history-taking
- Examination of the skin

The aim of all clinicians seeing a patient is to get them better. In order to do that it is essential to know what the patient has. Dermatological diagnosis is often seen as difficult, because there are so many different conditions, and because the terminology can be confusing, but in essence the process is no different from handling any other organ and its diseases: you need to assess the problems that face the patient and then create a management plan.

PSYCHOLOGICAL ASPECTS

Be aware that skin disease has a major impact on the well-being of the patient, both physically and psychologically: patients cannot easily work with severe hand or foot dermatitis; severe itch can disrupt sleeping and the rest of normal life; patients with skin disease find it difficult to cope in society because the visibility of lesions represents a deviation from the 'norm'. This is true for acne, facial eczema, psoriasis and other dermatoses on the hands, vitiligo (especially in pigmented skins), hair loss, port-wine stains and many other disorders. It is not easy to form close personal relationships when your skin is covered in scaly, red patches or you scratch so much at times that you bleed. Quality of life surveys indicate that chronic skin disease may be more disabling than diabetes or heart disease.

The doctor's actions must show that this is understood and that there is no need to apologize for seeking help. Touching the skin is a critical part of the consultation. Offering opportunities for the patient to discuss the effects of skin disease is also important; not everyone will accept the chance immediately and there need to be other occasions when the opening is made. It may be necessary to point out to accompanying friends and family the misery that skin disease can cause.

Patients with skin disease invariably feel better when they know that their doctor knows a little of how they feel.

DERMATOLOGICAL HISTORY-TAKING

The essentials of dermatological history-taking are listed in Box 23.1.

As with any other specialty, begin with the presenting complaint. Then define and qualify it, establish whether there are any other linked problems, and assess its severity.

There are some differences in dealing with skin disease:

- Patients often present with several problems (and 'While I'm here, doctor, …', is also common).
- Skin signs are obvious; patients (and friends, neighbours and relatives) often have strong opinions – this may affect the way they describe the problem.
- The visibility of skin lesion(s) often leads to early examination – before some of the standard history has been taken.
- Skin diseases present with itch; the phrases used by patients to describe the itch may need to be learned.

BOX 23.1 Essentials of dermatological history-taking

Presenting complaint	Where? How long? What symptoms? Itch, bleeding? What effect does it have on your life at work and at home? How and with what has it been treated already?
Past history	Skin disease (specifically eczema and psoriasis) Asthma Allergies and atopy General disorders
Family/close contacts	Any skin disease Any allergies or atopic diseases (e.g. hay fever, asthma)
Occupation and hobbies	Exposure to materials in the workplace or at home Exposure to alcohol
Therapy	Medical, systemic and topical (including other people's and old creams); over-the-counter products and those recommended by non-medical health professionals, e.g. pharmacists, specialist nurses, alternative/complementary practitioners Cosmetics and toiletries

- Skin disease has major psychological effects, especially when it affects the face – this may need to be drawn out.
- There are important genetic aspects to many skin diseases.
- Some skin diseases are infectious or contagious.
- There are important environmental aspects to many skin diseases.
- Patients frequently use multiple creams and ointments on their skin – these may have come from many sources.
- Patients frequently forget the names of the treatments they have used on their skin – it is helpful to be able to show patients examples of the creams they might have used.

EXAMINATION OF THE SKIN

It is very common for the examination to begin at the start of the consultation, and for the early findings to condition and guide the direction and nature of the history-taking and the rest of the consultation.

Skin examination requires some specific techniques and thought processes: it is very common for part, if not all, of the examination to begin at the start of the consultation, and for the early findings to condition and guide the direction and nature of the history-taking and the rest of the consultation. Skin examination, like dermatological history-taking, requires some new techniques and thought processes:

- It is considered 'best practice' to examine the whole skin every time; in practice, this is unworkable and unreasonable – no one wishes to be completely undressed for a wart on the finger or a scalp cyst.
- Palpate skin lesions as well as look at them – this provides useful information and also indicates that the doctor, at least, is not repelled or frightened by the rash.
- Measure lesions rather than try to describe them in terms related to coins or fingernails; draw tumours in their approximate location, with a note of their size in millimetres.
- Examine 'secondary' sites when certain diagnoses are suspected (e.g. nails in psoriasis; finger webs, wrists, nipples and scrotum in scabies).
- The results of the examination should be recorded using the terms outlined in the boxes.
- It takes time to learn which lesion(s) to focus on in a rash; all rashes are dynamic and contain both 'young' and 'old' lesions; only a proportion will bear the signs classically associated with the likely diagnosis.

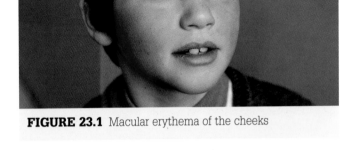

FIGURE 23.1 Macular erythema of the cheeks

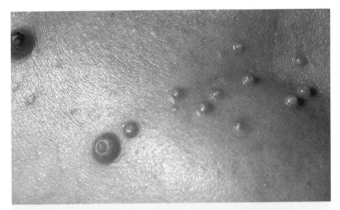

FIGURE 23.2 Molluscum contagiosum: typical cluster of lesions

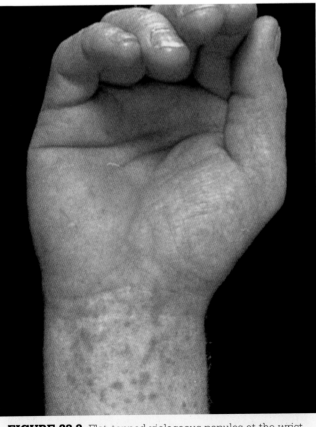

FIGURE 23.3 Flat-topped violaceous papules at the wrist

BOX 23.2	Characteristics of individual lesions
Macule	Flat skin discoloration (Fig. 23.1)
Papule	Elevated lesion <0.5 cm in diameter (Figs 23.2 and 23.3)
Nodule	Elevated lesion >0.5 cm in diameter (Fig. 23.4)
Small plaque	Elevated, flat-topped lesion <2 cm in diameter
Large plaque	Elevated, flat-topped lesion >2 cm in diameter (Fig. 23.5)
Wheal	Elevated area of cutaneous oedema
Vesicle	Fluid-filled lesion <0.5 cm in diameter (Fig. 23.6)
Bulla	Fluid-filled lesion = 0.5 cm in diameter (Fig. 23.7)
Pustule	Pus-filled lesion (Fig. 23.8)

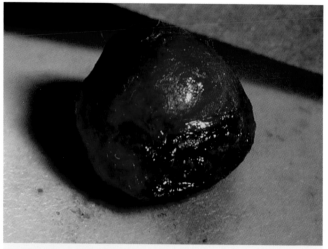

FIGURE 23.4 Large pyogenic granuloma

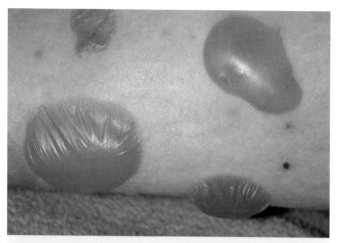

FIGURE 23.7 Bulla: fluid-filled lesion = 0.5 cm in diameter

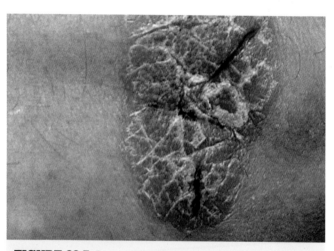

FIGURE 23.5 Diagnostic appearance of a plaque of psoriasis

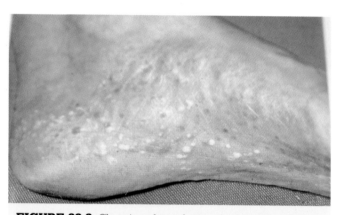

FIGURE 23.8 Chronic palmo-plantar psoriasis

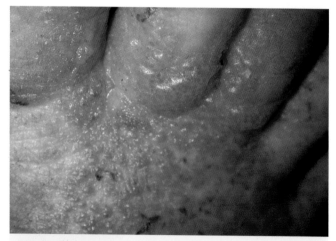

FIGURE 23.6 Vesicle: fluid-filled lesion < 0.5{ts}cm in diameter

BOX 23.3 Characteristics of the surface

Scale	Visible and palpable flakes of aggregated epidermal cells (Fig. 23.9)
Crust	Dried exudates (Fig. 23.10)
Horn	Projection of keratin (Fig. 23.11)
Ulceration	Loss of epidermis (± underlying dermis and subcutis) (Fig. 23.12)
Excoriation	Superficial ulceration as a result of scratching (Fig. 23.13)
Maceration	Softened, wettened epidermis (Fig. 23.14)
Lichenification	Flat-surfaced epidermal thickening, often with accentuation of normal skin markings/creases (Fig. 23.15)

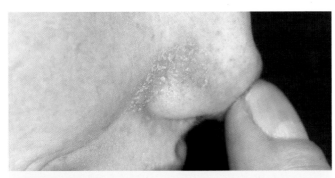

FIGURE 23.9 Seborrhoeic eczema: typical scale and erythema in the nasolabial fold

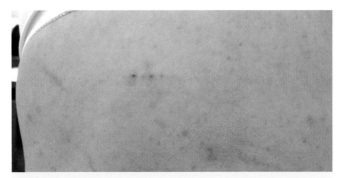

FIGURE 23.13 Linear excoriations with no underlying rash

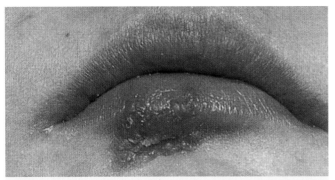

FIGURE 23.10 Herpes simplex of the lips (cold sore)

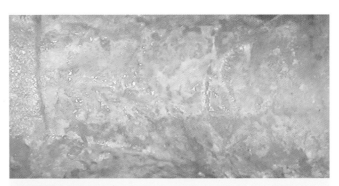

FIGURE 23.14 Maceration: softened, wettened epidermis

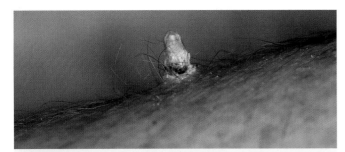

FIGURE 23.11 A cutaneous horn – these lesions are usually actinic keratoses, but may be early squamous carcinomas; they are best removed

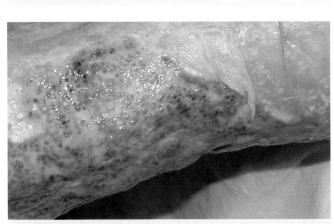

FIGURE 23.12 Leg ulcer

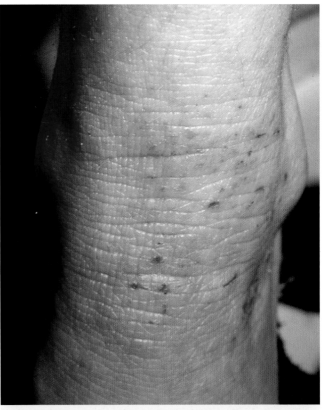

FIGURE 23.15 Lichenification in chronic atopic dermatitis

Special investigations

There are a number of special techniques for advancing the diagnostic process in skin disease, and some situations in which investigations represent an important part of disease management.

Dermatoscopy

Dermatoscopy involves the use of a surface microscope usually with a hand piece of similar size to an ophthalmoscope/auroscope (Fig. 23.16a) to obtain further information about pigmented lesions.

It has the potential in primary care to aid in the diagnosis of benign skin lesions such as seborrheoic keratoses (Fig. 23.16b), dermatofibroma, blue naevi and vascular lesions. This may reduce the need for unnecessary skin surgery or the number of patients referred to secondary care.

Various scoring systems have been developed for the diagnosis of melanoma using dermatoscopy and in experienced hands (normally secondary care) it appears to be useful in this regard, although it is by no means an easy process and special training is required.

Blood tests

It is often useful to perform a routine haematological and biochemical screen in any patient in whom the skin changes may be part of a more widespread, systemic disorder. The same is true for patients with an itch but no rash; such patients should also have their ferritin level checked. Immunological screens are helpful where autoimmune processes are involved (e.g. vasculitis, skin changes of lupus erythematosus), and also in elderly patients.

Some clinicians offer RASTs for allergic disorders. These require very careful interpretation. Organ-specific autoantibodies are common in alopecia areata and vitiligo, although this knowledge rarely, if ever, helps with management. Glucose estimations are important in necrobiosis lipoidica.

Several of the drugs used in dermatology require monitoring. This is discussed in the section on treatment.

Blood for indirect immunofluorescence

There are circulating antibodies to skin components in patients with pemphigus (most) and bullous pemphigoid (many). The laboratory needs to be equipped to undertake the test. Serum is required.

Skin scrapings and clippings

Skin scrapings and clippings can be used to aid in the diagnosis of fungal infections and mite infestations (scabies), and, occasionally, other conditions. In diagnosing fungal diseases, it may be sufficient to send samples to the local laboratory (although the quality of service and expertise in mycology varies considerably).

A quicker answer can be obtained by undertaking direct microscopy in the clinic, and this is required in pityriasis versicolor and in scabies.

It may well not be practical in primary care settings, but the following are needed if you wish to have a go:
- A good-quality microscope.
- A disposable scalpel blade, a pair of fine scissors, and a pair of forceps.
- Slides and cover slips.

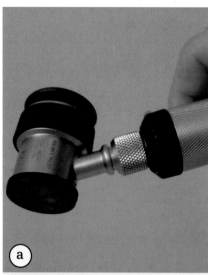
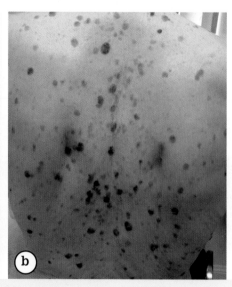
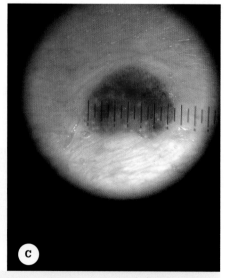

FIGURE 23.16 **(a)** Dermatoscope. **(b)** Clinical picture of seborrhoeic keratosis. **(c)** Dermatoscopic picture of seborrhoeic keratosis

BOX 23.4 Investigational techniques

Blood tests	For a wide range of disorders, for indirect immunofluorescence in immunobullous disease
Swabs	
Bacteriological	To ascertain nature of infecting organism, antibiotic sensitivity
Viral	To ascertain nature of infecting organism
Scrapes or clips	To obtain material for inspection for fungi, mites, molluscum bodies, giant cells (in herpes virus infections); to set up cultures for fungi
Biopsy	
Light microscopy	Pathological interpretation, including special stains and immunocytochemistry as necessary
Immunofluorescence	Bullous disorders; cutaneous and systemic lupus erythematosus; vasculitis
Electron microscopy	Especially useful in congenital and acquired blistering diseases
Culture of skin biopsies	The organisms causing TB, leishmaniasis and some rarer organisms are more easily, or can only be, cultured from skin biopsies
In-situ hybridization	Subtyping human papilloma virus; establishing definitive information on some genetic disorders
Patch tests	Investigation of allergic contact dermatitis (Fig. 23.17)
Prick tests	Positive prick test to latex (Fig. 23.18)
Testing for IgE hypersensitivity	Important in suspected latex allergy
Place in other disorders (e.g. urticaria, atopic eczema) less clear

- Potassium hydroxide (KOH) solution for epidermal scrapings, hair and nails (usually 10% KOH, but 20–30% is better for nails).

Some training and experience!

Samples should be taken from:
- The edge of cutaneous ringworm lesions.
- The blister roof of vesicular lesions (using a pair of scissors).
- Both scalp scale and hair in suspected scalp ringworm.
- Both infected nail plate and samples of subungual hyperkeratosis/debris, in suspected nail infections.
- A whole burrow in scabies

Samples of epidermal scale, and hair and nail are placed on a microscope slide with a drop of KOH solution and a cover

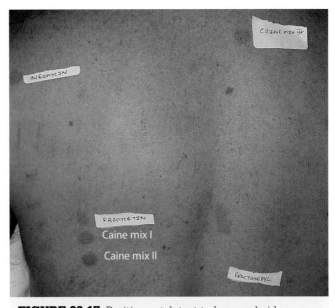

FIGURE 23.17 Positive patch test to haemorrhoid ointment (proctosedyl), framycetin and local anaesthetic mixes that contain cinchocaine with a cross-reaction between neomycin and framycetin

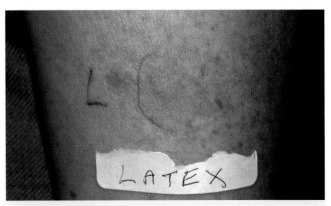

FIGURE 23.18 Positive prick test to latex

slip. After a few minutes (20–30 minutes for nails), the slide can be examined for the presence of fungal elements, seen as mycelial strands crossing cell boundaries. Scabies mites, eggs, egg cases or immature forms are easily seen under low power.

Culture for fungus is very useful for both practical and epidemiological purposes in knowing the source of the infection. Samples should be sent folded into paper (preferably black to make the scale easily identifiable) to a laboratory that is properly equipped to grow fungi. Culture results are usually available within 6 weeks.

Skin biopsy for histopathology and direct immunofluorescence

Whole skin samples can be examined in a number of ways to aid diagnosis:

- Light microscopy; this is now used for a wide variety of testing procedures, capable of defining many critical features of the disease process.
- Direct immunofluorescence; 'IMF' is still used to confirm the diagnosis in several skin disorders, notably pemphigus, pemphigoid and dermatitis herpetiformis.
- Electron microscopy; useful in some situations, especially congenital blistering diseases.

- Culture; it is occasionally helpful to send whole skin samples for culture, e.g. TB, leishmaniasis.

Two techniques are commonly used to obtain diagnostic skin samples: punch biopsy and elliptical incisional biopsy. These are illustrated in Figure 23.19.

The area to be examined or removed is anaesthetized, usually using injected lignocaine. In some instances (especially in children), the skin may be deadened first by the application of a topical anaesthetic cream for 30–60 minutes (90 minutes recommended if using EMLA). A piece of skin is then removed using the punch knife or scalpel, and the skin edges are brought together with a fine suture.

The site chosen for the sample is important:

- The skin lesion(s) should generally be fully formed.
- Late lesions should be avoided; in dermatitis herpetiformis and bullous pemphigoid histology may be altered by the passage of time.

For 'ordinary' light microscopy specimens simply need to be transported to the laboratory, fixed in formalin. Direct immunofluorescence, however, requires samples to be snap frozen. They are usually placed in normal saline *and must be taken straight to the laboratory.*

Similarly, specimens for culture should be sent fresh to the laboratory and those to be examined by electron microscopy held in special fixative during transfer.

If there is any doubt, it is always best to consult the laboratory concerned.

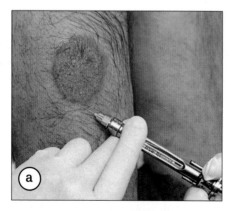
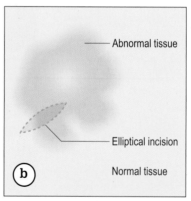
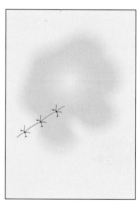
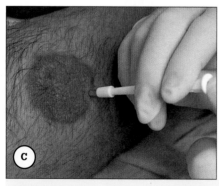
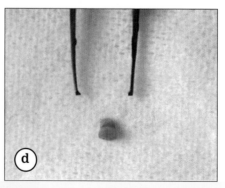

FIGURE 23.19 **(a)** Skin biopsy: the skin is anaesthetized. **(b)** Skin is removed either by cutting out an ellipse of skin with a scalpel or, **(c)** by means of a punch biopsy. **(d)** Punch biopsy specimen

Biopsies in bullous disorders

In the bullous disorders it is best to take two separate samples: the one for light microscopy needs to contain an early blister in pemphigus and pemphigoid, but a pre-bullous lesion in dermatitis herpetiformis. In pemphigus and pemphigoid the sample for IMF should include some perilesional skin; in dermatitis herpetiformis it needs to be from non-sun-exposed, normal skin – the buttock is often a good site.

Scalp and nail biopsies

It is sometimes necessary to obtain tissue from the scalp or the nail. These are probably the province of the specialist.

Basic interpretation of histology reports

Patch testing

The term 'patch test' describes an investigative tool that involves the deliberate application of materials suspected of causing allergic dermatitis, to the skin, under controlled conditions. This is most often carried out in specialist settings, but simple, one-off challenges on unaffected skin (e.g. inner forearm) may be useful. The suspect material should be applied to the skin under occlusion for 48 hours. This should not be done if the substance(s) being examined is irritant.

Full-scale patch testing is a complex business.

Suspected offending agents are applied to the surface of the skin for 48 hours before being removed; the site is examined for evidence of allergic dermatitis (Fig. 23.20); a further examination at 96 hours is also essential. It has been estimated that up to 30% of positive reactions will be missed if this is not undertaken because some compounds produce later reactions (e.g. lanolin, neomycin). In most instances, a battery of common test allergens is used and these may be modified and adapted for local circumstances or for particular problem areas (e.g. medicaments) or occupations (e.g. hairdressing). It is also often useful to test materials suspected by the patient of being responsible (e.g. cosmetics, materials handled at work). However, care must be taken not to place highly irritant chemicals on the skin. If there is any doubt, a specialized test should be used. If there is time, a visit to the patient's place of work may draw attention to tasks and contacts that were not apparent from the history alone.

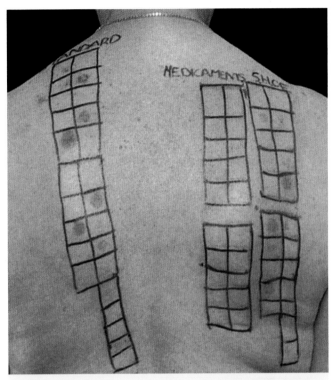

FIGURE 23.20 Finn chamber patch testing to the back – results after 98 hours: several positives in the standard and shoe batteries

There are commercial patch testing kits and it is tempting to use these in primary care settings. However, it is our firm opinion that they are best avoided unless there is access to a high degree of training and expertise. We say this principally because one of the key elements is knowing how to apply the results to everyday living and this is best done by a dedicated specialist.

Prick testing

This is a more controversial type of allergy test. It has gained a reputation for being misused by some practitioners, especially in the context of atopic dermatitis. The technique may be valuable, however, in immediate (type I) hypersensitivity. The most important example in recent times has been the emergence of latex allergy. Latex type I hypersensitivity peaked in the 1990s with dramatic increases in latex glove use throughout industry. Prick testing to purified latex extract is the most sensitive test for latex allergy. Prick testing should only be undertaken if there are adequate resuscitation facilities available in the event of anaphylaxis.

Chapter 24

Treatment Principles

Summary

- Treating skin disease: basic principles
- Prevention

TREATING SKIN DISEASE: BASIC PRINCIPLES

Broadly speaking, skin diseases may be treated using one of the following techniques:

- Topical application of a cream, ointment, lotion, gel, tape or spray.
- Local injection of active agents.
- Exposure of the skin to ionizing radiation (ultraviolet, X-rays, γ-rays).
- Ingestion or injection of systemic agents.
- Removal of tissue.
- Physical destruction of tissue by heat, cold, electricity or light.

The broad principles of treating skin disease are discussed below. Some of the most common therapeutic modalities and their key indications are included in the boxes. Note that therapeutic agents are often used in combination.

Many of these treatments are 'generic' in that they are used by several specialist groups, and the reader may well have encountered them before. However, it is worth noting a few specific points about some of the treatment modalities that are not used very frequently outside dermatology.

The bases of topical agents (and emollients)

All topical agents are 'held' in suspension in a base of some kind, which allows the patient to apply the material to the skin surface. Some bases are greases, oils or waxes (ointments); others are emulsions of oil, grease or wax in water (creams) or emulsions of water in oils (oily creams). There are also aqueous gel bases, alcoholic and aqueous solutions (used especially on the scalp to avoid matting the hair), mousses, and liquid and powder sprays. This rather bewildering array of preparations has been produced as a response to the different treatment needs of different disorders and patient requirements.

In general, the greasier a base is, the more occlusive it is. This also generally implies a greater degree of emolliency or moisturizer effect, as it prevents water loss to a greater degree. On the other hand, a lighter cream is much easier to use and is usually more cosmetically acceptable. Some of the more modern oily creams aim to achieve a balance between these two extremes, by providing a higher degree of occlusion and emolliency with a lower and more acceptable degree of 'greasiness'. Some agents designed purely to be emollients contain additional ingredients (such as urea, allantoin or aloe vera) which are claimed to increase the moisturizing effects.

The needs of each patient must be judged individually, although the old rule of thumb still has an element of truth to it:

> 'If the skin is dry, use an ointment;
> if it is wet and weepy, use a cream.'

BOX 24.1 Topical modalities

Emollients	'Dry' skin; eczema; psoriasis
Salicylic acid	Warts; psoriasis
Exfoliants	Acne
Tar	Psoriasis; eczemas
Dithranol	Psoriasis
Corticosteroids	Inflammatory disorders; vitiligo; alopecia areata
Calcineurin inhibitors	Eczemas; vitiligo; psoriasis, esp. face and flexures
Retinoic acid/analogues	Acne; psoriasis
Antiseptics/antibiotics	Bacterial infections; acne
Antifungals	Fungal infections; seborrhoeic dermatitis
Antivirals	Viral infections
Parasiticides	Scabies; lice
Vitamin D analogues	Psoriasis
5-Fluorouracil	Solar keratoses; Bowen's disease; superficial basal cell carcinomas
Diphencyprone	Alopecia areata
Capsaicin	Itch
Imiquimod	Warts (esp. genital); dysplastic states; emerging role in skin cancer management
Diclofenac	Solar keratoses
Local injections	
Corticosteroids	Alopecia areata; keloids; granuloma annulare; necrobiosis; resistant inflammatory disorders, acne; infiltrates
Ionizing radiation	
UVB phototherapy	Psoriasis; eczema
Psoralens (+UVA)	Psoriasis, eczemas; mycosis fungoides; vitiligo; some photodermatoses
X-rays	Skin cancers and dysplasias; lymphomas
γ-Rays	Mycosis fungoides

Box 24.1 continued	
Systemic agents	
Antihistamines: non-sedating	Urticaria
Antihistamines: sedating	Eczemas; itch
Antibiotics	Bacterial infection; acne; rosacea
Antivirals	Viral infections
Antifungals	Fungal infections; seborrhoeic dermatitis
Corticosteroids	Numerous indications in severe skin disease
Immunosuppressives	Severe inflammatory skin disease; bullous diseases
Methotrexate	Psoriasis
Retinoids	Acne; disorders of keratinization; psoriasis
Dapsone	Dermatitis herpetiformis; leprosy; vasculitis
Antimalarials	LE; polymorphic light eruption
Monoclonal antibodies	Psoriasis; pyoderma gangrenosum; ?eczema; ?mycosis fungoides
Destruction of tissue	
Cryotherapy	Warts; benign epithelial tumours; superficial dysplastic epithelial lesions; superficial basal cell carcinomas; lentigo maligna in the frail elderly
Diathermy or hyfrecation	Tags; spider naevi; pedunculated seborrhoeic keratoses; warts
Lasers	Vascular lesions; epithelial lesions; pigmented lesions; tattoos; scars
Removal of tissue	
Curettage	Superficial epithelial lesions; pyogenic granulomas; warts
Snip + diathermy or hyfrecation	Pedunculated lesions, e.g. tags
Excision	Lumps, cysts and defects

Salicylic acid

Salicylic acid 'softens' keratin and helps to remove scale from psoriasis and from other very scaly disorders, especially in the scalp. It is often added to mixtures of tar and steroids. Salicylic acid in higher concentrations is also used to treat viral warts.

Tar and dithranol

Tar is soothing when applied to itchy, inflamed skin. It is also a valuable adjunct in the management of psoriasis, where it seems to augment the effects of ultraviolet radiation. Dithranol can return psoriatic skin to normal. It can cause quite nasty burns, however, and it also oxidizes to a brownish-purple dye. It is used in creams and ointments and in a complicated, stiff paste known as Lassar's paste.

Topical corticosteroids

Topical corticosteroids are undoubtedly the mainstay of the treatment of most inflammatory dermatoses, and a number of other conditions. However, topical corticosteroids need to be handled with care.

There are a number of well-recognized side effects:

- They have the potential to cause significant skin atrophy if they are applied to the same area of skin repeatedly over many weeks or months.
- They reduce the skin's resistance to superficial infections.
- They can increase hair growth locally.
- They may induce comedones (blackheads).
- They may inhibit the pituitary–adrenal axis if sufficient quantities are applied to lead to significant systemic absorption.

Topical corticosteroids are by no means 'all the same': some are much stronger than others. The British National Formulary categorizes them into four classes or groups: Mild; Moderate; Potent; Very Potent.

Furthermore, several factors increase the potential for atrophogenicity and absorption:

- The base – ointments are stronger than creams, which are stronger than gels, which are stronger than lotions.
- The site of application – the face and flexures are much more vulnerable.
- The size of the patient – children have a higher surface-area-to-body-mass ratio and are more susceptible to absorption of steroids.
- The use of occlusive dressings over the steroid (especially polythene).

Topical corticosteroids need to be treated with respect. For acute episodes, it is safe to use high-potency agents for short periods. For longer-term treatment care must be taken to minimize the amount and strength of the agent(s) applied as far as possible – always bearing in mind that it is of no use using a weak steroid if no improvement follows.

Topical immunomodulators

Two agents that modulate immune function after topical application have been introduced, primarily for the treatment of atopic dermatitis: tacrolimus and pimecrolimus. Both exert their effect predominantly by calcineurin inhibition, which alters T-cell reactivity. Successful use has also been reported in facial psoriasis, seborrhoeic dermatitis and vitiligo. They do not cause cutaneous atrophy or any of the other steroid side effects. There is some (perhaps undue) concern about possible carcinogenicity with the long-term use of both agents.

Retinoic acid

Retinoic acid, a topical derivative of vitamin A, has been used for many years in the treatment of acne. More recently it has been shown that regular use can reduce facial wrinkles. It has also been used with some success in psoriasis.

Vitamin D analogues

Vitamin D analogues have quickly found an important place in the management of plaque psoriasis. Reports of improvement have also been recorded in other hyperkeratotic disorders such as pityriasis rubra pilaris, ichthyosis, porokeratosis and epidermal naevi.

Diphencyprone

The application of agents that induce an allergic contact dermatitis can encourage regrowth in alopecia areata, although the percentage who derive persisting benefit is small. Diphencyprone appears to have replaced some of the earlier alternatives because it is safer (not oncogenic) and is not found in normal everyday life. It is reserved for patients with extensive, unresponsive disease.

It may also be useful in the treatment of viral warts.

Ultraviolet radiation (phototherapy and photochemotherapy) (Figs 24.1 and 24.2)

The therapeutic benefits of light treatment in the management of psoriasis and vitiligo have been recognized for years, with an increasing range of indications in the last few years. Paradoxically, some of the photodermatoses are now treated with UV.

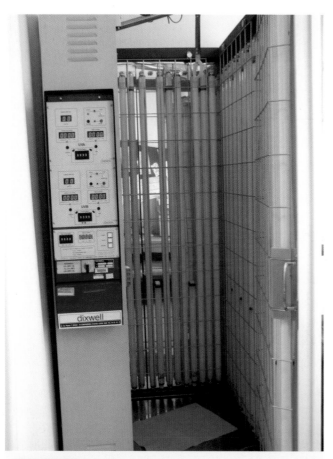

FIGURE 24.1 UVB machine

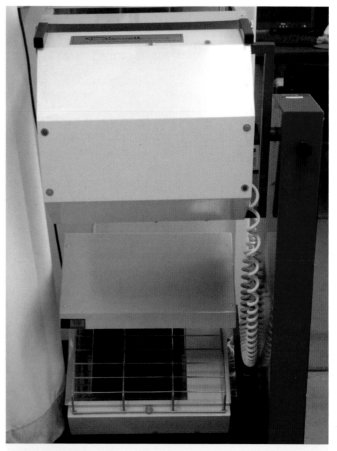

FIGURE 24.2 UVA machine for treating hand and feet

Two wavelength bands are used: UVB and UVA. UVB (medium wavelength) has been part of the dermatological armoury for many decades and forms a major part of the therapy of severe psoriasis, eczemas and mycosis fungoides. Recent work has shown that a narrow segment of the radiation spectrum (narrow-band UVB; TL-01) is the most effective and has a better safety profile.

Long-wave UV (UVA) can be used alone, but the addition of a *psoralen*, a chemical that interacts with DNA in the presence of UVA, has resulted in greater efficacy for some patients. However, there are risks: ultraviolet radiation is carcinogenic and PUVA is more so.

X-irradiation

Although once used for chronic inflammatory dermatoses, X-irradiation is now reserved for neoplastic disorders.

Methotrexate

Methotrexate, a folic acid antagonist, was first developed as an anticancer drug. Its use in severe psoriasis is well established, where it is one of the most reliable agents available. The drug is associated with some side effects, notably marrow suppression and liver fibrosis, but these can generally be avoided if patients are monitored properly. Avoidance of alcohol and awareness of drug reactions is important. Concomitant administration of folic acid (5 mg daily) reduces the incidence of side effects.

Dapsone

Dapsone is used extensively as a first-line agent in leprosy in many developing countries. It also has important effects on several other diseases with no apparent common features (apart, perhaps, from the pathological involvement of polymorphs): dermatitis herpetiformis, vasculitis, acne and relapsing polychondritis. Dapsone can cause haemolysis and a careful watch must be kept during treatment, with regular FBC *and* reticulocyte counts being essential. It is sensible to check for glucose 6-phosphate dehydrogenase (G6PD) deficiency before commencing therapy in at-risk populations.

Oral retinoids

There are two vitamin A derivatives that are useful when taken orally. Acitretin (which is replacing, or has replaced, etretinate) is used in the ichthyoses, Darier's disease and other disorders where keratinization is abnormal. Psoriasis often responds well and a combination of oral retinoids and ultraviolet B phototherapy is widely used for severe disease. Isotretinoin is very commonly prescribed for severe acne. Both drugs cause the skin to become rather 'dry' and give rise to a characteristic cheilitis. They both also raise lipid levels and can cause hepatitis, although this is rare. There has been much debate about the risks of depression with isotretinoin use. The consensus is that, although this may be a rare complication, much of the reported psychological disturbance is not drug related. Both drugs are teratogenic. Pregnancy must be avoided during use of both, and for 2 months after isotretinoin and 2 years after acitretin.

Immunomodulators

A number of systemic immunomodulators have been used for treating skin disease: azathioprine, hydroxyurea, ciclosporin, cyclophosphamide and mycophenylate mofetil. Azathioprine and ciclosporin have certainly stood the test of time. Their side effect profile restricts their use to severe skin disorders. Agents such as mycophenylate mofetil are still being assessed.

Following up patients on these drugs requires careful monitoring – see Box 24.2.

BOX 24.2 Monitoring systemic dermatological therapy

Steroids	General haematology, biochemistry; consider osteoporosis prevention programme for long-term use
Retinoids	Liver function and lipids
Methotrexate	Test dose: 5 mg with haematology at 5 days Haematology; biochemistry; P3NP (procollagen peptide) Intermittent liver biopsy (now very unusual, but may still be required if screening tests are persistently abnormal)
Ciclosporin	Creatinines (follow-up based on average of three pre-treatment levels: >30% rise = need to respond); BP monitoring Lipids
Azathioprine	Haematology; biochemistry; pre-treatment Thiopurine methyltransferase (TPMT) level
Dapsone	Haematology; biochemistry; haemolysis screen

For most drugs, monthly estimations are sufficient while assessing response and stabilizing. Thereafter, frequency depends on patient need.

Monoclonal antibodies (biologics)

The latest breed of immune modulator is a range of agents genetically engineered to target specific molecules or receptors involved in inflammation. At the time of going to press, two have become fairly widely used: infliximab and etanercept – both used in psoriasis with or without arthropathy. Many others are in the pipeline.

Curettage and cautery/diathermy

In curettage and cautery/diathermy, the skin is anaesthetized and a curette is used to scrape the lesion away. Bleeding from the raw, oozy base is then stopped by gentle diathermy or hyfrecation.

Cryotherapy

Many skin lesions respond to cryotherapy. The best agent is liquid nitrogen which, if handled and stored correctly, is very safe.

A simple rule of thumb is to ensure that a small rim of 2 mm white (i.e. fully frozen) skin appears around the treated lesion. This should then be maintained for 5 seconds for thin benign lesions, increasing if tolerated to a maximum of around 30 seconds for very thick lesions and plantar warts. Neoplastic lesions may need therapy at the more aggressive end of the spectrum – we advise treating only Bowen's disease and superficial basal cell carcinomas on 'safe' sites (i.e. not the face). The area should then be allowed to thaw and a second treatment cycle instituted.

There are two main methods of applying liquid nitrogen to the skin: using a spray (Fig. 24.3), or a cotton wool bud dipped in a flask (Figs 24.4 and 24.5). The latter may be more practical for facial warts or when treating young children. A commercially available version of cryospray – Histofreeze – can give good results if used properly.

Diathermy/hyfrecation

The application of heat or electricity to the stalk of pedunculated lesions is a very effective way of removing them and sealing off blood vessels in one go.

Excision

The technique for excision is essentially the same as for an incisional biopsy except, of course, that the ellipse passes around the whole lesion (Fig. 24.6). It is important to give any tumour a wide enough margin to be sure of complete excision.

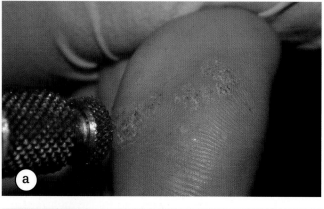
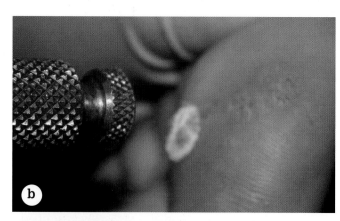
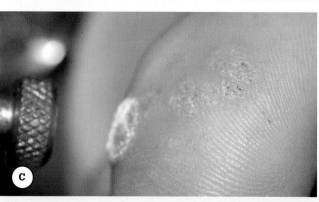
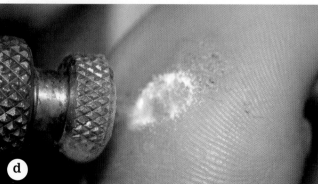

FIGURE 24.3 **(a)** Affected finger and spray nozzle. **(b)** Spray on toe. **(c)** Spray on finger. **(d)** Spray on finger

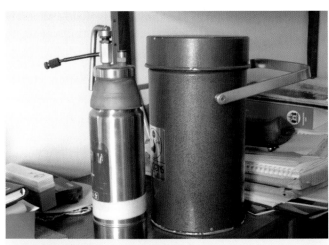

FIGURE 24.4 Liquid nitrogen flask

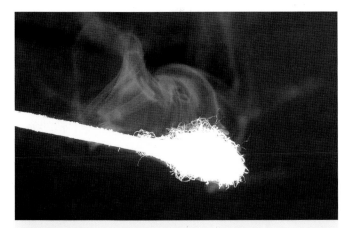

FIGURE 24.5 Cotton bud dipped in liquid nitrogen

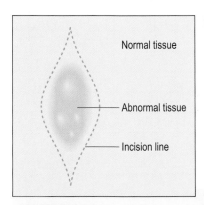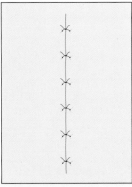

Normal tissue

Abnormal tissue

Incision line

FIGURE 24.6 The technique of simple excision

PREVENTION

In recent years, a great deal of attention has been paid to preventing skin disease.

There are three areas that have particularly attracted attention:

- Sun exposure and skin cancer:
  - There are two levels at which skin cancer prevention can operate – primary and secondary.
  - Primary prevention is aimed at reducing the chance of an individual developing skin cancer and essentially involves lifetime reduction of sun exposure (see Box 24.3 for key components of sun exposure reduction).
  - Secondary prevention aims to prevent avoidable morbidity and mortality by encouraging early diagnosis and treatment (see Box 24.4 for guidance).
- Fixed factors – family history and genetics:
  - There is no evidence that any environmental measures will prevent the development of psoriasis or atopic eczema, despite much of the folklore that surrounds these conditions; in particular, assertions that breast-feeding, avoidance of any foods by lactating mothers or in early infant feeding, or attempts at house dust mite reduction are without scientific support.
  - Families with a strong history of melanoma or other skin cancers should avoid sun exposure as far as possible (see boxes).

BOX 24.3 Sun exposure advice

Ideally avoid being out of doors between 11 and 3, especially in high summer

If out of doors:

- Seek shade wherever possible
- Cover up: wear long sleeves, cover the legs, put on a broad-brimmed hat and sunglasses
- Apply high-factor sunscreens frequently and in adequate quantities

---

BOX 24.4 Features giving rise to concern in a pigmented lesion

- New appearance
- Change:
  - In size
  - In colour
  - In shape – especially an irregular edge
  - Of the surface
- Itching
- Bleeding

- Occupation and care of the hands:
  - It is always a good idea to keep irritant exposure to a minimum, but this is more important in people with a history of atopic eczema or other chronic skin conditions.
  - Instead of soaps, patents should be encouraged to use non-soap cleansers and emollients.

- Certain occupations can prove a very severe challenge – hairdressing, catering, nursing, manual labour – and it may be sensible to offer advice about future career aspirations to anyone in whom there is doubt about how robust the skin barrier is.

Chapter 25

Treating Emergencies

Summary

- Angioedema and anaphylaxis
- Meningococcal sepsis
- Disseminated herpes simplex
- Erythroderma
- Pustular psoriasis
- Severe nodulocystic acne
- Toxic epidermal necrolysis and Stevens–Johnson syndrome
- Necrotizing fasciitis

It is rare to be faced with a true 'dermatological emergency'. However, this chapter will briefly address acute treatment of people presenting with a few skin problems, or symptoms thought to be due to skin problems, and appropriate referral if necessary.

ANGIOEDEMA AND ANAPHYLAXIS

The immediate issue is whether there is any obstruction of the airway. If there is, then emergency treatment should include efforts to secure the best airway access available in the circumstances. The patient should be given an injection of intramuscular adrenaline if possible, and transferred to emergency facilities where full resuscitation equipment is available.

If the airway is not compromised, it is safe to treat with oral antihistamines and prednisolone, starting (in an adult) at a dose of 30 mg daily. In a child it is good practice to refer to an appropriate information source to establish the dosage.

MENINGOCOCCAL SEPSIS

The meningococcus is a highly virulent organism that causes a severe and progressive meningitis and septicaemia. One of the consequences of the latter is disseminated intravascular coagulation, which leads to a highly characteristic eruption consisting of rapidly spreading purpura that does not blanch on pressure, except very early in the course of the illness. This clinical sign should alert any clinician to the impending disaster that may befall the patient if adequate investigation and urgent treatment are not instituted.

DISSEMINATED HERPES SIMPLEX

The commonest situation in which this is encountered is in a patient with atopic eczema. An example of the clinical signs is seen in Figure 25.1. In many patients these are preceded by a fever and malaise.

In most circumstances, the patient is best managed in hospital with intravenous antiviral medication. If there is no evidence of toxicity (the patient is afebrile and generally well), oral acyclovir, commencing at 400 mg five times daily, may be justifiable.

Topical steroids or any non-essential drugs apart from emollients should be stopped, and it is sensible to provide broad-spectrum antibiotic cover.

Another critical problem can arise with ocular involvement, for which an urgent ophthalmological review is essential.

ERYTHRODERMA (Figs 25.2 and 25.3)

The key to managing erythroderma is the establishment of the cause. Basically, there are four main disorders

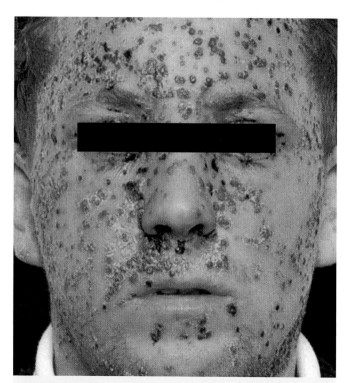

FIGURE 25.1 Extensive herpes simplex of the face in a patient with atopic dermatitis (eczema herpeticum/Karposi's varicelliform eruption)

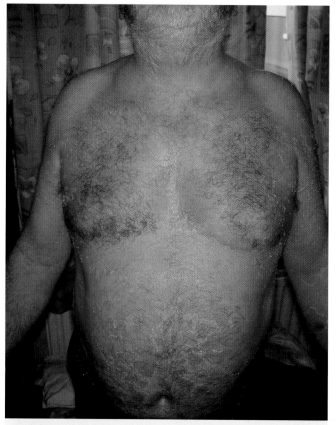

FIGURE 25.2 Erythrodermic psoriasis

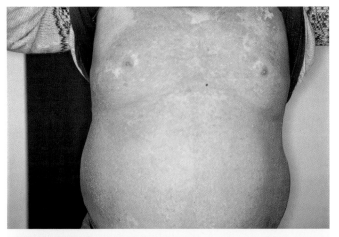

FIGURE 25.3 Erythroderma

to consider: eczema/dermatitis, sometimes arising from contact allergy; psoriasis; drugs; cutaneous T-cell lymphoma. While it may be tempting to start systemic steroids, there is generally no necessity for immediate on-the-spot intervention unless there is evidence of significant cardiac failure. Steroids, while usually helpful in controlling any of these diseases, may complicate further management of the patient, especially if the underlying diagnosis is psoriasis.

However, the patient must be kept as warm as possible, any obvious general medical problems should be addressed and then an urgent review organized, with a view to admission.

PUSTULAR PSORIASIS (Fig. 25.4)

A similar approach to that adopted in erythroderma should be taken in a patient suspected of having pustular psoriasis.

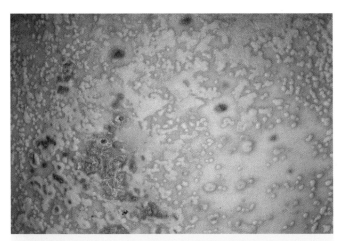

FIGURE 25.4 Acute pustular psoriasis: a dermatological emergency

SEVERE NODULOCYSTIC ACNE

Patients with very bad acne require very careful handling, but there is no need to act precipitately. The correct approach depends on a number of factors:

- The length of the history.
- The existing therapy, if any.
- The presence of systemic symptoms.

If the disease has arisen very rapidly, it is likely that the patient will require systemic steroids, usually together with standard oral anti-acne antibiotics.

TOXIC EPIDERMAL NECROLYSIS (Fig. 25.5) AND STEVENS–JOHNSON SYNDROME

(Figs 25.6 and 25.7)

There are criteria by which these disorders can be separated diagnostically, but in practice this is less important than ensuring the patient has access to a centre that can offer

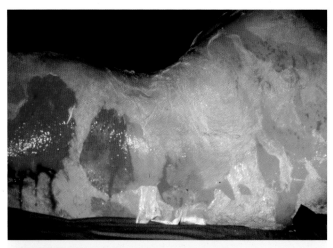

FIGURE 25.5 Toxic epidermal necrolysis

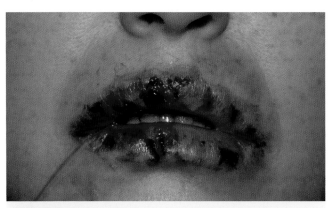

FIGURE 25.6 Oral ulceration in Stevens–Johnson syndrome

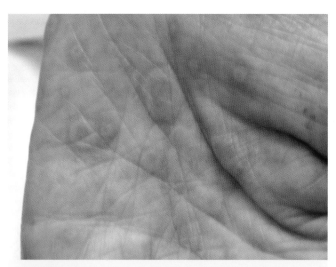

FIGURE 25.7 Typical target lesions on the hand in Stevens–Johnson syndrome

the appropriate level of care. This is often best provided in a unit with burns expertise or highly developed specialist dermatology nursing and with a general intensive care unit.

There is controversy about the best treatment over and above these general measures, but intravenous immunoglobulin and ciclosporin are options.

NECROTIZING FASCIITIS

This dreadful condition is very difficult to diagnose clinically. There may be very little to see on the skin surface, or there may be deeper spread from an area of cellulitis. The areas become very painful – often out of proportion to the clinical signs. If there is the slightest suspicion, however, urgent admission is required, because the only hope comes from a wide surgical debridement of all infected tissue, together with high-dose intravenous antibiotics.

Index

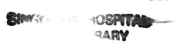